FIGHTING FAT

Canada, 1920–1980

While concern about obesity has seemed to reach an apex in the twenty-first century, our preoccupation with fatness has a long history. In *Fighting Fat*, Wendy Mitchinson explores the history of obesity and fatness from 1920 to 1980 in Canada. Bringing together discussions of body, medicine, weight measurement, nutrition, and identity and self-image, Mitchinson examines the attitudes and practices of medical practitioners, nutritionists, educators, the media, and those who see themselves as fat.

Fighting Fat analyses a number of sources to expose Canada's obsession with body image over sixty years. Mitchinson looks at medical journals, both their articles and the advertisements for drugs for obesity, as well as magazine articles and advertisements, including popular "before and after" weight loss stories, to reveal the cultural perceptions of and attitudes to body fat. Interviews with more than 30 Canadians who defined themselves fat during the period under study highlight the emotional impact caused by the stigmatizing of fatness.

WENDY MITCHINSON is a Canadian historian and a distinguished professor emerita at the University of Waterloo.

Fighting Fat

Canada, 1920–1980

WENDY MITCHINSON

UNIVERSITY OF TORONTO PRESS
Toronto Buffalo London

© University of Toronto Press 2018
Toronto Buffalo London
utorontopress.com

ISBN 978-1-4875-0357-4 (cloth)   ISBN 978-1-4875-2274-2 (paper)

Library and Archives Canada Cataloguing in Publication

Mitchinson, Wendy, author
Fighting fat : Canada, 1920–1980 / Wendy Mitchinson.

Includes bibliographical references and index.
ISBN 978-1-4875-0357-4 (hardcover). – ISBN 978-1-4875-2274-2 (softcover)

1. Obesity – Canada – History – 20th century. 2. Discrimination against overweight persons – Canada – History – 20th century. 3. Obesity – Psychological aspects – Canada – History – 20th century. 4. Obesity – Social aspects – Canada – History – 20th century. 5. Overweight persons – Canada – History – 20th century. 6. Overweight persons – Canada – Social conditions – 20th century. I. Title.

RC628.M58 2018   362.1963'98   C2018-901784-8

University of Toronto Press acknowledges the financial assistance to its publishing program of the Canada Council for the Arts and the Ontario Arts Council, an agency of the government of Ontario.

   Canada Council   Conseil des Arts
                       for the Arts   du Canada

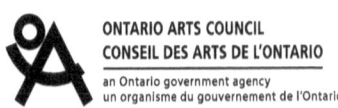
ONTARIO ARTS COUNCIL
CONSEIL DES ARTS DE L'ONTARIO
an Ontario government agency
un organisme du gouvernement de l'Ontario

Funded by the   Financé par le
Government   gouvernement
of Canada   du Canada

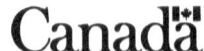

*For Michael Mitchinson
and
Donna Mitchinson*

Contents

List of Illustrations ix
Acknowledgments xi
Abbreviations xv

Introduction 3
1 Nutrition Policy: "Dietetic Missionaries" 26
2 About Obesity 56
3 Causes of Obesity 81
4 Treatment: "Stubbornly Resistant" 110
5 "Dietary Drugland" and Surgery 141
6 Infant, Child, and Teen Obesity 174
7 Body Image 207
8 Narratives of Fat Canadians 237
Epilogue 265

Notes on Sources 271
Journal Abbreviations 279
Notes 281
Index 399

Illustrations

Portrait of Daniel Lambert by Benjamin Marshall, c. 1806	15
"Here's Health with Milk" billboard, 1940	39
"Send in food, not Mounties," workers' protest, 1934	41
"Ration Time at Banff Indian Days, Banff, Alberta," c. 1930	47
Youth versus middle-age, a weighty matter: cartoon, 1967	64
A meatless Ukrainian Christmas dinner with the Danilowich family, 1954	68
Buying treatment for the man who ate too much: cartoon, 1963	85
The Honey-O concession at the Pacific National Exhibition (PNE), 1978	87
Women holding a bake sale in Taber, Alberta, 1953	88
Young women exercising at the YWCA, Edmonton, Alberta, 1926	112
The Darlene Slenderizing Glamour Salon Device, Pacific National Exhibition (PNE), 1950	116
A very small diet: cartoon, 1961	125
The unhappy fat man: Ionamin advertisement, 1963	162
The chubby cyclist: Ionamin advertisement, 1963	162
The ideal overweight patient: Dexedrine advertisement, 1957	165
A multi-use diet drug: Dexedrine advertisement, 1956	167
A broader therapeutic approach to weight control: Probese advertisement, 1962	169
Winner of the "Better Babies Contest" at the Pacific National Exhibition (PNE), c. 1920	175
The spectre haunting parents of thin, unhealthy young children, c. 1920	176
Teenage girls eating pizza at a pyjama party, c. 1960	185

Camp Slim-Teen, Calgary, Alberta, 1974	199
Champion weightlifters from the Vancouver Police Mutual Benevolent Association, 1923	210
Slender young women at an Ontario beach, 1925	211
"Her new Easter dress arrives": cartoon, 1927	225
Older woman in a bathing suit, Vancouver, c. 1925	228
New fashions for women, but men still wore suits: cartoon, 1970	235
The midway sideshow at the Canadian National Exhibition (CNE), 1913	238
"Big" Byng Whittaker and Peggy Lee on air at Radio CJBC, 1948	247

Acknowledgments

Fighting Fat would not have been possible without the financial support of the Canada Research Chair (CRC) Program, the Associated Medical Services in partnership with the Canadian Institutes of Health Research (CIHR), and the CIHR, which funded this project and the project that led to *Obesity in Canada: Critical Perspectives* (Toronto: University of Toronto Press, 2016). My seven years as a CRC in Gender and Medical History allowed me more time for the project than I would have had otherwise. The Dean of Arts and the History Department at the University of Waterloo supported aspects of two workshops (on body and medicine and obesity), which I co-organized. For a month in 2007, I was a fellow at the Bogliasco Foundation Study Center in Liguria, Italy. It was a wonderful beginning to the project, and gave me time to think about obesity and start looking at some of the medical literature on the subject.

Over the years of researching, I had graduate students or former students search through medical journals, various magazines, and Library and Archives Canada, looking for writings and photos on obesity. I am indebted to them: Adrienne Byng, Nicole Fera, Kristin Hall, Cheryl Hulme, Heather Marshall, Esmorie Miller, Sarah Morse (McNeil), Alisha Pol, and Danielle Terbenche. Renaud Séguin and Patrick Laurin worked on *L'Union Médicale du Canada*. My thanks to Suzanne Morton for suggesting Renaud; when he could no longer work on the project, Renaud recommended Patrick. Carol Cooper was my major research assistant over the many years of the project. She kept me up to date on the obesity literature, and her analysis of it always produced more themes to follow. I owe her so much.

Colleagues were generous. Heather MacDougall gave me a number of 1920s issues of *The Journal of Home Economics* belonging to her grandmother, Helen M. Wright, who used them teaching home economics in Toronto. Marlene Epp let me read a successful grant application to give me a sense of what a particular funding agency wanted from an applicant. For many years, Jane Nicholas kept her eyes open for obesity sources while she was researching her own work on the history of freaks. Julia Roberts and Greta Kroeker also showed significant interest in the obesity project, as did many others at the university.

My first essay on obesity was "Obesity in Children: A Medical Perception, 1920–1980," in *Contesting Bodies and Nation in Canadian History*, edited by Patrizia Gentile and Jane Nicholas (Toronto: University of Toronto Press, 2013), 269–85. Patrizia and Jane were helpful in giving me different perspectives on bodies. The next was "Educating Doctors about Obesity: The Gendered Use of Pharmaceutical Advertisements," in *Bodily Subjects: Essays on Gender and Health, 1800–2000*, edited by Tracy Penny Light, Barbara Brookes, and myself (Montreal & Kingston: McGill-Queen's University Press, 2014), 344–86. Tracy, Barbara, and one of the manuscript's reviewers encouraged me to expand my research on the legislation of drugs. The result can be seen in chapter five. Patrizia Gentile and Marlene Goldman were generous in explaining some of the literature on the concept of the affective turn, which I used in "The Media and the Ideal and Fat Body: An Examination of Embodiment and Affect in a Canadian Context," a chapter in *Reclaiming Canadian Bodies: Visual Media and Representation*, edited by Lynda Mannik and Karen McGarry (Waterloo: Wilfrid Laurier University Press, 2015), 5–32. Another essay on obesity was "Mother Blaming and Obesity: An Alternative Perspective," in *Obesity in Canada: Critical Perspectives* (Toronto: University of Toronto Press, 2016), 187–217. Jenny Ellison and Deborah McPhail were wonderful to work with as co-editors of *Obesity in Canada*, and both are pioneers working on the history of obesity in Canada. Our fellow authors in *Obesity in Canada* came from various disciplines, and each of them had different and challenging perspectives on obesity. They expanded my way of seeing the "obesity epidemic" in the present: Natalie Beausoleil, Jennifer Brady, Charlene Elliott, Michael Gard, Jacqui Gingras, Shannon Jette, Barry Lavallee, Darlene McNaughton, Moss Edward Norman, Elise Paradis, LeAnne Petherick, Jennifer Poudrier, Geneviève Rail, Carla Rice, Julie Rochefort, Andrea Senchuk, Jacqueline Schoemaker Holmes, Cynthia Smith, and Pamela Ward.

Others were also helpful. Camilla Blakely did a structural edit of an early draft of the manuscript. Dr Kathryn Bailey, a family physician working in southwestern Ontario, took time to read the manuscript of *Fighting Fat* and shared some experiences of obesity in her practice. Dr John Janik shared with me some of his work on obesity. Manuela Ferrari sent me a copy of her PhD dissertation, "Beyond Obesity and Disordered Eating in Youth" (University of Toronto, 2012), before it was in the public domain. Similarly, Heather Molyneaux allowed me to read her dissertation, "In Sickness and in Health: Representations of Women in Pharmaceutical Advertisements in the *Canadian Medical Association Journal*, 1950–1970" (University of New Brunswick, 2009). Jon Robison shared his work on obesity and children. Kelley Jo Burke lent me CDs of her "Fat Girls Sweet," a program that had been aired on CBC radio. Chin Jou and Todd Olszewski sent me their papers, on obesity and cholesterol respectively, presented at the 2009 American Association for the History of Medicine meetings. William G. Rothstein suggested literature for me to read on risk and epidemiology. Sandra Del Rosaria helped with translation. Dr Murray Enkin, who had read the manuscript of my earlier book *Body Failure*, and his wife Eleanor invited me and Rex to their home in Victoria when I was just starting the project and we had a lively discussion about obesity.

Alyshia (Ostrom) Bestard, a student at the University of Waterloo, already had experience in interviewing people who saw themselves as fat when she came into my office asking if I had any work for her. After reading some of her work, I was impressed by her sensitivity in interviewing, and I hired her to do interviews for *Fighting Fat*. She also helped find the people who agreed to be interviewed. Alex Matheson and Roswita Busskamp were contacts for two of the interviewees. Joan Kernohan, a friend's mother, had contacts in Taking Off Pounds Sensibly (TOPS), and through Carol Harper, another member of TOPS, Myrna Bennett, the regional director, TOPS Ontario, agreed that she would let members know about the project. I came across Rachel Buttery's name in an article on her bariatric surgery and contacted her to see if she would be willing to be interviewed. She didn't fit the project – not being fat before 1980 – but she posted my project to other friends who had had the surgery, and several contacted me and were interviewed. I owe a debt of gratitude to each of the thirty people who were interviewed and to others who talked to me about their weight.

Staff at the University of Waterloo have always been helpful. Andrew Barker in the Research Office directed me through many drafts of the CRC application. Angela Roorda, in my early thinking about obesity as a topic, helped me sort out which research group would be best for my project. Leslie Copp, also in the Research Office, helped me with CIHR grant applications. Jane Forgay in the Porter Library was always able to find the journals and articles that I needed. Keith McGowan, a computer expert, solved with remarkable patience the many difficulties my computer posed and poses for me. The staff in the History Department, Donna Lang (Hayes), Nancy Birss, Erin Cambell, and Anne Leask, were always supportive of what I needed. I've been fortunate to have worked in a department with good colleagues who gave me support, even though they might not realize it. Teaching always offset my researching, and over the years I understood that I needed to do both. Working with students was always "interesting" and challenging in the best way.

Archives allowed photos/images for the book: Glenbow Museum, Simon Fraser University Library, City of Vancouver Archives, Archives of Ontario, North Vancouver Museum and Archives (with the McCord Museum working on the photo), McCord Museum of their own images/photos, and the City of Toronto Archives. When copyright was needed but not found, the Copyright Board of Canada and the Canadian Artists' Representation Copyright Collective gave me permission to use some images. The Paladin Labs allowed me to use two copies of Dexedrine advertisements for the book. Len Husband, editor of Canadian History at the University of Toronto Press, was always helpful during the process of developing the manuscript of *Fighting Fat*. Also, a special mention to Lisa Jemison, managing editor, and Carolyn Zapf, copy editor, for their many helpful comments and sensitive editing of the manuscript, and to Noeline Bridge, who constructed an excellent index.

Friends were also supportive. At the beginning of the project, Bonnie Shettler kept her eye on literature about obesity for me. Rob Boyter helped me understand the chemistry of food and drugs. Gail Cuthbert Brandt helped with the translation of French text. Others simply reminded me that life is good: Mary Wybrow, Patrick Harrigan, Janice Dickin, Renée Bondy, Susan and Richard Reid, and many of those whom I have listed above. My brother Michael and his wife Donna are always there for me, and I dedicate the book to them. While I worked my way through readers' reports, my husband, Rex Lingwood, again read and edited the manuscript and helped to find the images. Rex is the centre of my life, along with Davis and Borg.

Abbreviations

BMI	body mass index
BMR	basal metabolism rate
CCN	Canadian Council on Nutrition
CMA	Canadian Medical Association
CON	Canadian Obesity Network
DSM	Diagnostic and Statistical Manual of Mental Disorders
FDA	Food and Drug Administration (US)
HCG	human chorionic gonadotropin
IARC	International Agency for Research on Cancer (WHO)
OHIP	Ontario Health Insurance Plan
OMA	Ontario Medical Association
PAAB	Pharmaceutical Advertising Advisory Board
TOPS	Taking Off Pounds Sensibly
WHO	World Health Organization

FIGHTING FAT

Canada, 1920–1980

Introduction

"'My weight is fine,' said the chubby man as he stepped off the scales. 'Only thing is, according to the chart I should be four inches taller.'"[1]

Obesity/fatness is the public health issue of the moment, and as a historian I'm interested in understanding how it became such a dominating one.[2] *Fighting Fat* is a study of Canadian approaches to obesity from 1920 to 1980 as revealed in English-language literature and a major French-language medical journal in Quebec. The sixty years between 1920 and 1980 were crucial. By the 1920s, the attractive body for both *young* women and men was slender. Even though older men – and, to a lesser degree, older women – could be heavier than the young, fatness wasn't acceptable. While physicians were concerned about thin bodies as a sign of possible malnutrition, some were starting to write about fat bodies and obesity. By 1980, physicians saw obesity as a major problem, and being fat became even more negative. Interest in obesity/fatness emerged in Canada during World War I as part of a larger health concern: the poor health of potential recruits. Officials and others were appalled at the high percentage of young men who could not pass the military's medical examination, although they should have been the healthiest group in Canada.[3] Health reformers had long been aware of the high infant mortality rates in Canada, but the substandard health of young men raised the spectre of a general decline in the health of Canada's citizenry. Once the war ended, the need to address the health situation escalated, especially for the most vulnerable in Canadian society. Subsequent events kept the concern at the fore. The Depression of the 1930s led to a lack of access to good food for many unemployed and their families. Nutrition became an important issue, and governments, the press, schools, and especially women's magazines and organizations undertook to educate Canadians about the healthy way to eat.[4] World War II was a repeat of World War I, with high rejection rates of potential recruits. As one article in the January 1943 issue of *Maclean's* declared: "20,000 young Canadians out of 50,000 rejected by the armed services in three months – Half a million children undernourished – Maternal death rate highest of 22 leading countries' – Our health front is a second front where we face a major battle which must be won."[5] After the war, improving the population's health remained a goal. Pundits pointed to the low fitness level of Canadians; even Prince Philip, in a speech to the Canadian Medical Association during his 1959 trip to Canada, stated that he found the fitness of Canadians quite unremarkable and challenged medical practitioners to do something about it. Seven years later, physicians helped create an organization devoted to sports medicine. In the late 1970s, the self-diagnostic Canadian Home Fitness Test was developed and popularized, showing Canadians that they were not fit.[6] If you were not fit, how could you be healthy? Such ongoing concern about health and fitness created the context for a rising interest in nutrition, and anxiety about the "weight" of Canadians was part of that interest. Indeed, what we read about obesity today is very much part of yesterday's obesity dialogue.

The Obesity "Epidemic"

For the last two decades or more, Canadians cannot open a newspaper, walk into a book store, or watch or listen to the news without being inundated by warnings about the obesity epidemic and what being fat is doing to increasing numbers of us. The word "epidemic" – some even refer to a "pandemic" – is utilized by physicians, government officials, public health advocates, scientists, popular writers, and the World Health Organization (WHO).[7] Using the word "obese" itself medicalizes those of us who are considered too fat, linking obesity to thirty or more specific health problems, including heart disease, type 2 diabetes (even in children), hypertension, osteoarthritis, several cancers, stroke, gallbladder disease, fatty liver, and early death. Recently, dementia has been added to the list. Debates exist over whether obesity is a disease itself, and, if so, what kind of disease. Some experts believe obesity is a mental illness.[8]

Beyond health problems are the perceived economic and social consequences. The annual direct and indirect health costs of obesity in Canada have been estimated at anywhere from $4.3 billion to $30 billion.[9] Warnings about the financial cost appeal to the market-driven nature of our society: the cost to the individual who is obese and the cost to the society in which obesity exists. Concern about obesity is reflected in the volume of literature produced, the studies undertaken, and the conferences held to discuss the topic. Obesity has become a metaphor for modernity, "a tracer condition for a broader social order gone awry."[10] In Canada, the panic-stricken response to obesity is also evident in suggested solutions such as increasing taxes on soft and energy drinks. The Fraser Institute has proposed that Canadians who are obese pay higher health premiums "scaled by the cost that individual's lifestyle choices imposes on others."[11] These responses reflect how we see our world – full of risk.

Worldwide obesity statistics are alarming. The WHO estimates that 650 million adults (eighteen years of age and older) were obese in 2016.[12] Approximately 25 per cent of adult Canadians are obese in addition to the 37 per cent who are overweight, rates that are worrisome for many, although the rate of increase has been declining. Obesity statistics separate people into groups based on race/ethnicity, class, gender, age, and place. Indigenous people, both adults and children, have among the highest rates of obesity in Canada. Low-income families have high rates as well, although how class works is somewhat complex. Obesity rates are 26.1 per cent for men and 23.4 per cent for women. Within those rates, however, a higher percentage of women compared to men are rated as class III obesity (morbidly obese). Canadians aged eighteen to thirty-four have the lowest obesity rates, and those aged thirty-five to sixty-four the highest. Location is also a variable, with the highest rates being in the Atlantic region and the North, and the lowest in British Columbia and Quebec.[13] There is little doubt that a real change in body weight has been occurring. Two theories to explain the causes of obesity dominate: environmental and biological. Neither one excludes the other.

Advocates of the environmental theory argue that modern society has become obesogenic: it encourages obesity by prompting us to eat (intake energy) and not to exercise (expend energy). Such a view implies that society rather than the individual determines what we eat and how much, and what kind of exercise we do and how much. Agency is largely denied to those who are fat, and yet the individual is expected to fight society's obesogenic culture.

Food is central. The contention is that we eat fattening food too often and are encouraged to do so. For example, advertisements for fattening foods are more numerous and conspicuous than those for healthy foods, pressuring Canadians to eat a diet with high sugar, fat, and salt content. The size of food portions served in restaurants and other eating places has also increased, and we are eating in those places more often than ever, rather than at home where portions can be monitored.[14] Canadians eat away from home an estimated five times per week; 40 per cent of Canadian families eat their main meal at home compared to 28 per cent of American families. Of course, meals at home may well consist of processed fast and fattening food. After all, supermarkets have increased their offerings of processed/fat food.[15] A 2005 Statistics Canada report revealed that low-income families tend to eat more fattening food (fast food) simply because it is cheaper. A contrary argument points out that home cooking is in fact cheaper than fast food, but overlooks the reality that low-income families and individuals often don't live close to food stores and don't have the time or money to travel to them. For those working long hours, the attraction of making meals at home pales.[16]

Lack of nutritional knowledge is presented as a factor that prevents us from eating well. How do we learn the principles of good nutrition, what to eat, and where to eat? While nutrition has long been part of the curriculum in Canadian schools, some schools no longer teach it. If schools are not educating young people about nutrition, what will happen to the family in the future? According to one study, Canadian mothers in the past could make sure their families were eating nutritionally. Now, there are so many other sources of food preparation that it is difficult to figure out who or what should be accountable for ensuring good nutrition.[17] Nevertheless, many people blame working mothers for poor nutrition, believing they don't live up to an idealized image of mothers from the past.[18] In addition, the market-driven food industry has resulted in a declining nutritional value in our food. If that is not enough to concern us, the use of high-fructose corn syrup and artificial sweeteners has raised our cravings for sweet food.[19] The slow/local food movement is a reaction to these developments, but it has not been able to offset the power of what has become the North American way of eating. Also, the variety of local food is limited during Canada's winter.

Advocates of a microbe hypothesis suggest that many food-related health problems are due to an imbalance in the number and variety of microbes in the gut. Because fat food is easily processed in the upper intestine, microbes in the lower intestine are starved and die off. These microbes, however, are important for many tasks, including breaking down high-fibre foods necessary for good health and converting calories to energy. According to research, people who are obese have a more limited variety of microbes and are missing certain microbes found in the gut of people who are not fat.[20]

The obesogenic environment not only encourages increased consumption and poor eating habits but also reduces the expenditure of energy. Recent statistics suggest that only about 50 per cent of Canadians are significantly active. Too many children no longer walk to school or play outdoors, often because parents are concerned about danger in public spaces. Many schools have cut back the time devoted to physical education. Sedentary activities such as watching TV or playing computer games are increasing. Studies indicate that such activities encourage snacking and expose children and adults to even more food advertisments throughout the day.[21]

Other studies reveal the degree to which an obesogenic orientation dominates the attitude towards obesity. Researchers have considered all sorts of risks for obesity, from having a friend or close relative who is overweight to genetic modifications due to stress, resource availability, climate change, artificial chemicals, and so forth. Some economic historians see obesity as a disease of modernity (or postmodernity).[22] That view sends the message: "Get used to it; it is our future." Our social context has also allowed us to deny what is happening. For example, clothing sizes have been scaled up, encouraging the delusion that the same size fits despite increased girth.[23]

While the obesogenic environment perspective provides a complex social/cultural understanding of the obesity epidemic, it doesn't offer solutions on a societal scale. Rather, studies of obesogenic factors assume that individuals are responsible for controlling their own weight. This assumption is certainly the message of Neil Seeman and Patrick Luciani's, *XXL: Obesity and the Limits of Shame*, in which they propose giving healthy living vouchers to people to be used at will. For example, the voucher would allow those who want to maintain a healthy weight to buy better food or pay for a gym membership. The underlying assumptions of an obesity voucher are twofold: first, that the search for a one-size-fits-all approach has not worked to overcome obesity; and second, that there must be a solution, even if it is an individual one.[24]

The biological view of obesity uses the obesogenic environment perspective to show why change occurs, but places its origin within the body to explain the difficulty in fighting off weight gain. Supporters of this view theorize that bodies are "hardwired" for survival and do not adapt to changing circumstances quickly. According to this argument, our bodies were designed to store energy (fat through feasting) so that we could survive periods of minimal food supply (fasting). Those who survived were those who were most efficient in storing fat, and, consequently, the "thrifty gene" became part of our DNA.[25] At the same time, energy expenditure was such that our ancestors expended a great deal of energy looking for food, but rested when satiated in order not to use energy needed for times of little food. In other words, our bodies are programmed both to eat when we can and to conserve energy. But we now live in a society where both are encouraged without having to face times of extreme food deprivation and times of extreme energy expenditure to find food as our ancestors did. The result for us is obesity.[26]

Another theory based on a hardwired concept is the "expensive tissue hypothesis." Acccording to this theory, our earliest ancestors had small brains that didn't need much energy to function. As the human brain became larger, energy-rich food was needed to maintain this larger brain.[27] The "set-point weight" is another hypothesis to explain the obesity epidemic. It suggests that an individual's body has a natural "set" weight controlled by genes and hormones.[28]

The hardwired theories are a macro explanation for obesity. Less grandiose is a genetic argument with a sex- and ethnic-based component: women have more body fat than men, and certain ethnic groups are fatter than others. Clearly, scientists are interested in the hereditary element at the familial level to explain the upsurge in weight. Part of the biological/genetic cause is also linked to how some people taste food. A significant minority of people are "bitter tasters," that is, certain foods taste bitter to them. As a result, they avoid certain foods and are more drawn to foods that taste sweet and often have a high caloric count. Other people may be extra sensitive to fat in food and eat less of it.[29] Recent studies have linked certain "new" genes to obesity. Other genes determine where fat is deposited – for example, on the thighs or abdomen. While these genes are linked to weight, this knowledge does not offer any insight into how to offset the weight gain.[30]

Some researchers, focusing on the biological/genetic causes of weight gain, estimate that genes account for 25 to 40 per cent of weight variability. Others suggest "genetic influence" accounts for up to 80 per cent of the excess weight for some people.³¹ The extreme statistical range perhaps reflects the complexity of genetics. But the genetic cause is only part of the picture. In the pithy words of Dr Scott Kahan, co-director of the George Washington University Weight Management Program in Washington, DC, "Genes load the gun, the environment pulls the trigger." For example, the two elements come together in a virus hypothesis about obesity. A virus attacks certain bodies (the biological argument), but a virus emerges only under specific conditions (the environmental argument).³²

Current interpretations of obesity hypothesize many causes. It isn't a surprise, therefore, that challenges exist for some of them. Challenges on two fronts are significant. The first front, what is usually called "fat studies," considers the subject to be fatness, not obesity. Indeed, most of fat studies literature gives voice to people who are fat, and that voice sees the concept of obesity as a moral panic. The second front perceives weaknesses in some of the obesity literature, challenging it on that basis.

Challenges to Fatness and Obesity

While feminists were active in challenging the pressure on women to be slender (underweight), many fat rights advocates noted that feminists were rather late in understanding the issues faced by fat women and society's rejection of fatness. At the same time, advocates (fat activists) were creating a positive view of fatness: fat people can be healthy; they can be fit; and fat women are beautiful and sexy. Some looked to biology: women naturally have a higher proportion of body fat than men, and fat protects them throughout pregnancy, childbirth, and breastfeeding. Fat is also what often defines women as female: their breasts, buttocks, childbearing abilities, and sexuality.³³

The 1983 book *Shadow on a Tightrope: Writings by Women on Fat Oppression* is an early fat studies work. It uses voices of fat women to illustrate how society sees fatness and explores the stigma that they face, the "medical crimes and the dieting ... [aimed] against women," and the problems of their everyday lives.³⁴ Other collections followed, presenting new subjects for scholarly research across different disciplines and perceptions.³⁵ Over time, authors clearly defined fat studies as "an interdisciplinary field of scholarship marked by an aggressive, consistent, rigorous critique of the negative assumptions, stereotypes, and stigma placed on fat and the fat body."³⁶ The 2010 book *Historicizing Fat in Anglo-American Culture* is somewhat different in that it looks to the past and employs a "cultural and historical analysis" of fatness. Editor Elena Levy-Navarro argues that, by the late nineteenth century, "fat" had become a "master term," just as had "race, sex, gender, and class."[37]

Other books focus more on theories. Some reject the "nature and life sciences" approach to understand the fat body and instead look towards the "realm of social and cultural criticism," advocating for fat people to take control over their own bodies.[38] Samantha Murray's 2008 book *The "Fat" Female Body* has a section, "Pathologising Fatness," which demonstrates that medicine's "seemingly" objective "science" is also informed by a moral view of fatness.[39] The 2014 book *Queering Fat Embodiment*, edited by Cat Pausé, Jackie Wykes, and Samantha Murray, probes "how compulsory heteronormativity works to regulate fat bodies and subjects."[40] It puts fat studies and queer studies together. Two articles from this book spoke to me as a historian. As a human geographer, Robyn Longhurst has a "sense of how place and space 'matter' to embodied subjectivity, especially in relation to sex, sexuality, gender … and body size and shape." To illustrate that concept, she looks to several aspects of queer theory: performativity, the closet, shame and pride, and body in "time and space."[41] Stefanie A. Jones' article raised the problem of what is fat and what are its boundaries.[42]

Canadian fat studies books are few when compared to the number published in the United States. Allyson Mitchell, a member of the fat activist group Pretty Porky and Pissed Off, wrote a dissertation entitled "Corporeographies of Size: Fat Women in Urban Spaces." In her thesis, she refused "the psychological and scientific discourses that pathologize fatness" – a strong theme in the literature on fatness – and accepted "a corporeal theory of corpulence that attends to the lived experiences of fat women."[43] Like Mitchell, Carla Rice is a fat activist; she belongs to Hersize, a group of women who experience "weight preoccupation." In her 2014 book *Becoming Women: The Embodied Self in Image Culture*, based on her dissertation, Rice combines "cultural imagery" and "personal narrative" in an original way, presenting narratives by those who are from different races, disabilities, body types, and age rather than from normative white, middle-class subjects. In doing so, she uses the concept of "intersectionality," acknowledging that "people live multiple layered identities and encounter shifting privileges and oppression" and making it clear that fat people are not alone.[44] I have utilized Rice's "cultural imagery" and "personal narrative" in chapters seven and eight.

The literature just mentioned is largely focused on women and the various theories used to understand the way society reacts to fat women's bodies. Most of the authors reject the word "obesity" and what it signifies – that obese people have a disease. Certainly, health isn't a subject much discussed in these works except to say that fat people are generally healthy and, if they are ill, their fatness isn't the cause. Those who feel ill because of their fatness are invisible in this literature. Are they without agency thinking that way? Kathleen LeBesco, author of the 2002 book *Revolting Bodies? The Struggle to Redefine Fat Identity*, has asked the question, What does a fat activist do if she wants (or feels the need) to lose some weight?[45] Despite problems with some of the theories, the major themes in fat studies are significant to the study of obesity/fatness. These themes include demonstrating that the obesity panic is a moral panic; revealing the prevalence of fat phobia and its stigma, which society uses against fat people; looking at fat body images as beautiful; and weakening the binary correlation according full citizenship to a "normal" body and denying it to an "abnormal" one. "Fat" as a master term will give historians and others another variable to think about – although when looking at obesity, "weight" is also a master term. While some authors reject medicine, others, such as Murray, understand that physicians have confidence in medicine but also view their patients through the lens of social and cultural perceptions. Even today, there is no consensus on fat measurement. As for fat boundaries, medicine uses numbers, while the cultural boundary is often based on attractiveness. Both change with age, time, place, and other similar identities.

If fat studies research concerns offsetting the cultural negativity of fatness, another section of the obesity/fatness literature increasingly challenges the way in which the concept of an obesity epidemic has taken over the discourse. The Canadian Obesity Network (CON) is "Canada's largest obesity association, made up of healthcare professionals, researchers, policy makers and people with an interest in obesity." Dr Arya Sharma, the scientific director of CON, along with others, "developed the Edmonton Obesity Staging System to assess health based on risk behaviours rather than on body weight."[46] It is a significant step. Over time, the network has fought the stigma of fatness (not obesity); in 2011, CON held a Weight (not Fat) Bias Summit. At the same time, CON is perceived as seeing obesity as a disease.[47] Fat and obesity can be classified within medicine. The book *Obesity in Canada: Critical Perspectives* is a collection of articles on both fatness and obesity. The book has four sections, each with a different objective: to analyse some of the science on obesity; to examine the concept of responsibility for obesity; to consider different responses to obesity; and to look at what might be coming in the future. Others in the humanities and social sciences have also questioned aspects of the dominant discourse.[48]

Concern about health and obesity has become fixated on a single measurement: weight. But weight does not measure body fat, and it is an excess of fat that is significant for obesity. We seem to be convinced by numbers, which are reiterated in support of either bad weight or good weight. By using body mass index (BMI), based on weight and height, we are put into classifications: underweight, below 18.5 BMI; normal weight, 18.5 to 25 BMI; overweight, 25 to 30 BMI; and obese, over 30 BMI. A weight gain of a few pounds can place someone in a new category. In the 1990s, when the US government accepted the WHO BMI classifications of normal weight, overweight, and obese, the American obesity rate increased by 61 per cent overnight.[49] In researching Canada's obesity statistics, Michael Gard notes that "obesity statistics change[d] very little from year to year ... even during the 1980s and 1990s when most of the increases in obesity prevalence in Western countries occurred" and questions whether such numbers signal a crisis. Compared to the United States, Canada lagged in collecting its obesity statistics. Perhaps because of Canada's healthcare system, its small population in a huge country, and its small scientific community, the obesity panic in Canada wasn't as strong as it was in the United States.[50]

As noted earlier, the panic about obesity centres on health. By the end of the 1990s, however, some experts suggested that being overweight by 10 to 15 per cent could be good for you. Certainly, dieting often doesn't work, and its failure can lead to greater weight increase. A more positive argument posits that being fit and overweight or obese (not morbidly obese) is a healthier state than being unfit and a "normal" weight. Concerns about the increase in sedentary lifestyles are predicated on the assumption that exercise is not only healthy but also effective as a way of controlling weight. However, those who do not like to exercise can take comfort from the argument that any kind of activity will do. Studies based on specific socio-economic groups found that increased exercise may not be necessary to maintain a stable weight. Certainly, the role exercise plays in weight gain is contentious. Recent literature argues that one-third of obese individuals are metabolically healthy and that they may actually become less healthy if they lose weight. Such a perception has been present in the literature since the mid-1960s, although not widely popularized. While this finding is good news, some studies suggest that the mortality rate of the metabolically healthy obese is the same as that of the obese with high blood pressure, high cholesterol, and high blood sugar.[51] Not all accept that conclusion,[52] however, and the inability of "experts" to agree is reflective of obesity/fatness studies in general – one study suggests one conclusion while another arrives at a contrary one.

Some of the theories put forward to understand the obesity "epidemic" are problematic. Critics of the thrifty gene theory argue that this theory is a form of racism because it is often used to explain the high rates of diabetes (due to obesity) in Indigenous groups, presenting them as "genetically 'thrifty.'"[53] The larger brain theory is intriguing, but it does not explain the current significant increase in weight when there is no evidence that the human brain has recently increased in size. This theory may explain our orientation to high-energy foods, but not why the fat epidemic is taking place now. It also overlooks the way in which tastes can change quite quickly, not only because of the body's reaction to certain tastes, but also due to social factors.[54] The set-point idea is also intriguing, but it doesn't take into account the environment in which people are living. All these hypotheses have enjoyed some popularity for a time, before their weaknesses were pointed out. The major weakness in all of them, however, is that they have not been able to suggest a solution to the obesity epidemic.[55]

Those who query the conventional wisdom about an obesity epidemic are raising questions that need to be answered. Is it not true that many connections made between obesity and health problems are confounded by other factors such as fitness, drug use, and the kind of food eaten? Can diseases cause obesity rather than obesity causing diseases?[56] Why don't news outlets query the rigidity of the BMI as a marker of obesity or, at least, suggest that a healthy lifestyle is more important than what a person weighs? Certainly, there are problems with the BMI. As used, the BMI is a tool of power and control, a tool that doesn't measure body fat, take into account where fat is located on the body, or distinguish between weight gain caused by muscle development and weight gain caused by fat. The BMI is also not a good measurement when applied to the young, the elderly, and certain ethnic groups. In addition, why are obesity statistics often conflated with statistics of those who are overweight, making the two statistics equally problematic and exaggerating the scope of obesity? Why does the weight issue so often revolve around women's weight, even though statistics show that the obesity rate for women in Canada is lower than the rate for men?[57] While a moderate stance on the issue of obesity is gaining more attention,[58] it is too often lost in what the media puts forward as science on this topic.

Are present-day attitudes towards obesity a form of moral panic, as the fatness literature argues, and are they, in part, socially constructed? It would not be the first moral panic that historians have traced. Early twentieth century Canadians feared the white slave trade. During World War II, Canadians were anxious about rising levels of juvenile delinquency. Both worries were actually aspects of deeper-seated fears: the first example reflected a fear of strangers and foreigners, who were seen as not respecting white women; while the second grew from a fear about the absence of fathers from Canadian homes because of the war. When historians looked for the white slave trade, they didn't find it, and juvenile delinquency had lessened. What about our current moral panic? It focuses on both social and cultural factors in our lifestyle, with a disparaging emphasis on individuals who are fat.[59] If fear of fat is constructed, who benefits?[60]

The Obesity Epidemic: Science, Morality and Ideology by Michael Gard and Jan Wright challenges the notion of an obesity epidemic. The authors don't dispute that people are heavier than in the past, but they do interrogate the concept of an epidemic and see much of the notional scientific work on it as reflecting "preconceived ideas and biases" based in morality and ideology. They even query whether scientific methodology can usefully be applied to concepts such as obesity. They also argue that the link between overeating and fat is still unproven.[61] What is clear is that obesity, and its context, is contentious and complex. As a result, most arguments about obesity are controversial to someone.

Historical Studies

While the obesity epidemic may be relatively new, concern about fatness has a history. Historians are well aware that body image and the body itself, and hence fatness and obesity, can be examined historically, since societies in varying times have seen corpulence in different ways.[62] Hostility towards significant fatness has been traced as far back as Hippocrates. That hostility lay closer to home in the late nineteenth and early twentieth century, when fat bodies were seen as unattractive.[63] But animosity was not the only perspective on fat over the course of history. Scholars agree that at times being somewhat overweight/ fat was positive, a sign of health and wealth, signifying a person who

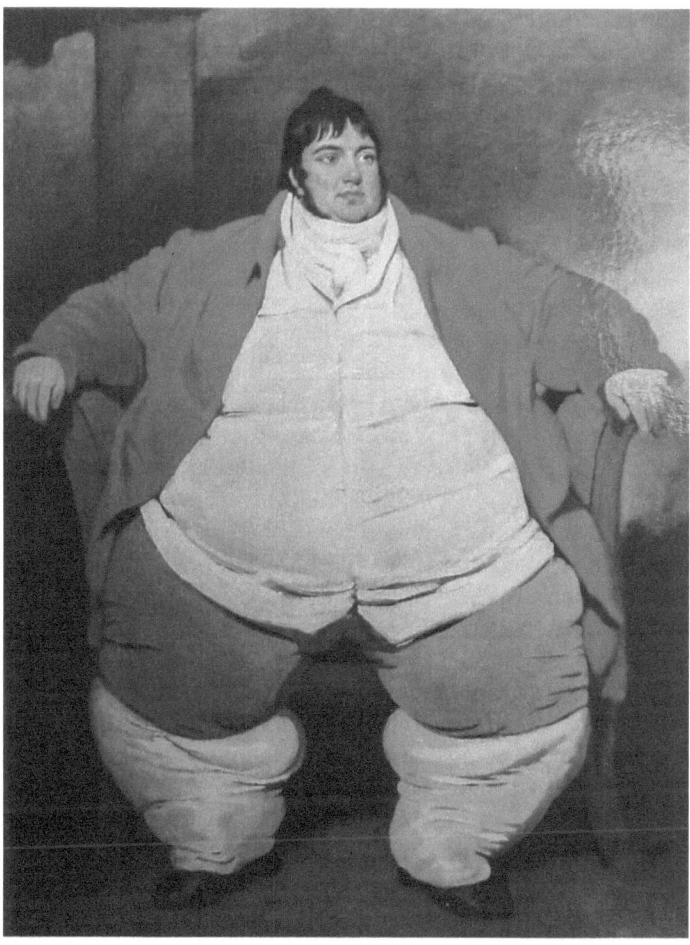

Daniel Lambert (1770–1809), shown here in a painting by Benjamin Marshall, c. 1806, was well known in England. His weight (700 lb/320 kg) became famous in the history of the body and obesity. Source: Benjamin Marshall (painter), Wikimedia Commons.

could afford enough food to be healthy and fat. As more people gained access to more food, the view changed. As the editors of *Bodies Out of Bounds* point out, *"fat ...* [became] a four-letter word."⁶⁴ Thus, any study of fatness entails a broad social approach to understand how those who were fat have been perceived and treated, and how being overweight or obese became an issue. The history of fatness has led to a history of obesity.

Hillel Schwartz, in his history of 150 years of dieting in the United States, *Never Satisfied: A Cultural History of Diets, Fantasies and Fat*, observes the contradiction between the image of thinness that has dominated American society since the turn of the twentieth century and the culture of abundance in which that image existed. Given the failure of dieting, more diets had to be tried. There has never been a perfect diet. In looking at *Never Satisfied*, we can discern central themes of the history of fatness: the stigma of fatness, the failure of diets, the mother-blaming for their children's fatness, the difference between the genders in fatness, and the measurement of fat. Other historians have followed Schwartz, as have some fatness advocates. For example, Amy Erdman Farrell, in her book *Fat Shame: Stigma and the Fat Body in American Culture*, sees fat women as being stigmatized more than fat men throughout the nineteenth century to the present. *Fat Shame* is part of the fat studies field that looks at themes important to fatness advocates (Farrell being one): images of fat bodies, obesity as a moral panic, and weakness in citizenship for fat people. Missing from the book are discussions of fat children and the different stigma for girls and boys. Because the book doesn't discuss fat children, mother-blaming isn't recognized, although mother-blaming is part of the stigma women have faced. Nevertheless, the book's strength is its rich research into the stigma facing fat women.⁶⁵

Peter Stearns' 1997 comparative study of the United States and France from the 1890s to the 1990s is an early history of fat. He chose to focus on the United States and France because America had many citizens who were "obese" at that time, while France had comparatively few. In *Fat History*, Stearns uses a cultural/social argument (a version of the environmental argument) to explain the differences between the two countries, at times using American exceptionalism to understand those differences. For example, he links the focus on obesity in America to a moral strain that turned health issues into something more significant. The exceptionalism argument culminates in Stearns' claim that the United States "led the world in excess poundage." Unlike Americans, the French continued to smoke, the result being "less need for compensatory snacking." The French also disciplined their children's eating habits, while Americans indulged their children.[66] Stearns' research notes that men's weight was the focus of concern in the later decades of the nineteenth century, after which the emphasis shifted to women. This focus continued until the mid-century, at which point Stearns refers to "important aftereffects" of discrimination that have lasted to the present. In looking at gender, Stearns criticizes feminist scholars for overlooking the early focus on men's weight and medical warnings to overweight men in the mid-twentieth century. What he doesn't say is that doctors were concerned about the health of white middle-class men and less concerned about women's health.[67]

Harvey A. Levenstein looks at fat in the United States and France slightly differently from Stearns. In his two books *Revolution at the Table* and *Paradox of Plenties*, covering respectively the 1880s to 1930 and 1930 to the early 1990s, Levenstein sees the consumption of food in the United States as more hurried and less involved in the ceremony of eating than in France, which could very well lead to a different consumption pattern. Eating is part of culture, and in his study of American eating habits, Levenstein argues that consumerism had significant influence, with much of the socio-economic underpinnings linked to and reflecting how food was seen, treated, and consumed. Margaret Willson's work also notes that the American diet has long been rich and abundant for most citizens.[68]

Sander L. Gilman's work on the history of fatness and obesity is noteworthy. He has contributed three books: *Fat Boys: A Slim Book* (2004), *Fat: A Cultural History of Obesity* (2008), and *Obesity: The Biography* (2010).[69] *Fat Boys* is about fatness in males – very fat males. Using cultural/literary history, his purview goes from classical times to the present. While looking at literature from the past, he also studies the medical view of obesity, seeing that "every classificatory system of medicine since Hippocrates has included the category of 'morbid obesity,' either as symptom or as etiology."[70] The discourse about "morbid obesity" led to his *Fat: A Cultural History of Obesity*. Most of the themes he addresses about obesity and fatness are not new – its moral panic; its "epidemic" status; its stigma; childhood obesity; and "obesity as an ethnic problem," including a chapter on "Chinese obesity." He also looks to medicine and how physicians determine that obese/fat people should be patients.[71] His book *Obesity* is largely about medicine's view of obesity, but his standpoint is that medicine and culture are in conjunction. The book starts with "the exemplary patient," a subject that most historians don't write about. His patient, however, is Joe from Dickens' *The Pickwick Papers*. Next, he chronicles obesity from the ancients to the Renaissance through to the Enlightenment. Other chapters examine aspects of the history of cure – morality versus science and a somatic treatment versus a psychological treatment. New causes of obesity and new solutions are discussed near the end of the book, followed by a section on struggles against obesity in China and finishing with "Globesity and the Public's Health." Throughout the book, Gilman goes from fatness to obesity and back to fatness again. With this structure, *Obesity* shows readers that the history of fatness and obesity can be viewed together.

Scholars have also started to study the history of obesity/fatness in Canada. In her study of fat activist women's organizations in the late twentieth century, Jenny Ellison sees in their members a retreat from dieting and what they experienced as a negative response to their bodies. The organizations were small, and ranged from those interested in fitness to radical groups fighting oppression. Finding and interviewing members of these groups was significant work. By looking into the activist groups, Ellison reminds us that in Canada "not just the national but the linguistic, social, and historical context in which fat activism has been articulated ... has shaped the movement's contours." Although some of the Canadian groups applied American ideas of oppression and fat liberation, most did not have a close connection with the American groups. Indeed, "few Canadian groups felt compelled to brand their activism as liberal, radical, socialist, and the like." While Ellison's work can be seen as a history of fatness, it can also be considered a challenge to the dominant perception of obesity.[72]

Deborah McPhail's dissertation, "Canada Weighs In: Gender, Race, and the Making of 'Obesity,' 1945–1970," and her book *Contours of the Nation: Making Obesity and Imagining Canada, 1945–1970* focus on the regulation of those who were fat. The context in those years included the Cold War fear, a shift in emphasis to service jobs for middle-class men, more women in the workforce, and changing demographics through immigration. McPhail sees her work "bring[ing] together feminist history ... geography ... political economy, and ... embodiment theory to explore discourses of Canadian obesity." It is part of the literature that doesn't see obesity as "purely" biological. McPhail views the history of obesity in Canada as one of middle-class white men and women who were "most affected by the scourge of obesity" and given treatment. Obesity experts differentiated between women and men, seeing women as having emotional obesity; with the increase of women in the workplace, the concept of mother-blaming was strengthened. Obese men (middle-class and white) were not seen as masculine, and, given the Cold War, obese men were not the citizens that Canada needed. McPhail's chapter on Indigenous and Inuit people in the North is especially important in that it emphasizes both the national design of Canada and the reality of its racism. McPhail argues that scientists and government officials saw obesity in the Indigenous and Inuit populations as a sign of being "almost-white," that is, the assimilation politics of the federal government were reflected in Indigenous bodies. These findings challenge the argument of other scholars who see the emergence of the "thrifty gene" theory in 1962 as a way of portraying Indigenous people as primitive.[73]

Statisticians sometimes look through a historical lens to understand the trajectory of obesity rates, seen, for example, in an article authored by John Cranfield, Kris Inwood, and J. Andrew Ross. They studied military men of both World War I and II, and created a BMI for them, although they did "ignore" some groups of men. Nevertheless, they concluded that Canadian obesity began to increase after 1945. Peter T. Katzmarzyk examined the 1953 Canadian Weight-Height Survey and its review of stature and body mass to create a baseline for subsequent studies. His work determined, among other findings, that the percentage of Canadians who were overweight was increasing, and that immigrants' weight was increasing in direct correlation to the length of time they had lived in Canada.[74]

Themes and Structure of *Fighting Fat*

Underlying this book is the belief that place matters.[75] Canada is a North American country, but it is not America. Some American authors have looked at race (black) and religion (fundamentalism) as factors in explaining high obesity rates in the United States. Canadian authors have tended to look at the high rates of obesity in Indigenous people; they don't seem to have looked to religion per se, but have looked to the French culture with its Catholic religion. Historically, consumerism was not as strong in Canada as in the United States, but it was growing. Canada's medical practitioners were able to keep up with international literature detailing results of studies, and they often attended the medical meetings of associations of other countries and invited leading

20　Fighting Fat

researchers to address their organizations. Within Canada, they wrote a significant amount on nutrition, weight, fat, and obesity.

Themes

The history of obesity fits into many subjects of historiography – body, medicine, weight measurement, food studies, fat studies, and identity (gender, class, race, and age) – which opens the way for variable approaches, methodologies, and themes.[76] The history of the body encompasses the way people describe, perceive, idealize, treat, abuse, and dress the body, and reveals much about societal values and relationships. As Joanne Entwistle points out, "Our body is not just the place from which we come to experience the world; it is through our bodies that we come to see and be seen in the world."[77] We live in a world in which the body is considered to be something malleable, something we can reshape, and, if we can't, then others will do it for us. Our body is very much tied to our identity; it is private and yet visible. Bodies differ in gender, ethnicity, age, class, and in weight and height. Weight and height together create an image that goes from thin to fat. Much of the scholarship sees the body as a discursive subject, but recently historians have returned to an interest in the material body, its various parts, and how they were seen and understood.[78] Obesity is about a fat body, a body that is understood through the discursiveness of practitioners, nutritionists, educators, and those who see themselves as fat. But for all of them, the material body that is fat cannot be ignored.

The word obesity comes from the Latin *ob* (over) and *edere* (to eat) Its meaning thus focuses on cause – too much eating. Blaming the individual is inherent in its definition, which is why many people who are fat often do not like to use the word "obese" to describe their bodies. Fat activists' rejection of the word "obese" is part of the linguistic turn, taking control of how they see their bodies, making "fat" a word of acceptance. "Obese" and "overweight," terms used by medical practitioners, don't suggest acceptance.[79] While practitioners were negative about obesity as a condition, even if their perspectives were not always narrow, there was no consensus about what being obese and overweight were, let alone what they meant.

One of the concepts used in the history of medicine is "medicalization," the way in which physicians have been able to link behaviours and certain bodies' actions to either physical or mental problems. Medicalization shifted what was not seen as a medical issue in one period to being a medical issue in another, expanding medical power. From 1920 to 1980, health professionals' authority increased through their advice about nutrition, dieting, eating, and exercise as treatment for obesity. The failure of such advice led to the use of prescription pharmaceuticals to control appetite and to allow Canadians to stay on a diet to lose weight. Medical treatment in the years under study shifted with the increase of pharmaceutical use – insulin, vaccines, amphetamines (originally used to keep soldiers awake during World War II), and psychiatric medications such as chlorpromazine, just to name a few. Drug treatment was considered modern, and it predisposed medicine to a partnership with pharmaceutical companies.

A history of obesity is, in part, a history of measurement and weight. Measurement is a tool for understanding; it gives information that we see as real and concrete. Measuring the body is an instrument of medicalization.[80] Weight is a measurement, but what a specific weight means shifts. For example, the definition of obesity is a comparable measurement to a "normal" or average weight. But what is the normal weight for any individual? How much over the norm or average weight indicates obesity? Over the sixty years of this study, the measurement of obesity varied from 10 per cent to 40 per cent over a changeable healthy weight standard, although 20 per cent over the standard was the measurement most often used. The word "overweight" became a "discourse of risk,"[81] the major risk being to health. It led to surveillance of Canadians' weight, not only by insurance companies' surveys but also by schools, various levels of governments, and other stakeholders. Countries today keep statistics on how many of their citizens are overweight, and they introduce policies to encourage the loss of weight – what Michel Foucault called the biopower of modern nations regulating citizens through body policies.[82] For those who are significantly fat, another concept, "healthism," underlies how some see them. Healthism places responsibility on the individual for chronic unhealthy conditions such as obesity, rather than focusing on social factors that could lead to government responses.[83] Both biopower and healthism can be seen in the reactions to obesity in the past.

Weight and its measurement is a way of keeping track of the body aesthetically. Medical and aesthetic weighing are reactions to cultural concepts of health and attractiveness. While this study focuses more on the former, it also examines fat bodies as portrayed in popular magazines, fashions catalogues, and through interviews. Measurement of fat is more than numeracy; it can be a verdict about the body with emotional implications,[84] a part of the affective turn that uses sensations and feelings as a focus.[85] In researching obesity and using the affective theory, we can see the fear, frustration, and concern about weight.

Food is central to a history of obesity, which can be seen as an element of food studies.[86] How Canadians ate, what food beliefs they held, and how their notions of eating and gaining weight came together are issues throughout *Fighting Fat*. Nutrition and eating well have a long history, although what is defined as eating well has changed over time. Canadians' failure to follow the "best practice" in eating led to frustration for individuals, nutritionists, physicians, and different levels of government. The tension between appropriate eating as a solution to obesity and overeating as its cause is ongoing.

The last theme is identity. In the historiography of Canada in the 1970s, class, gender (sex), and race were major concerns. Since then, ability, sexual orientation, and age have been added. In this study, gender dominates over class, race, and age in the literature on obesity and fat. Shannon Stettner and Tracy Penny Light contend that "women's bodies are a political terrain, such that, simply studying the historical treatment, regulation, and medicalization of them is itself a political act ... [with] women and women's bodies ... pathologized, psychologized, medicalized, and colonized."[87] Throughout most of the sixty years covered by this book, statistics suggested that women were more prone to obesity than men, although the Nutritional Canada Survey in the early 1970s was clear that obesity rates were similar for men and women. Physicians, who were largely male, regarded puberty in adolescent girls and menopause in older women as causes of adding fat to their bodies. At the same time, some doctors looked to the cultural and social pressures of being female or male to explain weight. Within the culture of body image, the gendered differences were emphasized. The normal/standard female body was more often than not a young and slender one, whereas men's bodies were portrayed as more varied in the media. Women lived in a world that saw their attractiveness as their entry to a successful life, while for men being overweight could be a sign of importance.

Health experts and those who wrote on obesity and the body didn't ignore class and ethnicity/race, but there was an assumption that the standard body in Canada was white and middle class. Practitioners worried about white middle-class male executives who were overweight and how their weight weakened their health and thus their citizenship. Body images through the media distinguished between the bodies of white-collar men's bodies and those of men who were employed in physical work. Class also emerged through a concern that those on relief during the Depression were malnourished. As for ethnicity/race, the medical literature used visible minorities as a foil to the dominant Anglo-Celtic white population. Indigenous and Inuit populations were of specific interest by the mid-century because of the problems caused by the introduction of a southern diet (carbohydrates, especially sugar). In determining why Indigenous people were not *choosing* to eat "good" food, experts placed the answer not on the cost of good food but rather on racial stereotypes, the "Indiannesss" of their living. As we have learned through the detailed work of Ian Mosby, nutritional experiments were conducted on Indigenous people to their detriment.[88]

The age of Canadians is important to consider in discussions of body image. For example, seldom were middle-aged women described as fashionable, while middle-aged men could be. Young women and men were always fashionable. In obesity literature, weight and aging went together. Elderly Canadians were rarely studied; when they were, the numbers were few. Young Canadians – infants, children, and teens – were seen as somewhat separate from one another and more so from adults. As a result, obesity experts had to recognize those differences when looking to the causes and treatments of their fatness.

Weight is a major aspect of identity. It is one that has not been looked at by historians until recently, with the exception of the literature on anorexia. Weight is personal, and many Canadians use it to construct their body image. The statistics of weight in a nation's population says something about the nation's health, the control of its population, and how others see it.

Structure

Fighting Fat begins with Canadians' concern about malnutrition. Chapter one traces the subject of malnutrition over sixty years as applied to either underweight or overweight individuals. The nutrition literature is a major source about weight and the need for Canadians to maintain what is deemed a healthy weight. Chapter two describes the concerns of health professionals and others who kept Canadians informed about the issues surrounding obesity. These professionals primarily focused on the definition of obesity, how best to measure it, and how to keep track of the obesity rate and its rise over time. Within the literature, debates took place on types of obesity and efforts to understand fat.

Over the years, an ongoing list of health problems linked to obesity developed.

Chapter three focuses on the causes of obesity. Underlying those causes was belief in an energy equation for a healthy body: energy intake (food) should balance energy expenditure (physical activity/metabolism). Despite energy expenditure being half of the energy equation, health experts in obesity tended not to emphasize the exercise aspect of energy expenditure. Rather, they stressed the intake of too many calories, asking why Canadians ate too much or ate the wrong kind of food. The next two chapters examine treatments. Chapter four begins with exercising. Although exercising was always listed as a treatment, practitioners were seldom interested in it; nor did they believe that exercise was a significant treatment for obesity. Instead, dieting was the treatment of choice, with continuous discourses over how to keep Canadians on their diets. One such debate was to understand the psychology of eating. Whether a psychological disorder caused obesity or was caused by obesity, patients needed to understand the reasons for how they ate. Chapter five focuses on the use of appetite suppressants, which emerged in Canada during the 1940s. Obesity was only one of many "medical problems" that led practitioners to use drugs to help Canadians, in this case to keep them on their diets. In examining the use of pharmaceuticals in obesity treatment, the chapter looks at advertisements in medical journals, illuminating how companies "sold" their products to Canadian practitioners. The chapter ends with a very short discussion of surgery treatment, one that Canadian practitioners seldom used before 1980. Chapter six looks to the fat problems of weight in infants, children, and teens, a dominant concern in the present day. Infants', children's, and teens' bodies were still growing, and because of their ages they could not be held responsible for the size of their bodies. The context of causation and treatment of obesity in the young, except for infants, reflected what was happening with adult obesity, but with some alterations for their youth.

One of my concerns in researching and writing *Fighting Fat* was the focus on the beliefs and voices of health experts. I could not envision the project without looking at the lives of those who were fat – whether overweight or obese – and the society in which they lived. Chapter seven introduces body image, with an emphasis on how large bodies were perceived by others through popular magazines and their short stories, advertisements, and articles. Eaton's catalogues from which they could order clothing for different body sizes, genders, and ages were important in the lives of many Canadians. Looking at the clothes, their sizes, how they were described, and the models wearing them is a small but significant entry into what fat Canadians experienced. Whether looking at advertisements, perusing advice articles on the body, or reading short stories in popular magazines, a reader received the same message: fat was not positive except in infants and very young children. For most teenagers and adults, being fat was negative. The stigma of fatness in Canadian culture was strong. The last chapter introduces some of the narratives and voices of Canadians who self-defined themselves as fat before 1980. There are two groups of narratives: the first is based on the magazine articles and advertisements showing fat people who had lost weight – the "before" and "after" stories; the second, the most significant, is based on thirty interviews conducted for this project. Their narratives provide different perspectives that offset those of the health experts. At times, their voices are full of the pain caused by being fat as children, teenagers, and adults. Chapters seven and eight give different perceptions of fatness and obesity.

In looking at the history of obesity in Canada, I am struck by how little has changed. Today the voices of fat people are louder than they were in the past, but for anyone who wants to lose weight, little has altered in causation or treatment, with the exception of the use of surgery. The details vary, but the broader perspectives have not changed. Like the current literature on obesity, all of the sources used in this study are self-interested to a certain degree, from the professional health literature blaming Canadians for not eating well or overeating that deflects from the failure of expert advice, to advertisers encouraging Canadians to buy products that promise a slender body. The medical perspective held that obesity was a health risk, which was going to weaken the future of individuals and the nation. The social/cultural perspective saw being fat as ugly. Often the perspectives merged.

1 Nutrition Policy: "Dietetic Missionaries"

"When people are leading boring, unhappy lives, they are not interested in healthy foods but prefer anything that is stimulating, cheap, and convenient."[1]

Nutritionists tell us to eat five servings of fruit and vegetables a day; statistics suggest that fewer than 40 per cent of Canadians do so.[2] Advice given but not followed has a long history. Before World War I, an understanding of the various components of food emerged, yet the poor health of potential recruits during the war brought the malnutrition of Canadians to the attention of health experts, concerned citizens, and various levels of government. While a major sign of malnutrition was being underweight – caused either by lack of food or poor food choices – nutritionists and other health professionals also came to recognize being overweight as a symptom of malnutrition. As such, nutrition is part of obesity's history. Indeed, the complex and contested nature of the study of nutrition is mirrored in the history of obesity.

In recent years, Canadian historians have been researching the history of nutrition at the federal and provincial levels, with some historians focusing on specific groups.[3] Very little in this literature, however, discusses obesity, even though nutritionists in the past saw being overweight as a sign of malnutrition. This chapter begins with the understanding of nutrition and nutrients, food standards, and the low quality of food that Canadians too often ate. Over time, the role of governments in nutrition became significant as citizens put pressure on them, especially during the Great Depression and World War II. After the war, Canadians expected governments and other agencies to continue overseeing the nutritional value of food. Throughout the decades, ongoing surveys of nutritional health and measurements of malnutrition were carried out, based on eating habits, what nutrients were lacking, and the weight of Canada's population. These studies allowed advice to Canadians to be seen as "science." The studies found that too many Canadians on the periphery because of class, race, and geography were at risk, unable to meet what experts considered optimal nutritional standards. The unevenness of eating habits due to personal taste and family dynamics could also compromise the health of those who did have access to nutritional food. Two groups of most concern were women, as wives and mothers, and Canada's young, children and teenagers. The health experts often blamed mothers for the poor eating habits of their children, wives for the poor eating habits of their husbands, and women in general for not eating well themselves. Children and teens were the future of the nation, and their nutritional health had to be given precedence. Other groups, such as the elderly and the Indigenous population, were mentioned but they didn't appear to be of significant concern or interest. However, some historians are now looking at how imperialism weakened Indigenous peoples' access to traditional food.[4] The chapter ends with a discussion of two sources of information, marketing and education, which advised Canadians about nutrition. The various claims of food companies in their advertisements and the various guidelines and advice issued by educators created a nutritional morass for Canadians to wend their way through.

Nutrition and Malnutrition

While *Fighting Fat* begins with the 1920s, nutrition as a subject has a significant history before that time. By the mid-nineteenth century, research had discovered food was composed of "protein, carbohydrates, fat, and water." It was becoming clear that some foods had more calories than others, and some provided different nutrients. As a result, nutritional regulation in Canada began. In 1874, the Adulteration Act created standards for both food and drugs. In terms of food, the act was intended to protect Canadians from fraud. In 1911, the Adulteration Act provided a "legislative framework for establishing positive food standards, and with the help of the Meat and Canned Foods Act and the Dairy Industry Act, the legal framework for successful adulteration prosecutions was finally in place." While the poor nutritional health of infants and children had long been an issue, World War I brought the health problems of young adult men into view because of the many potential recruits rejected for being unfit. The 60,000 Canadians who died in the war and the 50,000 who died from influenza after the war also made health a greater priority for Canadians. In 1919, the federal government responded by creating the Department of Health and, within it, the Division of Child Welfare. The Food and Drug Act, enacted by Parliament in 1920, attempted to control the veracity of claims made on food labels; in 1927, the Food and Drug Act was amended to allow control over food labels on items weighing over two ounces. Given the increase in availability of packaged and canned foods, this amendment was a significant change.[5]

Physicians, too, became interested in the science of nutrition and recognized the need for nutrition to be taught to the wider public. By 1921, three vitamins had been identified – A, B, and C – and vitamin D quickly followed.[6] Not surprisingly, articles and book reviews on nutrition abounded in medical journals. Physicians believed they were developing a better sense of what the body needed and what foods contained the substances required. While there was general consensus about nutrition, specific aspects were contentious. Not everyone in the health professions believed that physicians were up to date on nutrition, and debates in the medical journals revolved around which nutrients were of more significance and what was the best way to access them.[7] Some practitioners advised certain foods over others: butter over margarine and brown bread over white. *The Canadian Magazine* published an article suggesting that a proper diet could secure health and that by eating well an individual could put on or lose weight, sleep better, and look better. Other magazines told their readers about the wonders of drinking milk. However, much was still unknown, and not everyone even accepted the concept of a balanced meal. For example, Arctic explorer Vilhjalmur Stefansson in 1928 went on an all-meat diet for a year and remained healthy.[8]

Despite what was known about nutrition, Canadians didn't seem to be eating well. While rural families could have some control over their food (the food they planted or raised), Canada was becoming a more urban country; city families often didn't even know where some of their food came from. Sugar provided energy but no nutrients, and estimates indicated that by the end of the 1920s Canadians were consuming ten times more sugar than a century earlier. In an article on deficiency diseases, Dr Whetmore told his colleagues that Canadians also ate too much fat.[9] Added to these issues was the increase of refined foods resulting from the canning process. While canning might be able to maintain protein, fats, and carbohydrates, it limited the vitamin content of food.

Refining white flour removed minerals, vitamins, and roughage. For the food industry, however, the removal of nutrients helped to provide a longer shelf life for some foods.[10] The centrality of nutritious food for health meant various levels of government found themselves becoming responsible for food quality.

While studies in the 1920s reported that malnourished children could come from any class, during the Depression more health experts accepted the relationship between malnutrition and poverty. Others added disease and ignorance as culprits.[11] Food surveillance increased at the federal level as the economic downturn resulted in more food adulteration and false health claims as a marketing ploy to sell food products. In 1935, the League of Nations, through its Mixed Committee on the Problem of Nutrition, asked its member countries to assess the status of nutrition in their country. Canada's response was prosaic to say the least: "Public responsibility for food and health rests in the first place with the municipality, and in the second place with the Provincial Governments in supervising and the carrying out of such duties by the municipality. In the real sense of the word, it is not a national responsibility." One federal report claimed that no significant nutritional problems existed among Canadians.[12] Others disagreed. Leonard C. Marsh, a social scientist at McGill University, argued that too many Canadians lacked access to good food. Women's and other groups insisted that the federal government's assessment of nutritional reality lacked credibility. Despite the federal government's failure to see malnutrition in many Canadians, it did create the Canadian Council on Nutrition (CCN) in 1937 and adopted a dietary standard created by the Ontario Medical Association (OMA) for families on social assistance. In 1938, the CCN helped Canada become the first country to develop a national dietary standard against which nutritional survey results were measured.[13]

The federal government in the early 1940s introduced Canada's Official Food Rules, which established the norms of what Canadians *should* be eating, followed by new guides in 1944 and 1949. The purpose of the rules was to overcome what some saw as poor eating habits, a result of "lack of knowledge, lack of interest, [and] lack of adequate facilities for storage and preparation." Rules were fine, but for some Canadians there were no welfare measures to enable them to follow the food rules.[14] In 1941, Dr J.C. Simpson, retiring dean of medicine at McGill University, expressed concern about adolescent boys: "In the years to come boys of 16, 17, and 19 will be entering the university underweight, underdeveloped, without normal coordinations." His conclusion stemmed from the rejection, based on their poor health, of 80,000 recruits from the first 100,000 applicants to the Royal Canadian Air Force (RCAF). Others worried about the health of girls and women working in the war industries. Rationing of fats, meat, and sugar was also a part of wartime citizenship. But, as Charlene D. Elliott has noted, heavy Canadians could be "assumed to be undermining" the war's success by eating more than other citizens, especially the rationed foods. The war effort needed healthy people both at home and overseas, and public health experts linked health with citizenship and winning the war. Men who were accepted into the military were educated about nutrition, but the families of men in the armed services were not well served by the allowances provided, as they were based, regardless of the actual size of the family, on a family with only two children.[15] Given that the war was long – 1939 to 1945 – some military families didn't have enough money to keep healthy food in the home.

After the war, many Canadians wanted the government to continue its active involvement in controlling food prices. Women were especially sensitive to the cost of food, and the 100,000 members of the Housewives Consumer Association lobbied unsuccessfully for continued price controls on food. The government, however, was willing to involve itself in Canadians' lives more than it had done before the war. The push to make Canadians healthy through proper nutrition was part of the context that led to the creation of the Family Allowance in 1945. Also at the federal level, advertisement regulations for vitamins were tightened: the way in which vitamins were measured was regulated, and product testimonials to the public were prohibited.[16] An editorial in the 1945 *Canadian Journal of Public Health* pointed out that the focus on dietary deficiencies, especially vitamins, tended to make people overlook other nutritional problems such as obesity. As E.W. McHenry, Department of Physiological Science, School of Hygiene and Connaught Laboratories at the University of Toronto, warned, *over*nutrition was a cause of malnutrition and could result in health problems. Even popular literature reminded Canadians that those who were fat were malnourished.[17]

A summary of Canadians' dietary habits at the end of the 1940s by L.B. Pett, director of the Nutrition Division of the Department of Pensions and Health, Ottawa, reported that Canadians received 40 per cent of their calories from fats, whereas the recommended amount was 25 per cent. In addition to being concerned about the high fat intake, Pett worried about those who were not getting enough calories from fat.[18]

Not everyone had access to good food. Did Canadians even know what good food was? They were inundated with advertising about food products, with food faddists and quacks appealing to a "gullible" public. For example, McHenry complained that too many Canadians didn't eat cheese, believing it was "indigestible." Others wouldn't combine starches and proteins at the same meal, convinced that each food would have an impact on the digestion of the other. *Chatelaine* took to task the "old hand-me down notions about food": the dangers of cooking in aluminum pots or eating food out of cans and the possibility of developing "acid stomach" from eating oranges or tomatoes. Others criticized Canadians who believed that potatoes were fattening.[19]

The nutritional concerns of the 1940s continued into the 1950s, but with a significant shift. Unlike after World War I when the economy was poor for some years, after World War II the economy was strong. Following a decade of economic depression and half a decade of war, Canadians wanted to experience plenty. More efficient food production and the increase in frozen and packaged food helped Canadians to do so. Quantity and variety of food had increased. For example, Dominion grocery stores in the 1930s offered their customers 1,000 items; by 1956, they offered 5,000.[20] Many Canadians were also leading sedentary lives, while at the same time consuming more fat and less protein than they needed. Nutritional anaemia was on the rise due to iron deficiency.[21] With increased postwar immigration to Canada, some nutrition experts expressed concern about the way in which immigrants tended to adhere to their traditional foodways to the detriment of their health. Others, however, encouraged new Canadians to keep eating habits that were nutritional.[22] No consensus meant that nutritional advice to new Canadians wasn't clear; nor was it any better for the rest of the Canadian population. Nevertheless, many immigrant women had problems with Canadian food. For immigrant wives and mothers, making food for the family was part of their identity. Some food allowed them to maintain connections to the old countries; at the same time, Canadian food gave a connection to Canada. But that connection was difficult. For some immigrants, supermarkets and grocery stores were different from what they had known at home. For example, Rosa Valentti had only seen food in barrels in Italy, while in her new country food was in "prepacked forms" with labels in English or French. But immigrants were not the only groups that nutrition experts worried about: "Indigenous Canadians, Quebeckers, and other Canadians [were] considered deviant or dangerous in some way."[23]

Underlying the nutritional anxiety was a moral judgment. Blaming the individual for self-indulgence was accompanied by blaming the consumer for poor spending habits. For example, experts complained that Canadians spent too much money on meat, cakes, cookies, and soft drinks; however, many of these same Canadians found fruits and vegetables too expensive.[24] Nutritionists' frustration was palpable. They saw what was happening and believed they knew ways for people to save money so that they could afford good food. But in reality, nutritionists' idea of good food differed from the food many Canadians preferred to eat. Canadians liked their high-fat diet.[25]

Obesity as a form of malnutrition was becoming of more concern. The United Nations had already responded to the fear of overnutrition by revising caloric needs downward in its 1950 report. Pett described modern Canada as " automation at work ... more people riding cars than bicycles ... all the hours spent at 'do-it-yourself' projects, and other hours spent slumped in front of television ... all the calories from cocktails, and all the other calories ... ingest[ed]." Such a picture reflects a rather narrow segment of the population, but the point that the changes in society necessitated different nutritional responses was well taken. Statistics suggested that Canada ranked in the top ten countries for caloric intake, which could be seen as positive except that too many Canadians were taking in more than they needed. French-Canadian literature recognized the excess of food consumed during the Christmas/New Year period as well as at other "fêtes." By overindulging, both in drinking and eating, the health of Quebec's citizens could be compromised immediately or later.[26]

In the sixties, the society of plenty and consumerism worried physicians. *Chatelaine* quoted Dr Barbara McLaren, dean of the Faculty of Food Sciences at the University of Toronto, who suggested that Canadians were open to the "blandishments from advertisers," families seldom ate a meal together, and too many were on diets that were neither healthy nor of much help in losing weight. Too often Canadians spent their money on candy, soft drinks, and empty-calorie food, or overspent on expensive cuts of meat. As in other decades, there were complaints about food beliefs and Canadians' willingness to listen to food faddists. In response, McHenry published a book entitled *Foods without Fads*.[27]

In 1961, the CCN again approved adjusting Canada's Official Food Rules. The main shift was calling the document a "guide" to emphasize that Canadians had more flexibility in what they could eat, reflecting the increased variety of foods available. The word "guide" also appealed to a Canada in peacetime rather than wartime, when rules had been more accepted. The old rules (besides their inflexibility) were criticized because some of the quantities recommended led to overeating. Yet, even the new guide might have done the same, since serving sizes were not clearly specified. Also, the three-meal-a-day rule ignored the increasing acceptance by some nutritionists that many small meals were better than three larger ones. Other jurisdictions in Canada also created their own nutritional guides. In 1964, a diet manual was sponsored by the Ontario Health Association and the Ontario Dietetic Association, with the approval of the OMA.[28] Keeping track of all the guidelines could be problematic.

In 1970, an editorial in the *Canadian Medical Association Journal* (*CMAJ*) noted that Canada's Food Guide seemed to be recommending more protein intake for adults than what the CCN's dietary standard advised. Even different government departments couldn't agree on what food needs were optimal. Marjorie Harris, a staff and senior editor for *Maclean's*, aired her frustration with the many experts telling her what to buy and cook – manufacturers, the Food and Drug Directorate, the Department of Agriculture, dietitians, food chemists, and nutritionists. She was also unhappy about the quality of the food that came in packages, cans, and frozen forms. Taste and nutrition seemed to be disappearing.[29] Safety, nutrition, and the taste of food were often at odds. Food processing too often eliminated nutrients; the fad for vitamin megadoses was "plain dangerous"; and cooking oil in spray form was unsafe with its "fluorocarbon propellants."[30] The issue over fats was whether they were unsaturated or not, the former being the focus for health with most plant oils seen as healthier than animal fats. The Beef Information Centre, however, assured Canadians that beef and its saturated fatty acid was not a factor for heart disease.[31] The complications on the road to nutrition did not make it easy to travel, and that road is still difficult.

Nutritional experts argued that Canadians were not eating well: eating together as a family was declining; eating snack foods was increasing; and drinking milk was giving way to consuming more soft drinks, wine, and spirits.[32] An article in the *Canadian Consumer* blamed ignorance – "poor food buying and eating patterns." Thus, the individual was deemed to be at fault. Yet, stores with the cheapest food were not close to where the poor lived.[33] Schools sold "inappropriate" food to raise money for athletic activities or other school projects. And to top it all, some school lunches were nutritionally deficient, as were the contents of most school vending machines. Beverley Reichert, a registered dietitian, worried about Canadians being misled by books promising that eating the right kind of food could cure diseases such as cancer, diabetes, and arthritis; or being duped into thinking that doctors couldn't be trusted; or taken in by enticements to buy certain cooking utensils for weight loss. She vented about those who undermined the science of modern agriculture by instilling fear of chemical fertilizers and their effect on soil and the food grown on it. At the end of the 1970s, the government of Canada, once again, introduced a campaign to get Canadians eating better. Alison Cunliffe, writing for the *Toronto Star*, explained the situation to her readers: "The campaign will ... recommend calorie-cutting and limited use of salt ... But the findings of a government committee on diet and cardiovascular disease on which the government based its decision to launch the campaign have already come under attack."[34] If the government couldn't "get" healthy nutrition right, how could Canadians?

Measurement and Surveys

Nutritional advice to Canadians was based on knowing how well or not Canadians were eating. As McHenry pointed out in 1932, public health workers needed to know both how much Canada's citizens were eating and what they were eating. How else could their health be determined?[35] In the 1920s and 1930s, weight/height charts (using age and sex as well) were a quick way for physicians to determine the health of their patients. To find out the nutritional health of the population, surveys of groups began.

School children were a captive audience; consequently, an ongoing series of studies of children in schools began. In 1891–92, Franz Boas surveyed school children in Toronto to form a base for future studies.[36] In 1921, Drs Alan Brown, physician-in-chief at the Hospital for Sick Children in Toronto (1919–51), and G. Albert Davis, physician in the Out-Patient Department at the same hospital, reported on a nutritional survey of four Toronto elementary schools, chosen to represent different socio-economic groups and locations, plus a fifth school that had already had a mental health survey done on every child. The purpose of the study was to determine the health of children based on existing weight/height standards – indeed weighing in at schools was a way to teach children the link between weight and proper eating. Since experts in the field disagreed on the cut-off point for malnourishment, Brown and Davis used the two most popular benchmarks: the first established malnourishment at 7 per cent or more underweight for all children, while the second established it at 10 per cent or more underweight for children up to age ten and 12 per cent or more underweight for children aged ten to sixteen. The results of the survey of 2,843 children concluded that 44 per cent were deemed underweight by the first measurement, and 26 per cent by the second. This finding shows how, if there is no consensus on the measurement of malnutrition, the percentage of malnourished can vary significantly. If there is a consensus about the cut-off number – weight – the percentage is as accurate as the number chosen. Extrapolating from their figures, Brown and Davis concluded that just over 25 per cent of school children were "in a serious state of health." If that wasn't bad enough, malnourishment seemed to result in a "lack of physical and nervous energy which results in poor school work, and generally affects behaviour so that these children often appear listless and stupid." Malnourishment had become an explanation for much of what concerned society about its youth – poor health, bad behaviour, and lack of focus in school. Of course, there are other factors to explain poor health, bad behaviour, and lack of focus. Two positive findings from the study were a revelation: first, no matter how significant the malnutrition, it did not seem to affect the intelligence of the children; and second, malnutrition was not more prevalent among poor children.[37] While Brown and Davis used a measurement of underweight for malnutrition, it was pointed out by some that being overweight should also be considered a measurement of malnutrition.[38]

In lieu of a national survey, school studies continued. Keeping track of weight was important to the point that in the 1930s Dr McCullough, chief provincial health officer in Ontario, proposed that each school have weight scales and keep a weight chart on students every month.[39] Localized studies of families across the country also occurred, including, for example, a 1937 study of 100 "small income" families in Toronto. The families were not on relief, and thus they were not among the poorest. Yet, the study determined that, compared to the CCN's dietary standard, men were taking in only 77.5 per cent of the caloric standard and women only 70 per cent. Men consumed 86 per cent of recommended protein; women 73 per cent. In 1938, Marsh, in his book *Health and Unemployment*, suggested that 35 per cent of the unemployed were malnourished.[40] Using the concept of optimal nutritional standards preferred by the League of Nations, the federal government in 1939 had the CCN undertake dietary surveys of four regional cities – Toronto, Quebec

City, Halifax, and Edmonton – with reports on each made public in the early 1940s.[41] The Edmonton study of seventy-six families, whose yearly incomes ranged from $500 to $1,500, determined that 47 per cent of family members were deficient in caloric intake and 9 per cent were "grossly deficient." As in the 1937 Toronto study of low-income families, mothers were at risk.[42] Studies in rural Manitoba found that 20 per cent of the people surveyed were underweight.[43] If the various national food guidelines created a standard for Canadians, there were still no comprehensive Canadian statistics for weight, height, and age charts. The charts used to compare Canadian nutritional survey results were either out of date, not Canadian, or based on few studies. But plans for a national survey were in the works, with the survey scheduled to start in 1953.[44]

The desire for information about the nutritional state of Canadians escalated throughout the decades. With all the surveys and studies, the statistics of malnourishment engendered concern and were most likely meant to do so. In 1970, the federal government announced a nutritional study of the Canadian population as a whole. Nutritionists had been asking for such a survey, but the timing was ironic. The government departments in charge of nutrition had been cut back drastically, and the continued existence of the CCN, the advisory committee to the minister of health and welfare, was under review. The survey was to begin in the fall of 1970 and end in 1972.[45] Not surprisingly, the conclusions of the national study seemed quite familiar. Too many Canadians were deficient in iron, protein during pregnancy, calcium, vitamin D, thiamin (especially in men), and B12. Half of adults were overweight. The numbers were disturbing: 2,193,000 adults with high blood cholesterol; 1,585,000 men, women, and children deficient in iron; 1,823,000 children and teenagers who didn't get enough calcium; and 5,055,000 men, women, and children who didn't take in the "desirable amounts" of vitamin C. The Inuit were at "high risk" for lack of folic acid intake, while both Indigenous and Inuit women had a vitamin A deficiency during pregnancy.[46]

Not everyone took the survey as a reflection of Canadians' nutrition level. One critic pointed out that people who participated in the survey were probably those concerned about what they ate, and so the results of the survey should be seen as an "optimistic" view of the real situation. For his part, Pett noticed that the survey only had a 46 per cent response rate, and concluded that "the figures cannot justifiably be used to represent the population of Canada." Pett also noted that adequate diets had to be put into context and that food itself does not give a true picture of nutrition. For example, he queried whether the use of tranquilizers and contraceptives could create signs of malnutrition, even if those taking them were apparently eating an "adequate" diet.[47]

Malnutrition surveys were popular in the health professions, showing the concern about nutrition. The studies of the country, provinces, cities, parts of cities, rural areas, schools, families, the poor, and the middle class differed, but the conclusions over time indicated Canadians did not appear to eat well. There was always some group that needed to eat better.

Mothers, Children, Teens, and Others

The nutritional health of women throughout the sixty years covered in this study was consistently problematic. In the 1920s, maternal mortality in Canada was high – four deaths a day – and many of the deaths were caused by malnutrition.[48] And when the mother died, her infant had a lower chance of survival. Young women's eating habits were poor.[49] The 1937 survey of 100 Toronto families determined that mothers were the worst fed members of the family. The four city surveys also showed mothers to be at risk, and no wonder. Although the survey of the four cities was based on the concept of optimal standards preferred by the League of Nations, it did lower some of the nutrient requirements for women to reflect what the CCN saw as the lesser needs of Canadian women compared to European women. Many of the latter worked in the fields and therefore needed the energy intake assumed to be optimal for men. McHenry advised the lowering of the nutrient requirement for Canadian women, even though he was well aware from the 1937 Toronto study that the caloric intake for women was substandard. Over time, the CCN endorsed three national nutritional standards that decreased women's nutritional needs.[50]

Nutritional experts tended to blame women for their poor eating habits. In the 1940s, statistics on adults in Ontario indicated that 17 per cent were underweight and 16 per cent were overweight. It was suggested that a greater percentage of women compared to men were underweight in each age group due to "slimming."[51] Thus, women were blamed for their malnutrition. In 1951, an article in *Maclean's* informed readers that women between ages twenty and thirty-nine were at risk of "anaemia, thinness, overweight ... [and] protein and vitamin A deficiencies." Young, single women and older teenage girls fared even worse with their diets. For pregnant women, the results of malnutrition could be devastating – premature childbirth and/or the death of their babies. The reasons noted for women not eating well were varied: the high cost of food causing wives and mothers to put themselves low in the nutrition race; the desire of women to be slender leading them to adopt poor eating habits; and the consumption of too much sugar.[52] The National Nutrition Survey in the early 1970s determined that women's lower caloric intake led to poorer quality diets in terms of protein, most vitamins, and minerals. It was also noted that "serum cholesterol show[ed] 10 to 13 percent [in] adult men and 14 to 34 percent [in] adult women." Once again, the reason for women's poorer nutrition compared to men's focused on women being on weight-loss diets.[53]

Despite many women's poor nutritional health, women were a significant group in lobbying for nutritional reform, emphasizing their determination to expand their care for their families to others. Health experts, however, often saw mothers from a different perspective. Many health experts saw ignorance of nutrition as a major cause of malnutrition. More often than not, they blamed the ignorance of mothers for the malnutrition of their children and teens. Mothers were supposed to ensure that their children were neither overfed nor underfed; in the eyes of the experts, mothers failed.

During the 1920s and 1930s, experts were particularly concerned that too many children weren't getting enough to eat, or that what they were eating was not always nutritious. Malnutrition became a "troublesome condition."[54] In 1934, a study of Ontario schools surveyed 2,050 children, aged eight to sixteen, about their eating habits. Results showed the 20 per cent drank no milk at all, with those from poor families twice as inclined not to drink milk.[55] In 1937, McCullough worried that the image of chubby young children as healthy could result in the acceptance of children being overweight. Indeed, mothers saw putting weight on children as positive, a response to the death rate of children in the 1920s and 1930s. And it wasn't only mothers who saw chubby children as healthy: in some clinics for malnourished children, those who put on the most weight received a special treat or award.[56] As for adolescents, they needed more than 1,000 extra calories compared to a "moderately active" adult, and it wasn't always easy to get teenagers to eat extra calories and do it through nutritious food. Teenage girls especially did not eat well; yet, they needed more iron than their brothers because of the added stress of menstruation. That being the case, a mother's dilemma was to "coax" her daughters to eat

Nutrition Policy: "Dietetic Missionaries" 39

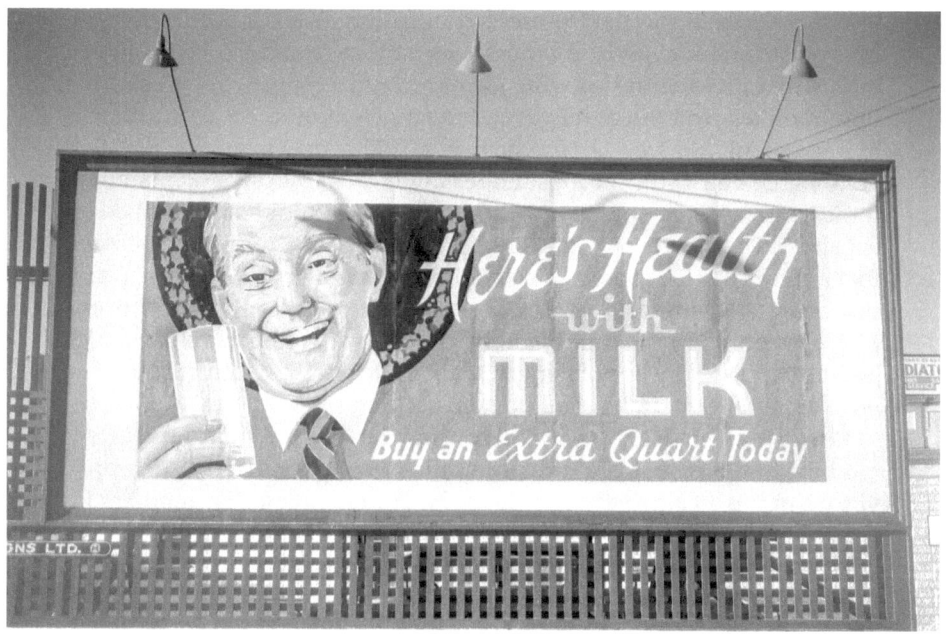

Nutritionists, educators, and doctors wanted Canadian infants, children, teens, and adults to drink milk for vitamin C. The idea behind this billboard design was to persuade older men to drink milk and to keep other adults drinking milk, as well as to show teens that milk was an adult drink and not only for children. Source: NB-55–907, 1940, Hook Signs Ltd., Calgary, Alberta, Glenbow Museum.

what they needed, not what they wanted,[57] as well as to make sure her sons were eating enough nutritious food. Certainly, mothers couldn't always control what their children ate. In an acknowledgment of child agency, F.W. Tidmarsh, physician in charge of Nutrition Services at the Massachusetts–Halifax Health Commission, noted that some children would rather drink tea or coffee than milk. "The morning cereal is refused," he said, "and candy is eaten at all hours with the result that there is no appetite for proper food at regular hours."[58] The agency of teens was even more of a problem for health experts. Teenage girls especially tried to maintain a popular body image by skipping breakfast and drinking tea or coffee rather than milk.[59]

While those in the field presented nutrition as a science in need of interpretation by experts, mothers were still expected to choose foods that would provide the growing list of recognized nutrients needed by their families. Too often, however, the advice to mothers was difficult to implement. Mildred D. Goodeve, in a 1935 article in *Health*, pointed out that breakfast was the most important meal of the day and planning for it was necessary so that a child could have a calm hour in which to eat and have a bowel movement before he or she went to school. Given that a mother might have several children, keeping track of them and providing a "calm hour" wasn't easy. Advice could also be contrary. McCullough told *Chatelaine* readers that lack of appetite in a child could just mean the child was not hungry, but it could also be a sign of illness[60] – not a comment that was going to help mothers.

Nutritional advice was available, and health specialists expected mothers to follow it, even if their families were poor. Nova Scotia provincial public health officer, William H. Hattie, noted that mothers in poor families didn't spend money wisely. A study in Brantford, Ontario, blamed housewives on relief for spending too much on sugar and other carbohydrates and not enough on milk and vegetables. Such mothers needed to be "clever" in their buying and cooking choices.[61] Yet, feeding a family on relief was not easy. As one mother wrote to *Chatelaine*:

> I am a Canadian Mother. The most noble calling in the world is mine ... My country realizes that my children are its greatest asset ... When depression comes, my country rushes to the rescue. But when the S.O.S. goes out, do Canadians cry "Mothers and babies first?" Is my name exalted when it appears on the relief list? Hardly ... I am provided with groceries. No milk ...When I appealed for milk for my twins I was allowed two quarts a day. Of this the babies took two thirds of a quart each, and I fed the rest to my other five children, a teaspoonful at a time as a medicine ... My children are starving and cold. That is fact, not theory. True, they have bread. They need meat and milk ... Canada is a rich country ... And her children are suffering for food, suffering a lack that the future can never remedy.[62]

Too many mothers could have said the same.

The Edmonton segment of the four city surveys showed that women and children represented 82 per cent of those whose diets were grossly deficient in protein and 90 per cent of those grossly deficient in iron. Of those grossly deficient in calcium, 74 per cent were children. The worst fed children were teenagers.[63] Variations on nutritional deficiencies and

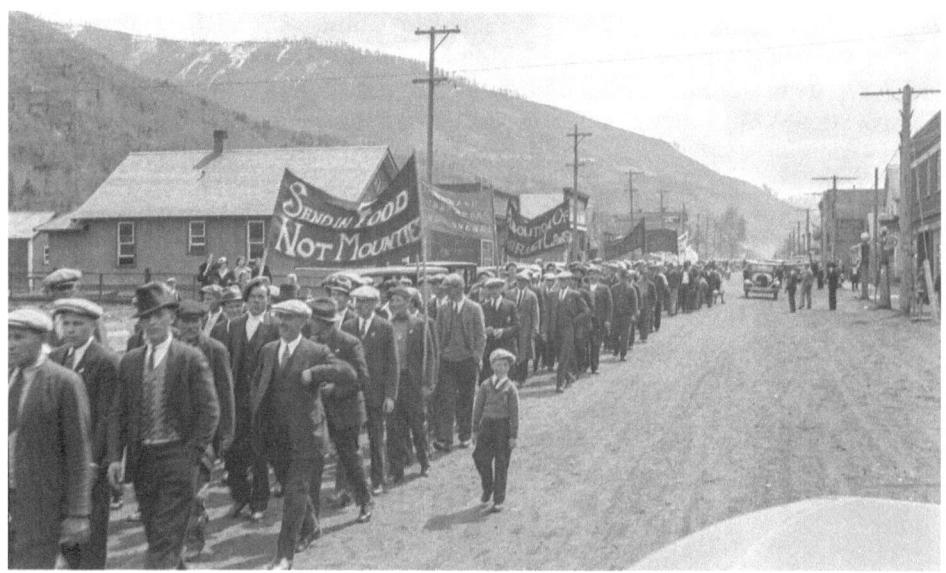

Food was scarce for many Canadians throughout the Depression, and many workers had difficulty feeding their families. This photo shows a protest by workers from both sides of the Crowsnest Pass marching down Main Street, Natal, British Columbia on May Day, 1934. The sign saying "Send in food not Mounties" is indicative of their concerns. Source: Photographer, Gushul Studio, Blairmore, Alberta; NC-54–2011, Glenbow Museum.

their types were also found in the Halifax, Quebec City, and Toronto studies as well. All four studies were clear that the father was the best fed member of the family, probably because his health was needed so he could work in order to buy food for his family. Instead of placing some responsibility for poor nutrition on the economic problems of the 1930s and responding to them, the government and many nutritionists blamed mothers for their children's lack of nutritional health;[64] that is, they blamed the family member who was among the worst fed. It was seldom recognized that mothers had difficulty getting their children and teens to eat, let alone meeting the demands of food rules.

During the war and after, children and teenagers (as well as mothers) were still at risk. For some, poverty was a factor.[65] In 1943, Dr Elizabeth

Chant Robertson, *Chatelaine*'s Child Health Clinic columnist, discussed the eating problems of some children, which she considered the result of parents forcing their children to eat more than they needed or wanted.[66] But parents still considered chubby young children to be healthy. In 1945, Alton Goldbloom accused mothers of forcing their children to eat certain foods; basing his advice on studies, he suggested leaving children to decide for themselves what they would eat. Such advice was easy to give, but difficult for parents to follow, especially mothers. The idea of children, some of whom had "violent likes and dislikes for various foods,"[67] and teenage girls with their fixation on being slender, choosing what they wanted to eat just wouldn't work in a family with more than one child unless mothers became short-order cooks. Advice from women's magazines was not any better. An article in the 1944 *Canadian Home Journal* advised mothers to tell their daughters that being thin was no longer fashionable.[68] The idea of a mother giving her daughter fashion advice might have appealed to the mother, but probably not so much to her teenage daughter. As a girl left young childhood, the shift to being slender was emphasized, a body ideal that many girls were trying to emulate. This body image led them to eat foods that experts rejected as unhealthy or to simply not eat enough. The body image for a boy as he left young childhood was to be bigger and more solid than girls. Those who did not fit this image, whether thin or fat, were seen as lacking in masculinity.[69] Gender played a role in nutrition. Beginning as young as the age of two, the total calories per day recommended by the Canadian Dietary Standard was 1,250 for girls and 1,400 for boys. The difference continued throughout childhood and adolescence.[70]

Governments were looking towards Canada's future and putting more money into education. Living in a democratic country in the 1950s, Canadian youth had to compare favourably with youth from communist countries. That could only happen if Canadian children and youth were healthy. Mothers continued to be told to make their children eat well. In 1953, G.T. Haig, author of "Suppose Tommy Won't Eat," described one mother who was worried that her two-year-old daughter hardly ate. The child looked healthy, had lots of energy, and seemed to be of normal weight and height. Haig talked to the mother further, asking what her daughter ate, which he determined was too much. As Haig told his readers, here was a healthy child and an overly worried mother, the latter because she simply did not know the food needs of a child.[71] She also had a specific image of what a healthy two-year-old should look like: a chubby child who looked vigorous. Since being underweight was historically a sign of malnutrition in children, it is understandable why mothers wanted to see their children with weight on them.

A new issue arose in the 1950s as a possible factor affecting child malnutrition: married mothers entering the workforce. In 1953, two schools in a middle-class area of suburban Greater Toronto and their students in grades 6, 7, and 8 took part in a dietary study. The study's goal was to determine food intake, in particular the consumption of cake, pastry, candy, sugar, and soft drinks; and to evaluate the impact of an employed mother on the nutritional quality of children's eating habits. Two conclusions were perhaps unexpected: eating sweets was not linked to other poor nutritional habits, and a mother's absence from the home did not affect her children's diets. The fact that those conducting the study raised the latter issue reflected the perception that working mothers could not be good mothers. Despite the positive nature of some study findings, however, the general summary was worrisome. Too many children took in less than the recommended amounts of vitamin D, milk, citrus fruit, whole grain cereals, and vegetables.[72] While sympathy for mothers was rare, Dr R.H. Johnson, in an article in *Health*, blamed too many experts in the field for confusing new mothers: they were overwhelmed by information from government agencies, private companies trying to sell them something, friends, and relatives, with each source proclaiming the expert nature of their advice. It is noteworthy that Johnson didn't blame the advice doctors gave to mothers.[73]

For decades, children had been surveyed and studied, and little changed in the 1960s. Researchers wanted to pinpoint the health differences among children, especially those on the margins of society, and to trace the changes in children's health over time. But, as with almost all the studies already completed, researchers found it was difficult, if not impossible, to come up with positive results. The bar for desired results was continually raised, and so failure was assured. Indeed, finding a negative result – a nutritional problem – seemed to justify the study. In 1968, a total of 508,519 school children in the province of Quebec were examined. Of those surveyed, 55,604 children were found to have deficiencies severe enough to endanger their development – most of them being forms of malnourishment.[74]

Given the concern about children's nutrition, it is no wonder that marketers often used an image of a child eating to sell food products to mothers. In 1963, Swift's Premium "franks" placed a telling and blatant advertisement in *Chatelaine*. The visual showed a chubby boy carrying an armful of weiners. Part of the text read: "No fair counting how many ... A youngster may be finicky about everything else, but somehow he managed to down four of these appetizing favourites without batting an eye. And that's A-OK, Mom! Because here is Meat Power from Swift – a good dietary source of protein."[75] The ad appealed to what almost any parent wanted for their children – eating something good for them. Certainly, from a mother's perspective, the goal was to get her children to eat. When the Nutrition Division of the Department of National Health and Welfare advised mothers to let preschoolers decide the amount of food they needed,[76] it was advice that Goldbloom had already given in 1945. The advice remained just as impractical for mothers in 1963.

The first wave of baby boomers were now reaching their teens. What teens ate, where, and with whom was part of teen culture, which had strengthened over the decades. If teens didn't seem to be aware of the empty calories they were eating, health professionals were. For some time, experts had speculated about the reasons teens didn't drink enough milk: teens saw drinking milk as childish, and teenage girls saw it as fattening.[77] In the world of teenage girls and boys, image trumped nutrition. What did change by the 1970s was that chubbiness in children ceased to be the ideal. Concern focused on those who were overweight, not underweight.[78] As for older children and teens, they were increasingly eating outside the home, in part because of "the affluence of Canadian society," "peer pressure," and "lack of parental guidance." As they had in the past, mothers still reaped the ire of commentators, especially mothers who were employed,[79] despite the 1953 study that had found little to worry about.

Nutritional experts continued to pay the most attention to women, children, and teenagers. Children and teenagers were the future of the country, and their health was significant. Women, when they became mothers, were responsible for their children's and their husband's nutrition as well as their own. Other Canadians were seldom discussed. After all, studies revealed men to be the best fed in their families. Yet, some men were of concern – not the poor but the successful. In 1920, J.E. Dubé, in an article in *L'Union Médicale du Canada* (*UMC*), complained about the way professional men continued to eat as much meat as their fathers had eaten, not cutting back to accommodate their changed lifestyle. The result could be diabetes and arterial sclerosis. By the end of the 1940s, practitioners were discussing the poor eating habits of executives. An article in 1950 on "busy business people" also put executives in the at-risk category. Assuming the "people" were male, the description depicted a man too tired either to eat or to pay attention to how much he was eating. Both could lead to malnutrition.[80]

The elderly didn't seem to be considered in the early decades. By the 1940s, however, some literature was appearing that suggested the elderly also needed balanced diets. In the 1950s, the elderly in Canada often faced living situations that didn't encourage healthy eating. A 1963 University of Manitoba study of housebound elderly in Winnipeg reported that 67 per cent of the seventy-four people studied had caloric intakes below the dietary standard for Canada and nutrient deficiencies – vitamin A, iron, and ascorbic acid. The National Nutrition Survey in the early 1970s provided a better sense of what the elderly faced. Seniors (over age sixty-five) were the most poorly nourished in the country. Reasons included limited financial resources, being alone, food fads, cultural habits, poor health, poor teeth, and failing taste buds. Elderly men were especially vulnerable. But for the elderly, being poorly nourished increasingly meant being obese. The Nutrition Survey reported that women were more likely than men to be obese, and one-third of the obese were over the age of sixty-five.[81] While cutting back on calories was one way to offset some of the diseases of the elderly, many elderly people were simply not eating enough to be healthy.[82]

Aboriginal peoples (Indigenous, Inuit, and Metis), more than any other group, were mainly absent in both the public media and the health literature. It took several decades before their malnutrition began to be addressed. Nutritional experts were concerned about Canadians who were poor and on relief during the Depression, but they didn't realize the extent to which the First Nations were deprived, dependent as they were on the federal government. From 1931 to 1934, relief expenditure for First Nations decreased by 16.5 per cent, whereas expenditure for Euro-Canadians increased by 367 per cent.[83] And the situation of First Nations populations remained dire. As Ian Mosby has noted, in the 1940s and 1950s "bureaucrats, scientists, and a whole range of experts exploited their 'discovery' of malnutrition in Aboriginal communities ... to further their own professional and political interests." In the 1960s, studies among Indigenous peoples and the Inuit determined an increase in weight that did not signal anything positive, as it was caused by a significant increase in sugar consumption and a decrease in animal protein intake. Neither did physical development in Inuit children signal improvement in nutrition.[84]

Indigenous youth in residential schools were at most risk. Ian Mosby, in his work on the history of nutrition during World War II, exposed the nutritional experimentation on residential school children that put nutritional theory before the health of the children. Neither did their risk lessen in the following decades. In the 1950s, food rules were taught in some residential schools, but they more often than not contradicted First Nations' customs and set up a situation whereby children saw their mothers as somehow lacking, weakening the bonds holding their culture together. And to what end? The food rules advocated foods the First Nations could neither have afforded nor even had access to. This kind of "education" remains in place today, as does the image of the Indigenous mother as a model of what a mother should not be – an unassimilated citizen.[85]

For the Indigenous populations, the National Nutrition Survey and its nutritional guides were seen in the context of the 1969 white paper to abolish the Indian Act and Indian status. While a white paper is simply a proposal policy tabled in the Canadian legislature, the Indigenous people saw it as a "White Paper" and an attempt at cultural genocide, and is still remembered as such, although the paper was discarded in 1970.[86] As noted earlier, the National Nutrition Survey reported that many Indigenous and Inuit people lacked significant nutrients. It also placed the Aboriginal peoples apart from other Canadians. The nutritional standards used did not take into account the cultures of various Indigenous and Inuit peoples, and as a result put them outside the normative standards, a situation they had long experienced in so many aspects of their lives, as had immigrants and the poor, only more so. For example, the food standard included how much milk should be consumed. It ignored the fact that many Indigenous people were lactose intolerant, and even if they weren't, that they would have had difficulty accessing milk or paying for it. Both the Inuit and the First Nations were increasingly subsisting on what nutritionists saw as a problematic diet – too much starch and sugar instead of the fish and game that had traditionally been their staple diet (with the exception of agricultural groups).[87] For health "experts," the result was obesity.[88]

Nutrition Policy: "Dietetic Missionaries" 47

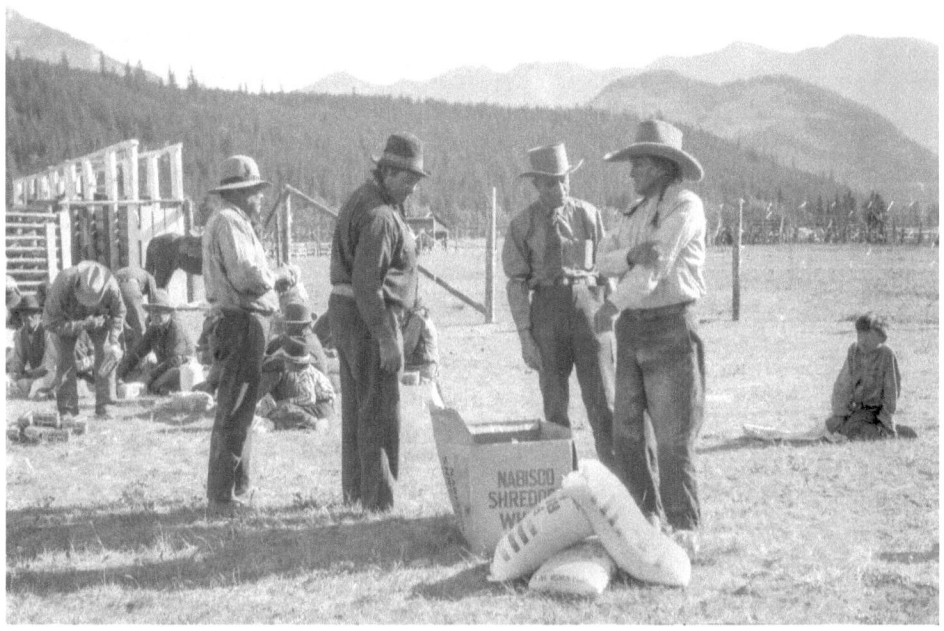

The federal government gave Indigenous people significantly less relief during the Depression as compared to others. This image, c. 1930, is titled "Ration Time at Banff Indian Days, Banff, Alberta"; Joe Big Plume, Sarcee (Tsuu T'ina), can be seen on the right. Source: Photographer, Arnold Lupson; NA-667–857, 1930s, Glenbow Museum.

Marketing and Education

From the perspective of health experts, Canadians failed to meet the nutritional regulations that existed throughout the decades. Various causes of malnutrition were listed: ignorance; poverty; disease; the inability of a mother to feed her children and husband nutritious food; the desire of adolescent girls and women to be slender; the youth culture that adolescents followed, which didn't encourage proper eating; the inclination of Indigenous Canadians to follow their own cultures; and food consumerism. Despite these multiple causes, many Canadians believed that nutritional education would overcome poor eating. The advice educators offered, however, shifted over time and did not always keep up with the most recent guidelines. And whose advice were Canadians to believe: advice from nutritionists and doctors, or advice in the major magazines? Or were they to believe the easily understood product marketing that surrounded them? Advertisements and articles in popular magazines were main sources of nutritional knowledge for Canadians. They provided information in a readable, non-confusing way, with clear directives, and often in the form of morality tales about the successes and failures of people who ate "right" and those who ate "wrong."[89] Governments put out pamphlets so Canadians could understand nutrition. Community education had the same goal, but with a personal aspect. Education about nutrition for adults, children, and teens was the approach taken to ensure Canadians would eat well.

Marketing

Advertisements appeared in both medical journals and the popular media. The former informed physicians that help was available to provide their patients with nutrients needed for sound healthy bodies. For example, the December 1921 issue of the *CMAJ* printed an advertisement for Frosst's Blaud Capsules, "an ideal form for the administration of iron." Such advertisements of stand-alone nutrients suggested that food might not always be sufficient to meet the nutritional needs of Canadians. Advertisements also informed practitioners that products such as Ovaltine could put weight on their emaciated patients.[90]

Almost any food product could be sold to Canadians in magazines based on its health value. Some marketers were very general in their appeal. An advertisement for the cereal FORCE emphasized its ability to supply "all the essentials of health." It was a "regulator" and helped with digestion. Other products emphasized the "food value" in terms of cost per calories and nutrients provided.[91] Deciding what food was best to purchase could be complex. Nutrients, too, were advertised in magazines. In *Maclean's*, an ad for McCoy's Cod Liver Extract Tablets appealed to men's desire to have "solid, healthy flesh" and to "feel well and strong," instead of being "nervous," "rundown," and "thin." Even their complexions would improve. For women, McCoy's claimed it could help them overcome their "hollow chest and run-down looks" that made them appear old and less attractive.[92] The gendered difference in the advertisements was telling. But for both men and women, body image mattered, and for both it was important not to be thin to the point of looking weak and unattractive.

To sell their products, marketers exploited parental concern that their children were not always willing to eat nutritious food. Parents were assured that by drinking Ovaltine a child's appetite would be stimulated in a "scientific way" so that the "natural sensation of hunger [would be] produced." Science would offer parents the solution to getting their children to eat. Neilson advertised their milk chocolate bars by appealing to mothers in a blatant way: ***Mothers Here Is the Perfect Chocolate for Kiddies, Neilson's Jersey Milk.*** The natural craving of your children for sweets should be satisfied ... Keep a box of Neilson's Jersey Milk Chocolate bars on hand and give each child a bar a day ... Nourishment and health for growing children in every bar."[93] Many themes emerge from such an advertisement: the perceived need on the part of mothers to know what to feed their children and to understand nutrition; the ability of marketers to use health concerns to sell candies; and the promotion of children's cravings for sweets as "natural" and a legitimate way to sell a product. If craving sweets was "natural," then mothers should meet that craving and not worry about it, a moral appeal to "nature." Just as vitamins were given once a day, here was a once-a-day chocolate bar, which provided mothers the comfort that it was good for children. And if the mother was not sure about what food was best, she could resort to the stand-alone nutrients, which seemed to increase in popularity each decade.

Marketing initiatives intensified during the 1940s and afterwards. In looking at nutritional advertising during the war, Alana Hermiston describes three frameworks employed: "instilling fear, inspiring patriotism, or a 'soft-sell' approach," which, while appealing to patriotism, also praised the role of women. Borden Company hit an advertisement bonanza for selling their milk products with Elsie the cow, Elmer the bull, and Beulah, their daughter. They created a cow family that Elsie cared for well. Fleischmann's Yeast touted bread as "a nearly perfect food" in an advertisement that appeared in *Maclean's* in 1940. The advertisement also asserted that the product made a "contribution to the advancement of Canada's National Health." The subtext could easily be understood to mean that bread made with Fleischmann's Yeast was part of the larger effort to win the war. By the end of the war, Fleischmann's advertisements shifted, focusing more on the speed with which Fleischmann's Yeast allowed women to bake, as well as on its nutritional content.[94]

Pharmaceutical companies consistently advertised supplementary nutrients in medical and lay publications. In addition to providing nutritional insurance, the appeal of such nutritional additives was that they were modern and allowed people to "eat and run." Thus, important people, who did not have time to sit and eat properly, could protect themselves by taking supplements. There seemed to be no end to who could benefit. After the war, Abbott Laboratories produced a series of advertisements focusing on specific types of people who suffered from undernutrition (nutritional deficiencies) and would profit from various of its nutrient products: the overweight woman looking for a diet that would work for her; the slender woman overlooking nutrition in her desire to keep her body thin; the professional man who ignored what he ate as he tried to save time; and those who were indifferent, smoking too much, drinking too much, or finding nutritional food unappealing.[95] Underlying such advertisements was the assumption that stand-alone nutrients were necessary. Even food companies were advising physicians on nutrition through their advertisements.[96] Food companies had become, or were trying to be, partners with medical practitioners.

The advertisements in the medical journals reflected the high status in which physicians were held and appealed to doctors to influence their patients. While historians of medicine often refer to the medicalization of society through the efforts of the medical profession, it is clear that private enterprise was, and is, a major supporter of these efforts. In the June 1959 issue of *The Canadian Nurse*, a Farmer's Wife (milk) advertisement let practitioners know that when they were in Edinburgh for the meeting of the Canadian and British Medical Associations, they could enjoy "club" privileges provided by Farmer's Wife. The privileges included club rooms, a mail and message exchange, fresh Canadian-style coffee, Canadian newspapers and radio programs, the Toronto Stock exchange quotations, and information on shopping.[97]

Marketing increased during the 1960s and 1970s, and practitioners became concerned. Alton Goldbloom, reacting to the cereal commercials on TV, pointed out that most cereals were fine to eat, but few were super foods. Indeed, much of their nutritional value was in the milk poured over them. He also made it clear that most Canadians didn't need to take vitamin pills. Eating well would provide enough nutrients for health. Evidently, however, many were not eating well enough: in Quebec, for example, favourite foods included potato chips or anything "sweet ... red ... [or] chocolate." Fleischmann's Oil, in an advertisement, assured medical readers that it would help to lower cholesterol, since it was made from corn. Carnation Instant Breakfast appealed to busy Canadians with the assurance that its "meal in a glass" had a variety of needed nutrients. A business called Nutri-Bio entered Canada, and through sales of vitamins and minerals employed 14,000 distributors across the country, selling $12 million worth of products a year.[98]

Education

While advertisements in the medical journals and popular magazines provided some nutritional information, albeit with the toal of selling products, more in-depth education came from other sources. Popular magazines such as *Chatelaine* and *Maclean's* published articles on what foods to eat to stay healthy and explained to their readers what nutrients were necessary. Literature such as Brown's *The Normal Child* (1923) instructed mothers about the kind of food children needed. The Child Welfare Council of Canada published "folders" on feeding children and teens up to the age of sixteen. The Child Hygiene section of the Canadian Public Health Association issued healthy diets for children.[99] Underlying this education was belief in the rationality of Canadians. After all, if people were not rational, what was the purpose of educating them? But, as David Smith and Malcolm Nicolson argue, the discourse about nutrition articulates "both a moralizing *and* a rationalizing impulse."[100] Giving nutritional advice is an attempt to control the body, specifically someone else's body.

The Depression in Canada emphasized the need for Canadians to become sharp shoppers and be able to wend their way through the competing advertising hype. Educational institutions took up the challenge, as did the medical associations and hospitals, the Red Cross Society, the Victorian Order of Nurses (VON), the Young Men's Christian Association (YMCA), the Visiting Homemakers Association, the Canadian Dietetic Association, the Canadian Home Economics Association, and the Housewives Association of Canada. As a consumer group, the latter was particularly concerned about nutrition during the Depression, focusing on the plight of those on relief, the high prices of some food, and the suspicion that government actions were not doing much to change the nutritional situation of Canadians for the better.[101]

With nutritional standards established, no matter what their flaws, the consensus remained that education was the key to better nutrition. In the 1940s, there were many venues for education. In Montreal, radio, press, magazines, meetings, and various organizations and clubs were used to put out the city's nutritional message. Public service announcements were one way to educate, as were a whole list of national, provincial, and local efforts. Films on nutrition were also available. Schools, too, were a main venue providing practical experience and teaching. School lunch programs did both: first, by making sure children had one good meal a day, and then, by doing so, providing an example of what a good meal should be.[102] Not all the advice given to Canadians was heeded. In 1945, Janet March told *Saturday Night* readers about the recommendation to save vegetable water for making sauces or drinking. Finding vegetable "broth" unappealing, she concluded: "I'll get my vitamins some other way."[103]

Most of the nutritional education was directed at women; if they failed to learn, it would be to the detriment of their bodies and those of their children and husbands. Yet, mothers were not the only ones needing education. Medical personnel needed to be kept up to date about nutrition too.[104] New vitamins such as vitamin K had been discovered, and it was predicted more would be found.[105] An article in *The Canadian Nurse* criticized physicians who were unaware of food prices and blithely ordered expensive diets for their patients. Doctors needed to be educated about how to eat well on less; otherwise, their patients would simply reject the doctor's advice, knowing they couldn't afford to follow it, or perhaps even worse, follow the advice at the expense of other family members.[106]

The results of nutritional education were never as positive as anticipated. The government of Canada acknowledged this weakness when it legalized adding vitamin D to white bread in 1953. While the government agreed with nutritionists that eating well was the best way to get all the necessary nutrients, the reason behind the enrichment of bread was the perception that not all Canadians ate well. Enrichment was insurance for those who didn't.[107] What to eat was a contested and competitive field. "Food fads" seemed to emerge every few years, were taken up, popularized, criticized by nutritionists, and then faded until new ones took their place. Canadians needed to become savvier about food, to be suspicious of extravagant product claims, and to eat well rather than take supplements unless advised by a physician.[108] Dr Chant Robertson was concerned about what appeared to be the increased consumption of fat. Fats were heavier in calories than proteins and carbohydrates, and thus she warned Canadians about becoming overweight. At the same time, fats limited the sense of hunger and helped the body absorb needed nutrients. Added to this was that all fats were not the same, each varying in nutrients.[109] It was all too much to keep up with. No wonder educating both lay and medical Canadians was an ongoing and contested process.

An innovative program was launched in Vancouver schools. A pair of rats was introduced to a classroom. One rat was fed according to Canada's Food Rules; needless to say, this rat thrived. The other rat, fed on sweets and soft drinks, did not thrive and became too thin. However, when the rat on the poor diet was introduced to a good diet, it became healthy. While the students liked the experiment, its intended message didn't seem to change what high school students were eating – teachers were even warned not to let teenage girls get the idea from the rat experiment that by eating a poor diet they could lose weight.[110]

Nutritionists for years had pushed the need for specific nutrients so strongly that J.E. Monagle, chief of the Nutrition Division in the Department of National Health and Welfare, complained that nutritionists were too fixated on specific nutrients rather than the overall nutritional picture. "Nutritionists are accused, in fact, of roaming the slums seeking the occasional case of nutritional deficiency to justify their existence."[111] An unattributed editorial in the 1965 *CMAJ* warned readers about the seriousness of being "overvitaminized." Vitamins had become so accepted that Canadians (both lay and medical) were forgetting that vitamins originally appeared only in certain foods and in certain amounts. There was a sense that by taking more vitamins you could improve upon nature.[112] The overvitaminization of society was never really resolved, simply because there was no one answer. In 1975, a session at the annual meeting of the Canadian Medical Association (CMA) presented two views on vitamins. One physician discussed the ability of megadoses of certain vitamins to fight specific diseases. A second physician sounded the alarm, not arguing against what was being said, but worrying that publicity about such propositions would work against protecting the public, who already seemed to be under the impression that vitamin megadoses worked to cure every ill, including the common cold and even schizophrenia.[113]

As a group, physicians didn't know enough about nutrition. In 1975, Dr Donald E. Hill of Toronto told the CMA Council on Community Health that while medical schools did a fair job of training physicians in nutrition, the training didn't extend to the postgraduate level or to nutrition counselling. As for practising physicians, most of them seemed "to rely on diet sheets provided by various sources, such as the pharmaceutical companies." However, such concerns had long existed in other areas of medical study. Medical schools had difficulty keeping up with new research, and once engaged in practice, physicians fell further behind. Dr Harding le Riche, professor of epidemiology at the University of Toronto, also pointed to the reluctance of professionals to be seen invading other specialties, in this case nutrition.[114] This reluctance reflected the narrowing of medical expertise that came with specialization. Yet, physicians needed to know about nutrition because their patients were interested in the impact of food on health. In 1976, Irmin Stephen, managing editor of *Canadian Doctor*, emphasized that patients were already experimenting with food and asking their doctors about the claims made for them by writers: "Can bran cure our digestive troubles? … Will brewer's yeast make us unfailing energetic?"[115]

Doctors were not the only health professionals with weaknesses in nutrition. Pharmacists weren't any better. Neither were nurses well trained in nutrition, with the result that courses began to be offered in newer nurse education programs. A turf war about who was best qualified to educate Canadians about nutrition, with nurses at times putting themselves above dietitians, didn't help Canadians.[116] When a survey of hospitals in Canadian cities found they provided substandard food, the Nutrition Committee of the Canadian Public Health Association was defensive and argued that the study and its interpretation of hospital food was "highly opinionated, inaccurate and poorly documented."[117] Nutrition had many stakeholders.

Teaching nutrition continued to be a growth area. Certainly, Canadians couldn't trust food advertisements, so parents needed to be educated in order to teach their children. As a result, the Regina Rural Health Region in 1972–73 introduced a nutritional program for parents, teachers, and consumers.[118] One Toronto bookseller reported there were 600 titles available on diet and nutrition. Eating may have been a positive experience in people's lives, but that didn't mean they understood what they were eating. How could they, given the debates about fast food, fat, salt, and "refined" carbohydrates? Food designations were becoming increasingly complex to the point that one *Chatelaine* article explained to its readers the meaning of dietetics, calorie-reduced food, low-calorie food, sugar-free foods, and carbohydrate-reduced food.[119] No wonder health food stores became popular in Canada, their numbers increasing from 220 to 250 in the early 1970s to an estimated 1,000 by 1979.[120] Despite the morass of the nutritional world, the belief in science and the power of nutrients remained strong. One article in *UMC*, for example, even suggested the possibility of balancing nutrients in such a way as to determine the sex of the child conceived.[121]

Conclusion

Little has changed in recent decades. Eating the "right food" is still considered a way out of any nutritional quandary, even obesity. The involvement of governments in health and nutrition is still strong, yet recent estimates indicate that 20 per cent of our population experience food "insecurity."[122] Looking at the 2011 Canada Food Guide, Bill Jeffrey, national coordinator for the Centre for Science in the Public Interest, notes that aspects of the guide are good in many respects, but it also "muddies the waters by under-emphasizing fruits, vegetables and whole grains and fence-sitting on the adverse health effects of consuming red meat, cheese, and refined grains." The guide overlooks the 45,000 premature deaths in Canada due to poor nutrition each year, 16,000 of them due to too much sodium intake. For 1,800 others, death came from taking in too much "trans-fat-laden partially hydrogenated vegetable oil."[123] As in the past, nutrition is contingent upon many stakeholders: different levels of governments, bureaucrats in various ministries, women in their role as mothers to their families and caregivers to their communities, educational institutions, dietitians, physicians wanting to offset some of the health problems of their patients, and Canadians who try their best to eat well.

Canadians saw malnutrition as a weakness in the body that should and could be overcome. Health experts focused on the cause that appeared to be the easiest to eradicate – ignorance. Education was considered to be the solution to the problem of malnutrition, reflecting a belief in rational citizens wanting to eat what was best for them and able to keep up with the latest ideas on nutrition. The central figure who needed to be educated, and the one who was regularly deemed to be failing, was the mother. The many difficulties a mother faced in keeping her family eating well were seldom recognized. Looking at the malnutrition of Canadians, practitioners recognized obesity as a form of malnutrition. But what did health experts know about obesity? How did they measure it? Who was at risk? And what risk did it pose?

2 About Obesity

"The biggest single problem – quite literally – that has to be tackled is obesity."[1]

When most of us think about malnutrition, we imagine an emaciated body, not a fat one. As noted in chapter one, Canadian health experts increasingly saw being overweight or obese as a form of malnourishment. As a result, obesity became a medical subject, with articles and books written about it, equipment marketed for obese patients, and anti-obesity food sold. While the measurement of obesity seemed obvious – a weight over a standard based on age, height, and gender – not everyone was happy with the weight/height charts. Nevertheless, physicians used the charts to understand which groups were more at risk of obesity: men or women, the elderly, Indigenous people, the poor or the middle class, immigrants (who towards 1980 were significant in numbers), or even people living in specific cities or regions. While weight was a factor of obesity, fat was also part of it. And if the weight that defined the obese was contentious, understanding fat was even more difficult. Fat had types, with some perceived to be good and others not. When too much fat and too much weight came together in obesity, physicians saw health problems.

The Rise of Obesity and Its Measurements

By the 1920s and 1930s, medical practitioners and Canadians had developed an interest in obesity. Medical journals were reviewing books such as *Obesity*, authored by W.F. Christie.[2] In 1923, a meeting of medical students at the University of Montreal had two presentations about obesity on its agenda. A year later, Montreal's Dr Edward H.

Mason raised the alarm to colleagues that obesity was "widespread." In 1926, a commentator in the *Canadian Medical Association Journal* (*CMAJ*) deemed "obesity ... one of the most common ailments."[3] The growing emphasis on dieting among Canadians reflected the attempt to maintain slender figures for women or lean figures for men. As a result, magazines wrote articles about Canadians being more overweight than ever. Advertisements for food products used the weight alarm to help sell their products. Hostility to obesity was common. In 1927, *Maclean's* reprinted an article from the British medical journal *The Lancet* designating obesity as a "crime." Being fat was "contrary to nature and unjustifiable." People who were fat were deemed by some to be mentally "sluggish" with "padding ... stretching the abdomen, obliterating the lines of intelligence on the face, producing a banana-shaped wad in the nape of the neck, and distorting all the curves of external comeliness." Fat was "unpleasant and ungraceful." Only seldom did those who were fat retaliate. A fat man in the joke "Why Weight for Him?" rose to the challenge:

> An incredible fat man got into a bus. He almost smothered a sour-faced little man when he sat down. The sour-faced man glared at him, and growled: "They ought to charge by weight in these buses." "In that case," bellowed the fat man, "it wouldn't be worth while stopping to pick you up."[4]

Even the workers' newspaper, *The Worker*, used phrases such as "gorged plunderers" to describe capitalists and "fat boys" to describe union leaders who were more interested in themselves than the workers.[5] Canadians were so concerned about being overweight that a 1935 editorial in *Maclean's* warned readers not to get too upset about weight and stress themselves.[6]

Nevertheless, both medical and lay populations did worry. As noted in the previous chapter, some experts in nutrition during the 1940s and 1950s suggested that all the attention given to undernutrition was covering a potentially more serious problem of overnutrition.[7] Books on obesity accumulated, reviews were written, and even the history of obesity with its "great" figures had become of some interest. Equipment for taking the blood pressure of oversized patients was advertised to physicians, indicating a specialized market noteworthy enough to generate a response from the private sector. The Detecto scale, for example, could weigh individuals up to 300 pounds.[8] Sessions for physicians to upgrade their medical education included obesity as a subject. Obesity had become a "modern epidemic," "undoubtedly the most frequent disease encountered" in medical practice, and "the number one scourge of man" in North America.[9] Physicians were often frustrated when treating fat patients. In the medical literature, obesity was deemed an "abnormality," making the person a "misfit" and "obnoxious." Dr E.W. McHenry, who wrote prolifically on nutrition, suggested that fat people should pay more for their streetcar fares since they took up more room than other people, a continuation of the "Why Weight for Him" joke.[10] This view was a foretaste of similar suggestions made in the current obesity epidemic. Being fat was not attractive. Signs of aging in women included "rolls of fat" on "too well-upholstered hips, a thickening waistline and flabby upper arms." The best that fat Canadians could expect was pity.[11] And if there was a panic, it was centred in medicine.

The alarm about obesity heightened throughout the 1960s and 1970s. The November 1967 issue of *Canadian Journal of Public Health* (*CJPH*) devoted considerable space to eight articles on obesity. One article by Maurice Verdy, assistant professor of internal medicine, Université de Montréal, described how obesity had once been a sign of wealth and beauty, but modern medicine now sees it as "le plus grand problème de santé auquel face notre société" [the biggest health problem facing our society]. In 1973, the Ontario Medical Association meeting in Toronto had obesity as a "major theme."[12] There was a booming business in anti-obesity products. Forty companies in Canada manufactured anti-obesity food and drink products, and spent a million dollars a year promoting them. Canadians were willing to spend $10 million on specialized food and $20 million on "appetite depressant pills, vibrators and other slimming aids."[13] The language around obesity became intense – Canada was facing an "epidemic problem" of "endemic proportions." Marc Lalonde, minister of national health and welfare, declared that more than half of Canada's population was obese, while Nutrition Canada stated that 50 per cent of Canadians were overweight, reflecting the confusion between being overweight and being obese.[14]

Determining obesity has never been easy, and yet today statistics on obesity drive the contemporary fixation on fatness. However, the statistics are less than accurate. The body mass index (BMI) measurement, based on weight and height, cannot overcome variables linked to age, ethnicity, and muscle mass.[15] Weight and height can vary depending on if they are self-reported or measured by an "expert," making it difficult to compare studies using different methods of measurement.[16] Whether the BMI is a signifier of health is more controversial. The real value of the BMI is that it is cheap, easy to use, and relatively accurate for large populations, but less so for individuals. Consequently, there is an ongoing attempt to find a better way to evaluate fat.[17]

Measurements are seen as concrete and act as signposts of so many aspects in our world: money, population, weight, height, age, calories, education, crime, rain, snow, and the like. Couple this view with a medical system that has accepted the concept of bodies being like machines through most of the twentieth century. Standardization became increasingly important in medicine to "protect patients. But once standards of health or illness are in play, they are difficult to shift."[18] In the nineteenth century, life insurance companies began using weight as a way to assess health risks among potential policyholders. The healthy weight was not an average weight, but a numerical construct based on perceived health and mortality statistics of policyholders. Weight was no longer simply a measure of a person's weight compared to others, but also a health factor. For much of the period under review, the major way of judging obesity was to use standard weight/height charts. The charts were a way of making a health judgment. But they were biased by gender (more men took out life insurance), class (generally those taking out insurance were middle class, not working class), and age (middle-aged and over).[19] Class would also encompass ethnicity/race. While insurance companies' statistics came from selected individuals, the data were most often used for large populations and then applied back to individuals. The charts were not uniform in terms of how weight was measured, who measured it, and what interpretation of obesity was followed. For many decades, the charts used in Canada were based on surveys of Americans.[20] It was for good reasons that physicians and others constantly criticized charts as inaccurate for assessing health and well-being. Despite such criticism, the charts remained in use for a long period.

In the 1920s and 1930s, weighing oneself was not part of a daily regimen since most Canadians did not have a scale in their homes.[21] Public scales were available, but when using them, individuals would remain clothed, which in winter could add significant weight. What Canadians could use to determine their heaviness or thinness compared to others was their ready-to-wear clothing size. Even when bathroom scales became more accessible and affordable, knowing your weight didn't let you know whether you were underweight or overweight. Popular magazines offered their readers mathematical equations so they could assess their weight according to a standard weight. In the 1920s, for example, some took the first 60 inches of height, multiplied by 2, and for every inch over 5 feet added 4 pounds. Therefore, a man who was 5 feet 8 inches tall should weigh 60 × 2 = 120 pounds plus 8 × 4 = 32 pounds for a total of 152 pounds. A woman was to weigh 5 to 10 pounds less a man of her height.[22]

A second method of assessment was to compare your weight to a weight/height chart. But, as the Metropolitan Life Insurance Company, the largest life insurance company in Canada, explained, a person first needed to get the chart from Metropolitan's pamphlet "Overweight and Underweight." According to the pamphlet, individuals over thirty years of age were advised to be 10 to 20 pounds under the average weight; if an individual was under the age of thirty, then 5 to 10 pounds over the average weight was best. Some of the charts used – although not those of the Metropolitan Life Insurance Company – allowed weight gain with age. But some doctors worried that with aging, heart and lungs would be under "wear and strain."[23]

Charts were often limited. To be accurate about weight and its effect on health, some physicians suggested "age, height, sex, chest circumference, and body build" had to be taken into account. Another problem was that not all weight was fat, so the amount of muscle and bone also needed to be considered. In 1936, Dr Walter R. Campbell, Department of Medicine, University of Toronto and the Toronto General Hospital, added "races" and "breeds" as factors. More significant, he pointed out that the charts measured averages, and practitioners worked with individuals.[24] The warning had gone out – physicians had to work with the patient in front of them. Trying to put any individual patient into a predetermined set of charts could overlook aspects of the individual that might negate the findings of the chart. How useful charts were to physicians was an open question.

Despite the problems of the weight/height charts, physicians used them in their practices. Dr F.W. Tidmarsh, a noted Halifax physician, defined malnutrition as a "condition existing when the body weight is above or below the normal standard for the individual, based on the height of that individual." His definition reflected confidence in the weight/height charts and their accuracy. Others (referring only to obesity) set the bar at 20 per cent over the weight/height standard, and some preferred "25 per cent above the normal average."[25] A fashion writer in *The Chatelaine* (renamed *Chatelaine* after May 1932) had a different perspective on what weight should be: what "makes us feel at our best and look our best." But not everyone at *The Chatelaine* was as flexible about weight. When a woman wrote to Annabelle Lee, the beauty expert at the magazine, Lee noted that the reader was 3 pounds over the recommended weight and advised exercises to help rid her of that excess weight.[26] Whether for malnutrition, obesity, or attractiveness, weight and weight/height charts were interpreted variably.

By the 1940s, with insurance companies in the United States looking closely at mortality rates, the willingness to accept young adults being overweight declined. The threat of tuberculosis and pneumonia among them no longer posed the danger that these diseases once had. For those twenty-five years of age and older, being slightly underweight had the best mortality rates, and so the Metropolitan Life Insurance Company began to use what it referred to as the ideal weight, the one that provided longevity. Canadians were told that the weight they were at age twenty-five was the ideal weight for the rest of their lives.[27] In 1958, Dr Howard N. Segall, former president of the Ontario Heart Foundation, agreed, although he provided some leeway by accepting that a man at age fifty-five who had weighed 150 pounds at age twenty-five and now weighed 160 pounds could still fit into the "normal" category. But an increase of 30 pounds needed to be addressed, and a gain of 50 pounds necessitated "the services of a physician." In 1942, the Metropolitan Life Insurance Company altered its weight/height charts for women and added body frame as a factor; the next year, it did the same for men.[28]

In 1959, a study by the US Society of Actuaries shifted the average weight – downward for women and upward for men – causing insurance companies to change their charts. Lowering the "ideal" weight for women, however, made no allowance for life experiences such as childbirth or menopause.[29] In 1956, L.B. Pett, a leading expert on nutrition from the Department of National Health and Welfare, and G.F. Ogilvie, a colleague from the same department, outlined the problems of weight charts using body frames. Too often these charts didn't specify what was meant by each body frame. While such charts usually had a low and high weight attached to each frame, Pett and Ogilvie queried how those judgments came to be. Charts using one ideal weight were also problematic – they gave some latitude above and below the weight, but that latitude varied from 5 to 20 per cent, which wasn't helpful. Even more problematic was the lack of Canadian weight/height standards. The "foreign" statistics used were often out of date and based on limited numbers of people.[30]

Within the medical profession, there was a growing sense that a more accurate determination of obesity could be made through "clinical inspection."[31] The goals of the insurance company charts and doctors' goals were different: the insurance companies focused on future health projections, while physicians tended to focus on present health. In 1946, Dr W.W. Bauer observed to the readers of *Maclean's* that normal weight was based on body structure, race, and family. He concluded: "The weight at which you look best and feel best is probably your normal weight, regardless of what the tables say [the definition used by *The Chatelaine*'s beauty expert in 1930]. If it is not more than 10% below or more than 20% above the figures in the table, you have additional assurance that it is probably a satisfactory weight for you."[32] It is noteworthy that Bauer still saw being underweight as more problematic than being overweight.

As mentioned in the previous chapter, the idea of a national weight-height-age survey based on Canadian figures had been approved in 1953. In addition to weight/height measurements, the survey also took skinfold thickness tests using calipers. Caliper tests were considered more adept at measuring fat, and the optimal choice was to use both weight and skinfold measurements. Using both overweight criteria plus excessive skinfold, the survey determined that 13 per cent of males and 23 per cent of females in Canada were obese (12 per cent and 10 per cent, respectively, were underweight).[33] But Pett warned colleagues that while charts based on a national study might be helpful to determine the particularities of adults, they wouldn't be as helpful for children. A child had to be compared to his or her own history.[34]

Canadians were using weight/height charts, but mathematical equations for measurement hadn't disappeared. In 1962, a popular health magazine measured women and men differently. A man was to take his height in inches, multiply it by 2, and add 15 per cent for fat allowance. For instance, a man who was 6 feet (72 inches) tall should weigh 165 pounds. The calculation for women was somewhat different: as their bones were smaller than men's, the fat allowance was not needed, and so was not added. Thus, a woman who was 5 feet 4 inches (64 inches) tall should weight 128 pounds. Notice that age was not a factor, so the ideal weight for an adult was to be the same at any age. In 1966, *Maclean's* described a new way of figuring out fat, the "ponderal index": "divide your height in inches by the cube root of your body weight in pounds ... Below 11.7 the person is ... obese." In 1969, Dr Barbara McLaren, dean of the Faculty of Food Science, University of Toronto, suggested an easier calculation of ideal weight for both women and men – 100 pounds for the first 5 feet in height and 5 pounds for every subsequent inch.[35]

Critiques of weight/height charts continued in the 1960s and 1970s. Dr H.D. Oliver was mindful that charts were just "statistical monuments" and not designed to "measure any one individual's obesity." Other body fat tests also existed and were more accurate, but none were as adaptable to the doctor's office as the charts. Even the skinfold test required "considerable training and experience." R.G. Stennett and Dr D.M. Cram, both at the Ontario Board of Education, were more optimistic with the advent of computer analysis, and they looked forward to more detailed factors being input and plotted to give a better sense of norms.[36] In 1973, Daniel Cappon from the University of Toronto described other ways to measure fat. X-rays could help assess bone density and size. The somatyping technique, developed by American William Herbert Sheldon, used photographic measuring based on one of three body shapes an individual fit into: endomorph (soft and rounded), mesomorph (muscular and solid), or ectomorph (leggy and lean). But despite such efforts, Cappon concluded (perhaps with his tongue in cheek) that "none of these methods comes close to the accuracy of a European technique developed for the bacon industry," in which a sound wave directed at a hog could be used to determine the thickness of the animal's fat.[37] No wonder doctors used the weight/height charts.

With different ways of measuring fat or weight, it is not surprising that the threshold weight at which an individual could be classified as overweight or obese varied. One food manufacturer understood being overweight as a weight 30 per cent over the norm, whereas the Canadian Medical Association suggested 12 per cent; others identified the threshold in pounds – 5 to 15 pounds over. An article by General Foods explained that normal body fat for men was 17 per cent of weight, whereas it was a bit higher for women at 23 per cent. When men went over 20 per cent fat and women over 27 per cent fat, then they had the "condition" known as obesity. In a study of older women workers in a Toronto department store, being 10 kilograms (22 pounds) over the "ideal weight" designated them as having "a substantial degree of obesity."[38]

Charlotte Young from the Graduate School of Nutrition, Cornell University, pointed out in the *CMAJ* that the different ranges of obesity weights used by physicians and others ranged from 10 to 40 per cent above the standard weight. A consensus on how to define obesity had

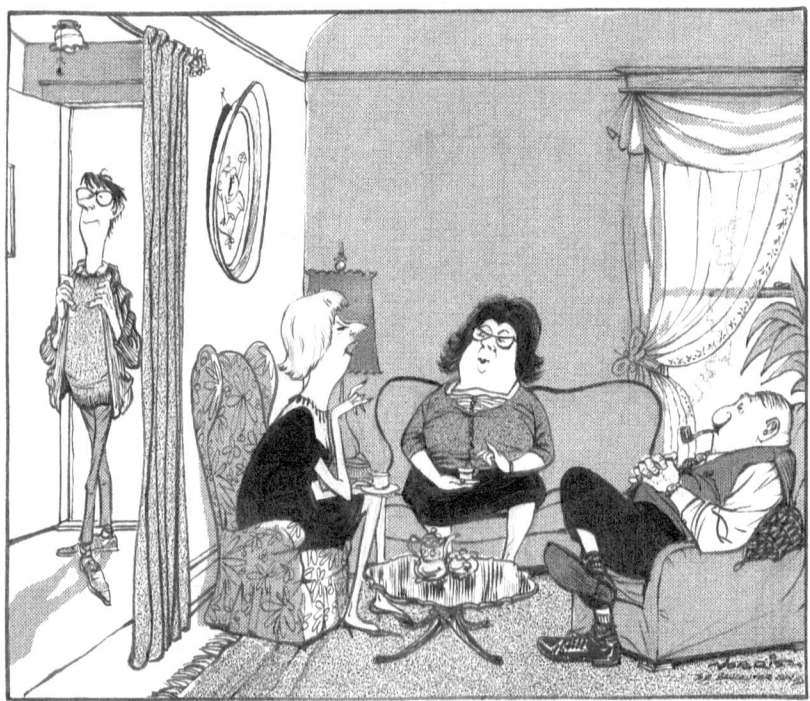

Health professionals thought older Canadians should maintain the same weight they had in their youth at age twenty-five. This 1967 cartoon contrasts the slender youth with overweight adults, reflecting the reality of the weight difference between young and middle-aged Canadians. The cartoon's caption reads: "He's now a teaching assistant ... and while he doesn't actually RUN the university ..." Source: MsC 25–776, 1–1967–03–22, SFU Special Collections, Len Norris Collection, Simon Fraser University Library.

not been reached, although 20 per cent seemed to be the most popular. James A. Collyer in the *Canadian Family Physician* was open about the definition of obesity. In an article with the telling title "The Unhappy Fat Woman," he defined a person with obesity as "any person who came wanting to reduce, and in whom the doctor found obvious signs of excess weight (i.e., fat at waist or hips, or forearms, and obvious abnormality of lb./inch ratio)."[39] The idea of weight being stable over time became stronger and sometimes appeared strange. One 1978 text on obesity known to Canadian practitioners held that weight should not vary from when an individual was thirty or even twenty years of age, at least until the person became elderly. As proof, the author referred to the Zulu people of Southern Africa, who at age sixty had maintained the same weight throughout their adulthood.[40] Dr David Sackett, professor of clinical epidemiology and biostatistics at McMaster University, questioned what was meant by normal weight. Is it the average or the ideal (and if so, the ideal of what)? For Sackett, "the normal range [was] the point beyond which intervention of some sort begins to do more good than harm."[41] The meaning of the measurements was still not easy to assess.

A 1979 article in the *CJPH* explained to its readers that the terms "overweight" and "obesity" were not synonymous. Obesity referred to body fat, whereas overweight "may be due to variations in body composition apart from excess fat."[42] The experts had known that was the case for years, but too often practitioners continued to use weight/height charts to determine the best weight for the patient. In an article in *Maclean's*, Dr R.W. Shepherd, resident psychiatrist at Montreal's Jewish General Hospital, clearly stated that he didn't like using the word "obesity." He seemed to prefer "fat" when referring to those above the normal weight. As he explained: "There are more fat people than obese people, since obesity is a medical term implying sickness, whereas many of the heavies are constitutionally or psychologically that way, and prefer to live free and fat rather than slim and for ever on a diet." He had no problem with this preference.[43]

Who Are Obese and What Is Fat?

Measuring obesity is a means of assessing the prevalence of obesity within populations. To understand obesity in patients, practitioners looked to who were considered obese through surveys, charts, and by other doctors. Before the 1920s, William Osler, a Canadian physician and the first professor of medicine at Johns Hopkins University, noted in the first edition of his well-known text, *The Principles of Medicine* (1893), that obesity usually developed after middle age. In his 1912 edition, he identified gender as a significant factor, which continued to be included in later editions. Women were considered more prone to obesity than men because of pregnancy, breastfeeding, and menopause, aspects of women's bodies that Osler closely tied to "internal secretions." At the same time, his 1912 text criticized women for being obese and losing their "good looks," as did the 1925 and 1947 editions.[44] Christie, in his 1938 text *Ideal Weight*, also saw fat as gendered. Women naturally had more fat on their bodies than men, which resulted in a body with "contours rounded," a body that he found attractive. Men were to have a different body surface, "'cut up' by grooves and furrows, especially on contraction of the underlying muscles." But both needed fat. According to Christie in his text *Obesity*, weight gain in men began when growth stopped, at around twenty years of age, and they began to work in sedentary environments, eventually settled down, and married. He claimed that women began putting on weight earlier since their growth stopped at puberty, as did the beginning of their sedentary life. One Montreal physician claimed that 60 per cent of the women who were obese had become so before reaching thirty years of age, and 75 per cent by the time they were forty. For men, it was 25 per cent and 50 per cent, respectively.[45] At times, the gendered description was a cultural belief, not one based on "science." For example, Osler saw fat women as unattractive, and Christie believed a sedentary life started at puberty for women. Yet, in the 1920s and 1930s, young women in Canada could be seen playing sports: the first Edmonton Grads women's basketball team won the world championship in 1924 and continued to dominate the sport until they disbanded in 1940, and Canadian women participated in the 1928 Olympics. Certainly, the idea that women were living sedentary lives through World War I and during the Depression is a fantasy. But it was a belief long held by many physicians and others.[46]

In the 1940s and 1950s, the risk of obesity remained very gendered, with some practitioners estimating women to be more prone by a ratio of ten to one. Estimates of the number of Canadians who were overweight and/or obese varied, depending on the survey. Consequently, health experts wanted a national study like the one finally held in 1953, which determined that 13 per cent of men and 23 per cent of women were obese. Obesity appeared to be a trait of middle age or older: women between the ages of thirty and fifty, and men between forty and fifty. For men, class was a focus of obesity. Physicians saw white male executives, whose work was deemed stressful, as patients at risk of obesity.[47] But if the life of an executive was deemed a cause of obesity for some men, the cause for women was thought to be their psychology and physiology. Dr Antonio Martel from Quebec City even introduced an iatrogenic aspect, which few physicians recognized, claiming that giving women estrogen to lessen menopausal symptoms increased their weight gain.[48]

In the 1960s and 1970s, the Canadian obesity profile became more detailed. The elderly had to watch their eating, particularly their tendency to overeat fats and carbohydrates.[49] Although the Indigenous and the Inuit populations had been ignored for decades, by the 1960s studies had determined that the southern diet had become the normative diet for people in the Canadian North, causing malnutrition and rising obesity. In effect, the southern diet was believed to be changing the very body that had been shaped over eons.[50] In Canada's centennial year, it was not surprising that studies compared French Canadians in Quebec to English Canadians in the rest of the country. The French and the English in Canada were somewhat separate in their cultures, their politics, and even in their weight. Minimal differences existed when whole populations were examined, but for those between thirty-five to forty-four years of age, skinfold test results were lower for French Canadians compared to English Canadians (4.9 mm compared to 8.2 mm).[51] Other regional differences in weight were also of interest. In 1978, a poll determined (from self-reports) that 50 per cent of adults in the Maritimes were overweight, 37 per cent in Quebec, and 35 per cent in the Prairies. Most respondents were 16 pounds overweight, except in Quebec, where it was 37 pounds. Commenting on an American study that connected race with weight, a 1971 *Chatelaine* article made reference to the eating practices of immigrants from the "Old Country," which could apply to Canada. After all, the number of immigrants and refugees was increasing. Traditional food could be calorie heavy, and when connected with lower economic status, it was a trigger for "active obesity." Daniel Cappon, in his book *Eating, Loving and Dying: A Psychology of Appetites*, focused on immigrants who brought with them rich carbohydrate diets in "disregard for [Canada's] ... attitudes to obesity."[52]

Gender remained the major focus. More women were thought to be obese compared to men, and studies in the North suggested that middle-aged Inuit women were especially putting on weight. But no woman seemed exempt. In her 1965 article, Charlotte M. Young

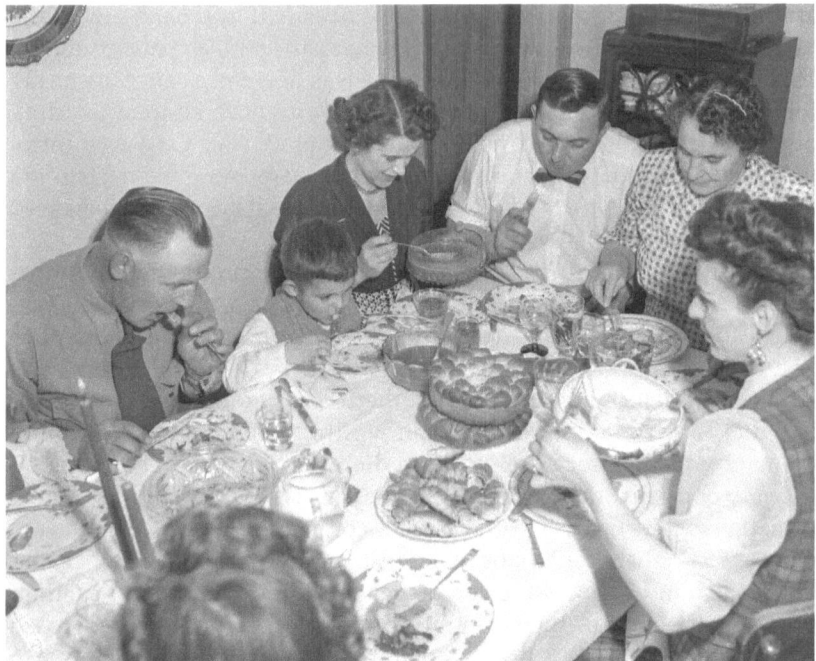

Many health professionals believed that immigrants to Canada didn't know how to eat well. Indeed, the professionals were trying to educate foreigners to eat as Canadians did, despite the fact that many Canadians did not eat well either. Ukrainians like the Danilowich family pictured here didn't eat meat for their Christmas dinner. Unlike the health professionals, *The Albertan* in January 1954 praised the Danilowich family's dinner as "12 delicious meatless dishes." Source: Photographer, Jack De Lorme; NA-5600–7498a, Glenbow Museum.

pointed out that some estimates on gender differences in body fat were significant. Older women were 1.5 times fatter than men, and young women were 2.5 times fatter. Yet, using a different measurement, Young concluded: "While women have increased 55% in body fatness from the third to seventh decade, men have increased 187% in roughly the same period." One of the reasons for the focus on women was that women outnumbered men by significant numbers in many, if not most, obesity studies. This imbalance was not because women were necessarily obese more often than men (although some statistics would suggest this), but because women sought help for their weight problems and were therefore convenient study participants. Commentators sensed that men were less likely than women to admit they had a weight problem.[53]

The relationship between gender and other variables became more nuanced and complicated. In 1970–72, statistics showed that 9.7 per cent of adults were obese – 7.6 per cent of men and 11.7 per cent of women – quite different from 1953, when obesity in men and women was found to be 13 per cent and 23 per cent, respectively. Most of that difference could be accounted for by the different methods of measuring obesity. If overweight were added to obesity in 1970–72, the statistics would be significantly higher: 40 per cent overall for adults, but 46.1 per cent for men and 31.7 per cent for women.[54] Within class, gender was a factor: affluent men were heavier than affluent women. Interestingly, women from the upper and lower economic groups were similar in weight until age fifty. At that age, women in the lower economic strata became heavier. Studies of young men suggested that the lowest income men had the highest energy intake (food), even though there was more obesity in young men with higher income. For young women, the obesity rate was higher in the low-income group, even though both groups took in roughly the same amount of calories. The majority of elderly women were overweight, and 30 per cent were obese. The Nutrition Survey of Canada revealed an age discrepancy between lower and higher economic strata in men, with the latter being heavier, especially in their fifties. Among the Inuit and Indigenous peoples, the young were more often overweight. In a 1978 self-reported poll of thirty-one Canadian cities, 53 per cent of men between ages forty-five and fifty-four reported being overweight. The average for this category was 17 pounds overweight, perhaps not that significant. For thirty-five to forty-year-olds, 48 per cent were overweight by an average of 41 pounds.[55] All the surveys about weight and who was overweight were attempting to get to the essential factor – fat. But what did Canadians know about it?

Fat is complex and can be classified into several types: brown, white, visceral, subcutaneous, and what some call "belly fat."[56] Food fats are divided into categories, including unsaturated fat, saturated fat, trans fatty acids, and omega fatty acids. Fat is more than fat! Fat is necessary for health and makes eating enjoyable; its consumption makes us feel full, that is, it satisfies our hunger.[57] By the late nineteenth century, fat was defined as an energy equivalent that had twice the energy of protein or carbohydrate, which meant that it took twice the energy to work it off. By the turn of the twentieth century, fat was assessed by weighing and comparing it with the weights of other food elements.[58]

In the early decades of the twentieth century, health experts in Canada learned about fat through the international literature. But Canadian doctors soon began to write about fat/obesity themselves. Looking at the extremes of fat, doctors saw obesity as caused either by exogenous factors (outside the body) or endogenous factors (within the body). In 1924, Edward Mason reminded *CMAJ* readers that exogenous obesity was caused by an excess of energy intake (food) compared to the expenditure of energy, and endogenous obesity by some "endocrine or other pathological disturbance."[59] Christie, in his well-known 1937 book *Obesity*, reminded his readers that fat was "primarily ... a source of nourishment ... a reserve of fuel" and that there were two types of fat – free and fixed. Free fat was the fat in a body that could be lost; fixed fat could not, no matter what the weight of a person. For example, abdominal fat (what Christie called "hard" fat) was very difficult to lose. Foreshadowing the interest in fat cells, he noted that fat cells never disappeared but were "adaptable repositories for varying amounts of fat, and also ... for the fat-soluble vitamins A, D and E."[60] Others noted that some fat was necessary for the body to utilize other foods and let nutrients do their work. It was suggested that fat was not inert but active.[61] Inert fat could be seen as "anonymous," but active fat seems more personal – it is not just fat, it is *your* fat. Canadians J.T. Phair and N.R. Speirs, in their 1945 book *Good Health*, reminded readers of the importance of fat: it took more energy to burn fat than carbohydrates, and thus more heat was produced. New was the interest in certain fats that had cholesterol.[62]

The discussion of fat intensified in the 1950s. Like many, German-American Hilde Bruch, an expert on obesity in children, had adopted the active view of fat. She also referred to brown fat as more resistant to metabolic use and able to survive starvation better. In *Nutrition for Today* (1951), Elizabeth Chant Robertson, in a neutral tone, told her readers that fats had many uses and set out what was essentially a primer for practitioners and others. Fats gave meals pleasurable flavour and were a "compact source of calories," much more than carbohydrates or proteins, and thus were good for people who did hard physical labour. Fats were slow to digest, limited hunger pains, and restrained people from eating unduly. They also helped the body to absorb vitamin A and carotene. She was quite open about the fact that different populations ate various amounts of fat in their diets, pointing to the Japanese who consumed 1 ounce a day, the British who ate 4 ounces, and the "Eskimo" who ate 10 ounces, based on 1930 records.[63]

The negative view of fat was also noted. In 1955, Alan Phillips, a regular author for *Maclean's*, published an article on heart disease and pointed to the work of Ancel Keys, an American scientist in biology and physiology, who was suggesting that "a fat called cholesterol" in the blood of the arteries in the heart was problematic. Two years later, Pett and Elaine Collett (from the Chatelaine Institute) wrote an article in *Chatelaine* that also made the connection between increased fat intake and heart disease. The result was a flurry of responses. A letter by Dr Alick Little, a researcher on atherosclerosis (plaque building in the arteries), noted that not all researchers would agree with Pett's dismissal of fat foods as bad for the heart. Even Pett had admitted that "the kind of fat may be important." E.W. McHenry, University of Toronto, also differed with Pett. McHenry saw low-fat diets as harmful in that they "limit one's intake of energy, fat soluble vitamins, and essential fatty acids." He also suggested that living in cities was linked to heart disease more than fat intake, proposing an environmental cause rather than a dietary one. The 1957 to 1960 Framingham study in the United States did not find any "relationship ... between blood cholesterol levels and the consumption of total calories, dietary cholesterol, animal fats, total fat, and percent of calories from fat" for either sex.[64] This line of investigation led to contentious debates about diet, and how significant the correlation was "among dietary fat, cholesterol, and atherosclerosis." Keys supported the dietary fat theory; indeed, his reputation was based on it.[65] That meant he embraced a low-fat diet and advocated reducing saturated fat.

The focus on fat continued in the 1960s, but in a changed form. In 1963, the Canadian Heart Foundation's board of directors approved the following description of what it knew about cholesterol:

> Cholesterol is a fatty substance which can be made by the body and it occurs normally in the tissues of man and animals. It has been shown that saturated fats, usually fats of animal origin which contain cholesterol, are particularly liable to increase the level of cholesterol in the blood stream. On the other hand, unsaturated fats, usually fats of vegetable or margarine origin, show a slight tendency to decrease the level of blood cholesterol.

Keys's theory about dietary fat was accepted by the directors. The description also said that obesity was a "significant contributing factor in the production of coronary heart disease."[66] While studies did not confirm a cause and effect relationship between heart problems and the consumption of dietary fat and high blood cholesterol, the "possibility" of such a linkage was seen as strong.[67] It was clear that the concern about cholesterol remained in the Canadian medical literature, with drugs on the market promising to help control it.[68] What health experts didn't know was that the Sugar Association (in the United States) paid researchers at Harvard University for a literature review on food and heart disease. The review was published in the *New England Journal of Medicine* in 1967. Apparently, "the researchers overstated the consistency of the literature on fat and cholesterol, while downplaying studies on sugar according to the analysis." Because of the review, American nutritionist Marion Nestle notes, many health experts focused on saturated fat, not sugar, as a factor leading to heart disease.[69] Now, it appears a leading factor might be sugar.

Without the information about sugar, concern about dietary fat extended into the 1970s. Of interest was cholesterol's link with a certain type of diet (high in fat) and a certain kind of fat (saturated). Cholesterol was seen as a men's problem, with certain women's hormones fighting it off.[70] By the end of the decade, there were suggestions that food cholesterol was not as bad as purported and wasn't harmful unless the patient was "disposed to high blood cholesterol." Indeed, clinical trials had revealed that "low-fat, low-cholesterol, polyunsaturated diets" did not offset cardiovascular disease. Nonetheless, Canadians were still advised to eat less fat and less saturated fat, and to eat more fish and poultry and less red meat – even by those who were querying whether the harm of cholesterol was significant. In 1977, the province of Quebec set a goal of reducing fat consumption by 50 per cent.[71] The issue of fat consumption was so prominent that even humorists became involved. A cartoon in *Health* depicted a big hippopotamus asking a slender bird, "Poly unsaturated?" The bird doesn't say anything, but its face looks somewhat conceited about its body.[72]

Research on fat was not only focused on cholesterol. In 1965, Young pointed out that "clinical obesity" was becoming more prevalent at younger ages in all groups; as fat increased with age, the fat became "inner" fat, which was more dangerous to health than subcutaneous fat.[73] Why fat appeared more in some people than in others was also queried. Some researchers thought that fat cells could grow in number and size, especially in babies and young children, which increased their susceptibility to obesity in later years. It was thought that such cells never disappeared – only their size changed, but not their number. In the late 1970s, however, some researchers suggested that if a person became obese enough and the fat cells had no room to expand, then the number of cells could increase.[74]

Research on brown fat was also ongoing. In 1979, Jean Himms-Hagen, professor of biochemistry at the University of Ottawa, reported: "Recent studies on brown adipose tissue have shown that a defect in this tissue is one probable cause of obesity." It was also now determined that four different types of energy expenditure were involved in burning extra food energy: "the basal metabolic rate, physical activity, the thermic effect of food, and facultative thermogenesis (cold-induced nonshivering thermogenesis and diet-induced thermogenesis)." To complicate the discussion, Himms-Hagen noted that obesity itself could most likely no longer be considered "a single disease entity."[75] This new research was perhaps more information than most practitioners could take in. It was just easier to understand that Canadians' food consumption contained 45 per cent fat rather than the 35 per cent recommended by Health and Welfare.[76]

If obesity is about fat, the health of fat people is the concern. According to Sander L. Gilman, medicine has viewed obesity as "pathological" since early Rome. It was an indication of disease. In the mid-nineteenth century, William Harvey, a British physician and Fellow of the Royal College of Surgeons, felt that obesity could be treated as a disease.[77] Today, the World Health Organization sees obesity as a "global ... epidemic."[78]

Health Issue

Obesity is an issue today, and was in the past, because of health concerns about fat and the dislike of fatness. The latter is culturally based, the former "scientifically" based. For science, the health/weight dyad is largely built on two conceptual methodologies. The first is correlation, a statistical tool focused on relationships that came to prominence at the turn of the twentieth century. As William Rothstein argues: "All researchers who use quantitative data gathered in natural environments now think in terms of correlations, even if their ultimate goal is causal inferences." Correlations "alert" practitioners when a pairing exists between a problem and some other factor. The pairing introduces the second concept – risk.[79]

At one time, risk was a neutral descriptor of probability, but it now seems to be negative. As Rothstein explains, with respect to medicine and health, the risk factor and "its statistical methodology," epidemiology, was applied around 1960. It provided a different understanding of disease and causation. Unlike looking for an external cause, risk factor is based on "multiple factors internal and external to the individual [being] involved in the etiology of every disease," that is, the correlation/risk factor approach tends to focus on individual responsibility rather than on a broader look at the socio-economic characteristics of society.[80] Epidemiology shifted the focus not only to the individual, but also away from creating a hierarchy of risk factors in favour of concentrating on those that can be altered.[81] Statisticians and epidemiologists try to determine how much something is a risk factor. For example, it has been hypothesized that obesity is a risk factor in 34 per cent of those with hypertension and 28.6 per cent of those with diabetes.[82] Many anti-obesity scholars and researchers are very careful not to apply the word "cause" when using risk factors. Instead, they use phrases that indicate correlations, such as "associated" and "indirect" relationship.[83] Unfortunately, not all are so careful (such as the media) and many reports don't differentiate between a risk factor and a cause.

The obesity field is premised on the assumption that being overweight/obese poses a health risk. For example, a listing of problems "associated" with obesity named at a national meeting of researchers, practitioners, and policy makers in November 2007 in Calgary included "hypertension, serum lipid imbalance ... abnormal fasting blood glucose ... insulin resistance, type 2 diabetes [non-insulin dependent], major depression and suicidality, stroke, coronary heart disease ... several cancers, [and] premature mortality." If that were not enough, "sleep disorders, orthopedic disorders ... hiatus hernia, gall bladder disease ... endocrine changes/reproductive disorders ... [and] impaired immunity" were added to the list.[84] Obesity is also linked to fertility problems in both sexes, decline in brain function, higher mortality rates, and a threatened reduced life expectancy for a younger generation. Too much weight gain during pregnancy leads to health issues for both mother and infant, and to future obesity in both.[85]

In recent years, there have been challenges to whether obesity is really the health problem it has been described to be. Take mortality. Looking at national statistics on weight and health shows that the developed countries with high obesity rates also have high life expectancy and vice versa.[86] A 2010 report based on the 1994/1995 National Population Health Survey – a study of Canadian adults, BMI, and mortality – stated: "Obesity class 1 was not associated with a significantly increased risk of mortality ... Obesity class II + was a significant risk factor for men, but not among women." Nevertheless, doctors could be seeing more people who are obese with morbidity.[87]

The linkage between fat/obesity and poor health has a long history. Osler's text in 1893 drew a link between overeating, arteriosclerosis, and "fatty heart." The 1912 edition acknowledged that some obese individuals could undertake vigorous physical activity, but others might suffer from "shortness of breath, embarrassed cardiac action, difficulty in walking," in addition to heart issues. The 1925 edition was much more vehement about the "danger" of obesity, associating it with a range of other ailments: diabetes, dyspepsia, and cancer, as well as problems of the heart, back, kidney, liver, circulation of blood, and breathing.[88] Of more immediate concern for practitioners, obese patients posed "a grave surgical risk ... because [they were] prone to unfortunate complications such as infection, the tardy healing of wound, and fat embolism." A 1927 article in *Maclean's* explained to Canadians that all organs were at risk as a result of too much body fat.[89] In his 1924 article on obesity, Mason indicated to his medical colleagues that those who were obese "may" suffer from an "incapacity" that could be "extreme," an incapacity that could make "it practically impossible for them to function as useful citizens." He recounted one patient, a Jewish woman, aged twenty-nine, who weighed 241 pounds when she entered the hospital on 19 May 1921. Six years before, when she married, she weighed only 160 pounds. At the same time as she was putting on weight, she developed irregularity in her menstrual cycle and difficulty breathing when she exerted herself. She wished to have children, but had not been able to become pregnant. Placed on a diet in hospital, she lost weight; after being discharged, her menstrual cycle became regular, she became pregnant, and gave birth to a "normal child."[90] In her case, useful citizenship was linked to being able to have a baby. Her ability to have a baby was a reflection of the "cure" for her obesity, as was the birth of a "normal child," although it was unclear just what would have been considered an abnormal child.

Nutritionists used mortality studies by insurance companies to urge those who were overweight to change their eating habits and lose weight.[91] Such studies gave an appearance of proof since they were always accompanied by detailed statistics. One article noted that for men who were 5 feet 7 inches in height or shorter, between forty and forty-five years of age, and 20 per cent overweight, mortality rates were 30 per cent higher than the norm. For taller men, over 5 feet 10 inches, the figure was 40 per cent.[92] The level of detail supports an unstated message that the science of statistics can determine a person's health based on their age, height, and weight. What isn't examined is how life expectancy differed between the groups. But a 1930 article did admit that for "those under the age of 45 years the penalty of overweight was by no means so marked." Only in the older group were mortality rates of the overweight determined to be significant.[93]

In the 1930s, obesity continued to be seen as the "cause" of "certain common diseases," "ill health," "bodily discomfort," and being "physically unfit." It was associated with sore feet, shortage of breath, diverticulosis of the colon, gallstones, and backaches to the point of needing an abdominal support to offset the pain.[94] Given the descriptors of obesity used, how could anyone look at an obese person and see that person as healthy? Yet, Christie reminded his colleagues not to go too far over on the fat-hating spectrum. Some diseases were mitigated by having fat reserves, for example, wasting diseases such as tuberculosis and recovery from a recent surgery for cancer. He even noted that some surgeries were easier if the patient was fat.[95] But his voice was a rarity within the literature on obesity.

By mid-century, the issue of weight was brought even more to the fore. The spectre of an early death remained for those who were obese, especially for those whose abdominal size was significant.[96] Some advertisements for appetite suppressants promised that the drug could overcome "headaches, giddiness, faintness, amenorrhea, rheumatic symptoms and edema of the lower extremities."[97] Worry about obesity in the elderly revolved around wearing down their hearts and contributing to the development of diabetes.[98] Canadians learned that if men didn't control their weight, they might experience a "decline of sex enthusiasm." The focus on men's health was reflected in "Watch Your Husband's Waistline," an article by Joan Phillips in *Canadian Home Journal*. The cartoon that accompanied the article showed a slender wife taking the waist measurement of her husband, who was wearing only his pyjama bottoms. In the article, Phillips pointed out that it was a wife's job to help keep her husband healthy, as if he didn't have any responsibility for his own weight and health problems. As noted earlier, special concern was given to male executives, described as "a well fed, somewhat constipated group which has faulty habits of rest and recreation and among whom the incidence of cardiovascular disease, hypertension and peptic ulcer is relatively high."[99] While industrial workers were also prone to heart problems, they didn't get the same kind of attention in the medical literature that was accorded white middle-class men. Going to a doctor was expensive for workers, whereas the salary of "executives" gave them ready access to doctors. Women complicated the issue of fat and artery disease. Supposedly, more women were obese than men, yet the perception was that women were less likely than men to develop fattening of the arteries. Estrogen was considered to be an advantage for women until menopause.[100]

During the Cold War in the 1950s, the fitness of populations was considered a reflection of the strength of democracy. Obesity posed a problem as it did not bode well for a healthy citizenship. Statistics of problems "caused" by obesity were used to increase fear. According to Dr I.M. Rabinowitch, two-thirds of all diabetics were overweight, although he admitted not every fat person would become a diabetic.[101] However, his phrasing suggested that the vast majority of them would develop the disease, which was not the case. Given the list of problems linked to obesity, it was not surprising that physicians and others believed that obesity also led to depression. Indeed, one article in *The Canadian Nurse* linked mania and/or depression with "a short, tubby person."[102]

On occasion, challenges to the doom and gloom scenario did occur. In *L'Union Médicale du Canada*, Rosario Robillard questioned the relationship between obesity and diabetes. In 1954, an editorial in the *CMAJ* suggested that the connection between obesity and "coronary disease" had perhaps been exaggerated and that controlling obesity would probably not affect mortality rates from heart disease to any "marked degree."[103] While such exceptions were interesting, they never stimulated much discussion. The mantra of obesity and health problems dominated, and it continued to do so throughout the 1960s.

Certainly, the relationship between obesity and mortality rates continued to be an issue. In 1965, while maintaining that even "minor excesses in weight" were "associated" with higher mortality rates, Young admitted that researchers didn't know if those rates were a result of weight, overnutrition, or fat. What was clear was the way in which mortality figures were put forward to overwhelm.[104] Assuming those who were obese could avoid an early death, their obesity continued to link them to hypertension, atherosclerosis, high blood pressure, depression, diabetes, coronary heart disease, musculoskeletal disorders in the back and lower legs, renal disease, liver and gallbladder problems, work-related injury, intensification of problems of pregnancy including toxemia, not to mention psychological "disturbances," infertility, car accidents, breathing problems, and strokes.[105] For some health problems, the linkage was two pronged. Obesity was seen as a "predisposing factor" in diabetes but also a result of diabetes itself. There could also be more than a two-pronged linkage, for example obesity in conjunction with hypertension, hypercholesterolemia, and smoking, which could predispose an individual to heart disease.[106] But most commentators didn't seem to list other predisposing factors. In the literature on obesity, obesity appeared to be the only factor. And it affected every aspect of life. For example, fat men on the factory floor had more difficulty dealing with summer heat than those who were average weight. At least such workers could now think about going to a doctor without financial penalty – Canada's Medical Care Act came into effect in 1966.[107]

The scenario still looked bleak in the 1970s for those who were obese. At times, the "health risk" presented by obesity was somewhat vague, just hovering over the health field. A 1972 note from the "Overseas Journals" section of the *CMAJ* mentioned the higher risk of being 10 pounds overweight compared to smoking twenty-five cigarettes a day.[108] What did such a statement and others like it mean? Surely 10 pounds on a 200-pound man did not have the same significance as 10 pounds on a 115-pound woman? However, the statement was easy to understand. You didn't have to be bothered with charts and percentage risks. It was the medical equivalent of a sound bite. Similarly, an article in *Harrowsmith* made the statement that 50 per cent of Canadians were overweight and followed it by the statement that 50 per cent of deaths in Canada were heart related, as if the two were connected.[109] Entrenched beliefs were difficult to change.

The insistence on a relationship between obesity and ill health and disease was overwhelming. For decades, physicians and researchers had been telling one another that this correlation was true. The tendency to quantify meant that correlations could be run off with ease. Correlations, linkages, and associations became the watchwords of the field. So many links existed that proof of cause seemed to prevail. In Helen Christie's summary of papers on obesity presented at the Ontario Medical Association meeting in 1973, several themes emerge.[110] First, the reader is overwhelmed by the list of linkages between obesity and death – 142 per cent higher mortality rates. Even if that statistic was an exaggeration, there would still be a willingness to believe that a significant linkage existed. And it was exaggerated, because any figure of that magnitude would have to be based on the extreme end of the obesity scale. Second, if premature death was not bad enough, the list of diseases and conditions would suggest that those who were obese led a poor life. Third, despite recognition that in some cases a clear linkage between obesity and ill health did not exist, this finding was lost in the flow of the inexorable list of problems. Obesity had become more than simply a problem of weight (fat) gain. It was a "cause" of so much ill health. Rid society of obesity and some of the major health issues of the day would be eradicated.[111] Worse for some commentators was the cost of all this ill health to society as a whole. Guilt, too, was part of the alarm. The overindulgence that obesity supposedly symbolized, and the wealth represented by such indulgence, needed to be shared with other countries and less fortunate peoples.[112]

The 1970s ended with challenges to weight charts and their meaning. Dr Magda Vranic, psychiatrist with the rehabilitation unit at the Toronto General Hospital, argued that the charts being used were "unrealistic" and resulted in Canadians who were only a bit overweight being made to feel "ungainly."[113] In some cases, there was nothing wrong with these people. They were just not slender. At the Canadian Nurses Association convention in 1974, nurses took part in a study to assess their physical fitness based on a test by Recreation Canada. The results were "puzzling"; the nurses scored high in fitness, but they had a high percentage of body fat. Instead of using this to challenge the obesity/ill health dyad, an attempt was made to explain the results in a way that would not challenge what had become rigid linkages. At the annual meeting of the Canadian Dietetic Association in 1977, Dr Winick, professor of nutrition and pediatrics at Columbia University, was queried about whether those who were obese should lose weight, especially when being overweight had been their normal condition for a long time. The question itself was intriguing, a challenge to standard thinking. Dr Winick replied that health risks were higher in people who were obese, but he admitted that those risks really depended on factors other than weight, for example, "glucose levels or blood pressure." An obese person could be healthy and fit. Dr W. Gifford-Jones noted in *Maclean's* that there was no point in worrying someone because he or she was 20 pounds overweight. Weight gain was something that came with age, and by raising the anxiety about weight, another health issue could be created. No clear cause and effect existed between most of the health problems linked to being overweight. Neither was there any weight that could guarantee health.[114]

Conclusion

The concern in the past, as it is now, was the coupling of obesity and health problems. Learning about obesity led Canadians and practitioners to refer to weight/height charts. As with nutrition guidelines, the charts were tools that were easy to use but somewhat flawed. While obesity is considered measurable, the statistics for obesity in the past have not been reliable. Just think about Pett and Ogilvie pointing out the problems presented by body frames in some of the charts. Also, a statistical trend over a larger population may not be much assistance to a doctor trying to help an individual patient. Nevertheless, weight surveys were able to create many statistics about those who were at risk of obesity based on gender, age, class, race, regional location, and other similar factors. Gender was a major factor; when physicians looked at men and women, it was through the perception of bodies, but also through a social/cultural awareness of gender. Underlying obesity is fat, and in the history of fat there were many debates about the science of fat, with one point of view dominating for a time but eventually being superseded. The causes that gave rise to obesity in the past are the focus of the next chapter. It will be evident that the contentiousness that surrounded trying to understand the role of fat extends to understanding obesity's causes.

3 Causes of Obesity

"The path ... of obesity in the individual depends on the physiology of hunger, the psychology of appetite, the psycho-physiology of activity and of weight adjustment-reduction; against the general matrix of ethnic, genetic and constitutional endowment, the socio-economic background for the availability of food, the cultural customs and values regarding eating and corpulence; and against the particular matrix of individual inheritance and constitution result in body build and of the family interpersonal dynamics and personal customs and values."[1]

Underlying many studies of causation and treatment of obesity in the past and today is an energy equation. To maintain a stable weight, energy intake should equal energy expenditure. Obesity is an imbalance in the equation, that is, the person is taking in too much food or the wrong food and/or not expending enough energy. Not everyone, however, accepts the energy equation. A 1988 discussion paper by Health and Welfare Canada argues that the energy equation is incapable of taking into account "individual differences in the efficiency of energy utilization, the role of genetics and the effects of interaction between heredity and environment on body size."[2] Despite the problems with the energy equation, it has had a long history, with Canadians (and others) and physicians seeing it as an easy way to understand weight gain or loss. Balance between energy in and energy out is good; imbalance, bad. Accounting for the imbalance, however, has proved to be difficult and contentious, and individual Canadians are often blamed for that imbalance.

Five proposed causes of obesity dominated the medical and popular literature from 1920 to 1980: eating too much (or eating poor food), psychological problems, heredity, metabolic/endocrinal factors, and lack of exercise. In one way or another, all are still being listed, with some causes now considered to be aspects of others. Each had a place in the energy equation. Energy intake revolved around eating, with overeating being the major cause of obesity. But what caused an individual to eat too much? By the 1940s, health experts were looking at psychological complications to understand overeating. Heredity, too, was part of the intake component. The difference between heredity and a psychological cause for overeating was that the latter often blamed the individual, whereas the former was not something the individual could control. Heredity did not lead to blame. The metabolic/endocrinal cause focused on body abnormalities that reduced energy expenditure. It, too, was not something the individual could easily control. Not being active was.

Overeating

Much of the literature on obesity today focuses on overeating as *the* cause. But understanding why people overeat is complex. Some look to an obesogenic environment: the type of food grown, the processing of food, its composition, its marketing, the size of portions, the places where we eat, the policies of governments, and the advice of nutritionists. The result is that we eat too much (often too much of the wrong food) and thus take in too many calories. Others focus on early humans, hypothesizing that the human brain became hardwired to eat whenever possible to offset times of famine. Still others examine the role eating plays in our lives: what we eat, when we eat, how we eat, with whom we eat, and how much we eat. In many respects, eating defines our identity.[3] Class, race, and gender also determine what we eat and how much.

In his history of the American diet, Harvey A. Levenstein argues that in the 1920s workers gained access to more food variety than before, resulting in weight gain, characterized by some as an "obesity ... problem."[4] Canadian nutritional experts did not see the 1920s this way. Their concern was largely for Canadians who were underweight. Nonetheless, they acknowledged what happened when energy intake outstripped energy expenditure – fat was stored in the body to the point of obesity, a result of "overnutrition" and consumption of the "wrong" foods. For example, a 1925 article in the *The Canada Lancet and Practitioner* entitled "What We Eat and Why" noted a relationship between "stout" people and their consumption of fat meat and lots of bread and butter.[5] In 1936, Walter R. Campbell, Department of Medicine, University of Toronto, pointed to Canadians enjoying eating varieties of food; since the cost of living had plummeted during the Depression, food costs were not prohibitive for those who were employed. Campbell, however, worried about those hurt by the Depression and the kind of food they ate – too many cheap carbohydrates rather than protein.[6] Not surprisingly, the popular press also fixated on eating as the cause of being fat. The press emphasized how consumption at almost any level was a key to weight. If you were not able to control what you ate and how much, then it was your fault if you became fat,[7] not the fault of being bombarded by food advertisements.

In the 1940s and after the war, the focus on overeating increased, especially concerning the type of carbohydrates Canadians were eating – "sweet" foods. Canadians' ability to limit their appetites was offset by marketers to a greater degree than in the 1920s and 1930s. Even a Westinghouse oven advertisement in *Maclean's* called on readers to "BRING ON THOSE BIG APPETITES … husky appetites."[8] Henry A. Christian, editor of the 1947 edition of *The Principles and Practice of Medicine*, accepted the energy in/energy out equation. In doing so, however, he described some of the complexity of obesity, arguing that individuals who were obese never went beyond a certain weight no matter how much they ate. Christian's explanation was that the surface of the body expanded as the body became larger, thus increasing "the basal heat production" (the metabolism). But if stability eventually resulted, at what stage of obesity did this happen? Most physicians didn't accept an individual who was obese as being stable in health, so they fell back on the reasons people overate: the gratification of various foods and flavours, the comfort aspect of eating, the relief eating provided "from anguish caused by intellectual, social or sexual failure," and the refusal to alter eating habits as they aged.[9] In their advertisements, some pharmaceutical companies concentrated on the temptation of food. The visual of an advertisement in the *Manitoba Medical Review* for Desoxyn (methamphetamine hydrochloride) showed a fat woman eating desserts in a restaurant being served by a half-man and half-snake waiter. Tired of dieting, she couldn't resist temptation. Others queried whether there was some kind of underlying hunger "mechanism" not working. If that were the case, practitioners could comfort themselves that they just had to find it and fix it. Until then, they concentrated on food consumption as the problem,[10] making overeating both the symptom and the cause.

After World War II and into the 1950s, obesity in Europe was an "anomaly" due to lack of food during the war years and for many years afterwards. In North America, however, obesity was an issue. Daniel Cappon, a member of the Department of Psychiatry, University of Toronto, even noted that eating references permeated the vocabulary in Canada and the United States: "can't stomach him," "could eat her," "honey," "like a peach," "sour face."[11] Certainly, societal changes made getting more to eat easier. More Canadians had more money to spend on food because the economy was strong, and they had more leisure time to eat. Packaged foods were becoming more popular, as were fast food/chain drive-ins.[12] The Metropolitan Life Insurance Company warned of overeating in its advertisements, stating that 95 per cent of obesity cases were due to eating and drinking. Culture, too, could direct eating. The French-Canadian medical literature acknowledged that eating and drinking were important to the culture of Quebec, especially the eating of sweet food and drinking of sweet liquors. As one French Canadian concluded: "Nous vivons dans une période de cocktails et de bridge ou de canasta. Les réunions sociales sont nombreuses" [We live in an era of cocktails and bridge or canasta. Getting together socially happens all the time].[13]

But could you blame Canadians? Magazines that constantly published articles on dieting and the need to cut back on calories also filled their pages with visions of shopping for food or families surrounded by a cornucopia of fattening food at meal time. Canadians were eating more fat than ever: in 1935, 114 grams (4 ounces) per day; in 1955, 134 grams (4.7 ounces).[14] As noted, nutritionists argued Canadians didn't seem to know what food was good for them. Some men, not wanting to accept responsibility for their own weight, pointed to their wives as the culprit. A March 1952 serial column in the *Globe and Mail* entitled the "Tubby Hubby Diet" saw wives' cooking as the origin of their husbands' weight gain, but also as the solution if the wives changed their cooking habits.[15]

In a review article in the 1950 *Canadian Medical Association Journal* (*CMAJ*), doctors D.E. Rodger and J. Grant McFetridge and dietitian Eileen Price, all from Saskatchewan, accepted that intake of calories was the only cause of obesity. Food intake was key, so the challenge, once again, was to explain overeating. For the three authors, the explanation

Causes of Obesity 85

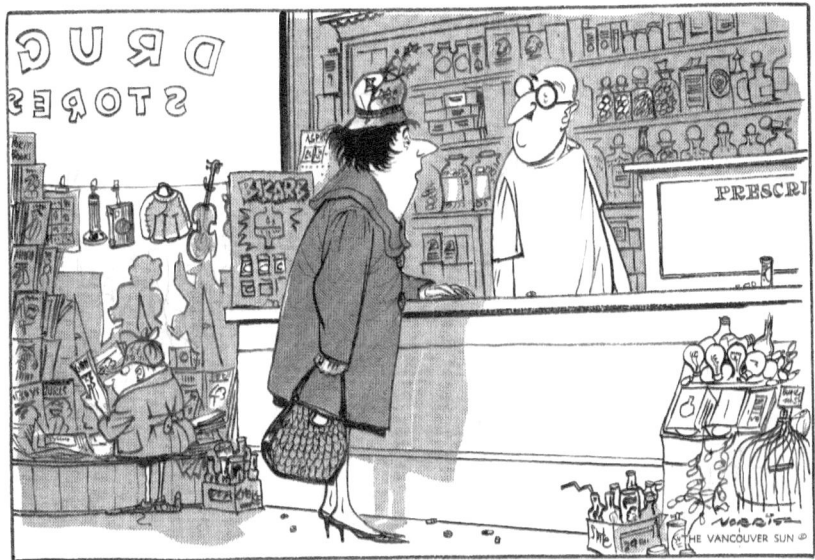

"... I'd like something for the man who ate everything."

Eating, according to the medical literature and popular magazines, was the major cause of obesity. Too many Canadians were eating too much. This 1963 cartoon shows a wife at a pharmacy to buy treatment for her husband – he ate too much. As she said, "I'd like something for the man who ate everything." Source: MsC 25–871, 1–1963–12–27, SFU Special Collections, Len Norris Collection, Simon Fraser University Library.

lay with the importance food had in society, both its availability and its taste. For most, food had gone beyond being only a means for survival. Eating was enjoyable, and so was the satiety it provided. Food made a person feel better, not only physically but also psychologically. Eating was an escape.[16] In the words of L. Bradley Pett of the Department of National Health and Welfare: "Food may ... be a symbol of friendship or even of love. Many hostesses ... are insulted if guests fail to gorge, or wives who cater to their husbands' likes rather than good nutrition."[17] Overeating had become a cultural marker for the good life, a way of caring for people. And the marketplace of packaged mixes and easy-to-make recipes pandered to that desire in a decade that emphasized domesticity. For many, eating well embodied a reward for having survived a decade of economic depression followed by a world war. It was not surprising that for many Canadians eating was a way of literally experiencing a full life. Only a few were willing to challenge the acceptance of overeating as the reason for obesity by pointing to thin individuals who ate a lot without putting on weight.[18]

By the 1960s, middle-class, mostly white Canadians were increasingly living in what they considered to be a modern world, but much of what made it modern also made them fatter than in the past: large refrigerators to keep food; appliances that made cooking easier; and easy access to snacks, which had become part of many Canadians' lives. With packaging and shipping, foods that Canadians would not normally be able to eat were now available all year long. The impact of seasons had been altered.[19]

Those in the field of obesity studies in the 1960s and 1970s recognized that for some people the urge to eat was overwhelming. You could be an "active overeater"; a "sedentary overeater"; or a "night" eater, who after the last meal of the day would get up during the night, feeling the need to eat. Others were "compulsive eaters."[20] But it didn't matter what kind of eater you were, physicians saw fattening food as the problem, especially carbohydrates – potatoes, bread, and the "cakes, biscuits, cookies and other sweet foods."[21] Carbohydrates were easier to digest than proteins; they resulted in a faster accumulation of fat; and, for Canadian consumers, they were also cheaper and thus tended to be eaten more. In reaction to the criticisms of carbohydrates, it was noted that they were "good sources of calories, contributing to total nutritional health and well-being." Eating too much protein and its fat "produces toxic substances" called ketones. Carbohydrates "burn" the ketones. The problem was that people were consuming more refined carbohydrates, which didn't have the positive qualities of unprocessed grains. The carbohydrate of most concern was sugar. Even populations that had traditionally been protected from sugar, such as the Inuit, were eating too much of it. Canadians' affair with sweets eventually led the federal government to "require manufacturers to declare the total amount of sugar and other sweeteners as a percentage of total weight of each cereal on package labels."[22] As the labelling was a move against obesity, some wondered if banning sugar altogether was the next step.

Causes of Obesity 87

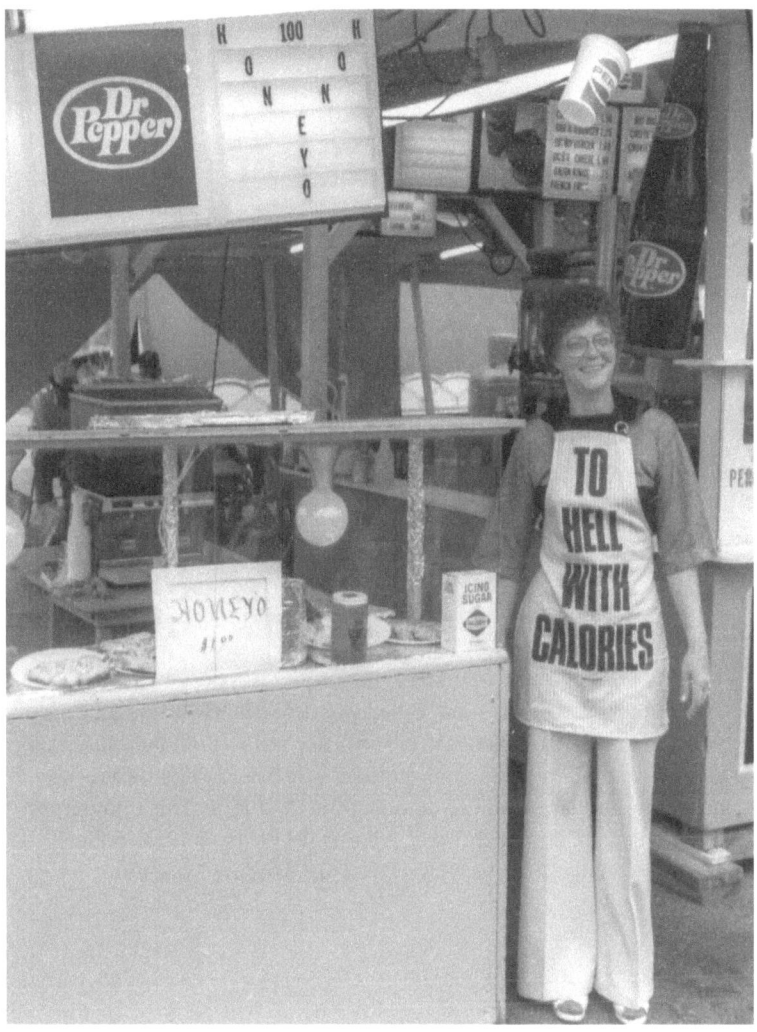

Canadians believed that eating too much would make them fat. But many didn't want to count calories, especially sweets. The Honey-O concession at the Pacific National Exhibition (PNE) in Vancouver, 1978, featured a woman wearing an apron with that message: "To Hell with Calories." Source: Photographer, Bob Tipple, 1978; AM281-S8-: CVA 180–7527; © COV, City of Vancouver Archives.

88 Fighting Fat

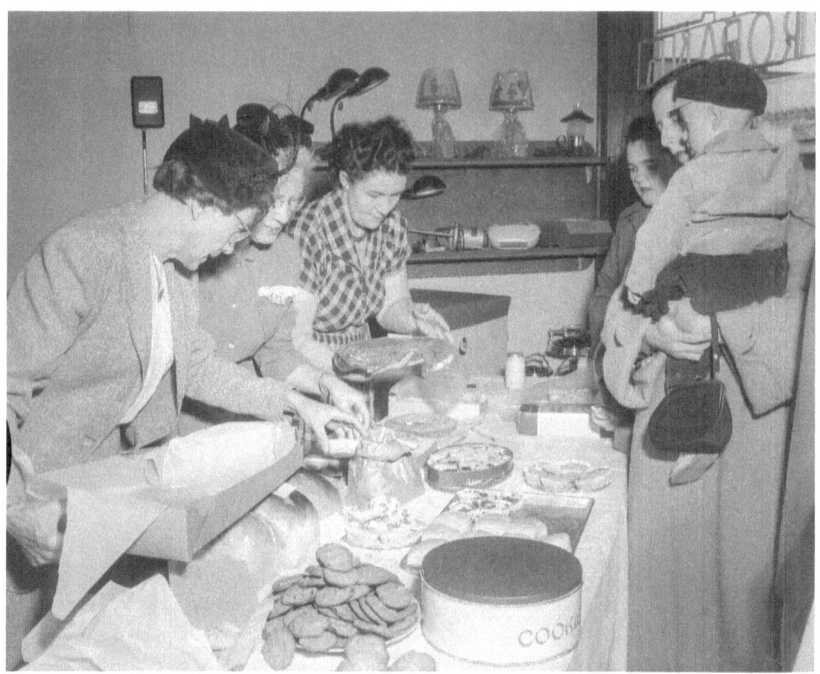

Most Canadians loved sweet food, especially desserts. However, nutritionists were trying to get Canadians not to eat so much sugar. Still, families liked to eat dessert, and many wives and mothers saw baked desserts as a way to make their families happy and to demonstrate their love. This photograph shows women at a bake sale in Taber, Alberta, 24 October 1953. Source: Photographer, Orville Brunelle; NA-4510–230, Glenbow Museum.

Experts did not always agree about eating and obesity. In the 1970s, some were questioning whether "fatty diets" were as problematic as the doomsayers suggested. R.J. Shephard, professor of applied physiology at the University of Toronto, noted that there was very little difference in eating habits between those who were overweight and those who were not. Others were rigid about what foods and how much could be eaten.[23] Vigilance was needed. The elderly especially had to watch their eating. A study of fifty older people living on their own or with families reported that eight people in the study were over the 10 per cent mark of normal weight for their height. They "consumed a snack at least once daily."[24] Such findings raise two questions. Is being overweight by more than 10 per cent truly harmful for an older person? And did nutritionists really think that one snack a day was harmful?

Overeating was deemed the number one factor causing obesity, but understanding overeating was still complex, as it was connected to social, cultural, and psychological factors; iatrogenic issues; hypothalamic injury; and the fat cell notion. In 1974, A. Angel, Toronto physician and professor at the University of Toronto, described studies that compared those who were obese with those who were of average weight, based on how they responded differently to "the appearance, taste and sight of food and, in addition, respond[ed] more readily to external cues, such as clock time, than to internal cues ... e.g., gastric contractions and hunger." Others were enamoured of the set-point weight concept, the idea that a body had a preferred weight and needed to eat in order to reach that weight. Ironically, despite all the focus on eating, its nature had not been studied. Indeed, one overview of obesity in the late 1970s pointed out that sixty years of research "had failed to provide any clear indication that fat people eat more food than normal weight individuals, and had provided no information at all on eating pararmeters such as the duration of meals, speed of eating and size of mouthfuls."[25] The only consensus was one that had survived the decades: obesity was a sign that the energy equation was not in balance, that more energy was consumed than expended, which is essentially a tautology that gives no explanations for how or why balance is so elusive.

Psychological Problems

Overeating was assumed to be *the* factor in understanding obesity over the decades. But how could the need to overeat be explained? The comfort and joy of eating reflected an emotional relationship with food, not just a survival need. These pleasures were part of the psychology of eating. But when Canadians thought of psychology with respect to obesity, they were thinking of a psychological disorder, disturbance, or stress. Those advocating fat rights today argue that the negative view of people who are fat tends to be expressed through psychological discourse.[26] Indeed, some of the anti-obesity experts see obesity as a mental or brain disorder that should be listed in the *Diagnostic and Statistical Manual of Mental Disorders* (*DSM*). Yet, others contend that fat people do not necessarily have psychological problems or low self-esteem, and neither do they suffer from mental distress more than other people.[27]

In Canada, psychology emerged as a discipline in the 1940s, and the psychology of obesity was not widely considered until then. In 1946, Edmonton physicians Leonora Hawirko and P.H. Sprague reported on studies on "upset appetite-regulating mechanism" caused by "dissatisfaction with life." The dissatisfaction led to mood alteration, which in turn could cause appetite to be "upset." In this area, as in so many others, the focus was on different levels of causation. Eating too much caused obesity. But what caused a person to eat too much? "Dissatisfaction." End of discussion. But what caused the dissatisfaction, and why did it affect some individuals more than others? Some researchers focused on what they saw as insecurity in those who were obese. Canadian practitioners would learn from a well-known book on obesity that for girls obesity was a means of defence against suitors. Still others listed boredom, family issues, and depression. Being obese could also be a way to avoid activities that the individual found "unpleasant." The irony is that even today physicians are repeating this perception as if it were a new insight.[28] The popular media in the past linked the newborn's need for love and security with food, a connection that could continue into adulthood.[29] Such psychological overtones would be familiar to many readers. The reverse relationship between obesity and psychological problems was also recognized, that is, that obesity caused psychological problems – a typical chicken and egg situation.[30]

As Canadians became interested in psychology, the relationship between a psychological problem and weight gain continued to intrigue and intensify during the 1950s.[31] Advertisements for mood-altering drugs to help people keep to their diets often focused on the depressed state of those who were obese, although such advertisements were not always clear whether depression was a result of obesity or a cause. Some saw depression as the result of having to be on a diet, not the result of obesity itself. No matter what the story, a depressed state became part of the obesity syndrome. Indeed, psychological factors could be open ended. According to Cappon, what a person weighed was an aspect of modernity, of being "statistically conscious." Yet, such awareness could "be a bad thing" leading to "self-consciousness," then to "anxiety," which led to overeating.[32] General practitioners were not experts in psychology, and they didn't have time to trace psychological problems in their patients. And most patients couldn't or wouldn't pay their doctors to do so.

Psychological stress could also be gendered, painting women's world as the domestic one and men's as the world of work outside the home. The review article by Rodger, McFetridge, and Price speculated that women dealt with "frustrations and tensions" through eating, perhaps accounting for the higher rate of obesity in women, or at least, for those middle-class women who were the majority of subjects in obesity studies. Men, apparently, had more outlets to relieve tensions. Women were often diagnosed with "emotional obesity," with many fitting into the postmenopausal group of women who were perceived to gain weight in a way that was difficult to counteract because of both physiological and "psychosomatic factors." An editorial in the 1955 *CMAJ* referred to "emotional instability" linkage with anorexia and obesity, both of which were connected to women. The editorial's author also queried why some people "chose" one type of symptom rather than another, assuming that anyone with emotional instability could *choose* the way to express their instability. He seemed to be seeing both anorexia and obesity as volitional to a certain degree, and he was interested in why some stopped or restricted eating and others overate. Despite the recognition of emotional instability, the editor seemed to be looking for some kind of control underpinning the choice made.[33] Cappon took a different approach and speculated "a girl's overeating [could] result from penis envy." Not all agreed with using a Freudian perspective. Hilde Bruch did not. The German-American analyst admitted there were pregnancy and impregnation fantasies, but she didn't see them as germane to obesity in adolescents or adults. For others, the cause of overeating was the fear of sex or pregnancy on the part of women and their desire to be fat to offset any male attention.[34] Men were not exempt from the psychological gaze. Pett, in his discussion of the symbolic importance of eating, referred to the psychological associations that went with men and eating. "Some men are aware of the need to cut down on their food portions but they just cannot do it because it seems to lessen their feeling of being big or important."[35] Looking at differences between women and men in obesity was a reflection of how psychologists viewed gender (or sex). But changes in the 1950s were significant: more women were going to work, even married women, and while middle-class men had good jobs, their masculinity fell short of the men who had gone to war.

Psychological causes of obesity were intriguing, and not surprisingly the popular media spread the word. For example, an article in *Maclean's* informed Canadians about the creation of psychodietetics, "a science that attempts to explain such things as gluttony, food allergies and lack of appetite." Dorothy Sangster introduced Canadians to the work of Cappon, and the *Globe and Mail*'s Josephine Lowman explained "emotional obesity" as a term used by physicians and psychologists.[36] Canadians took much of the literature on obesity in the popular media to heart, to the point that a 1959 editorial in the *CMAJ* suggested that patients coming to practitioners had internalized the psychological view of obesity and were demanding help for their "anxiety" or "insecurity," which they believed led to their overeating. Yet the editorial's author indicated that the psychological view had done little to respond to patients' needs. His frustration was palpable. Others didn't think there was much they could do except acknowledge the emotional aspect of eating. After all, the "malaises sociaux" [social problems] encouraged obesity.[37] Cappon's conclusion about obesity's cause was telling: "Too many people are too fat because they eat too much and probably because they exercise too little."[38] Even for a Freudian psychiatrist, all the complexity boiled down to the causes health experts had long pronounced.

In the early 1960s, Dr Doris L. Hirsch, instructor in psychiatry at Dalhousie University, and Dr W.I. Morse, associate professor of medicine at the same university, referred to the previous twenty years in which emphasis had been on "emotional factors" as an element in obesity causation, an exaggeration, but one that had some validity within the psychiatric and psychological communities. Hirsch and Morse described their work with seventy-four patients at the Victoria General Hospital, Halifax. They found problems counselling patients when they used psychiatric methods. According to Hirsch and Morse, it wasn't their methods that were obstacles but the patients who came from the clinics and thus from "the lower socio-economic groups." The authors pointed out:

> Clinic patients are unprepared to think in abstract, reflective terms about themselves and tend to expect the physician to do the investigation, contributing only concrete answers where possible ... Secondly, these patients, in contrast to many patients who attend psychiatrists, came not for psychiatric help but ostensibly for reducing diets and were, therefore, not highly motivated to search within themselves for possible emotional factors contributing to their weight problem. A further difficulty was, of course, that the patients were evaluated psychiatrically by only one examiner without control of the examiner's bias ... [I]n addition, no control

group of normal-weighted people was interviewed. The essence of these difficulties is that this type of psychiatric evaluation is relatively superficial and fails to get at possible deeper dynamics which might be of value in correlation with metabolic studies.[39]

Hirsch and Morse found "no specific personality type" in their group, and while dependent personalities were common, the finding was not significant. Most of the patients were women, and, as noted by Hirsch and Morse, "in our culture women are expected to be somewhat dependent." They observed that the patients who were dependent often had basic metabolic rates lower than others and higher serum cholesterol concentration, which the authors linked to "small differences in thyroid function." As we will see, the thyroid and its function was considered a metabolic/endocrine factor. In linking a specific personality to a thyroid function, Hirsch and Morse connected the psychological or the psychiatric, as they preferred to state, to the biological. Not wanting to end the description of their work in a negative way, they put forward the "discovery" that "moods" affected eating habits, although a response varied with the mood and the individual so that no generalization was possible.[40] The article provides an insight into the failure of psychiatric/psychological methodology to determine causation and the limitations of whom it could help. That people who were obese were blamed for not being "reflective" suggested a weakness in the process of investigation, a negative attitude to workers, and the expectations of psychiatric methods of the time. The gendered assumptions of dependent personality revealed the attempt to find a common personality trait to account for obesity. Despite the study not being particularly useful in its findings, the authors' conclusion tried to sound positive.

The open-ended discussion, evident in the preceding medical literature, reflected the way the psychological/psychiatric approach could see emotions as the origin of overeating. "Tension and frustration" led to a delayed sensation of fullness after having eaten enough, leading to more eating. The hypothesis posited that the ennui of modern life with its "boredom," "loneliness," and "social pressure" also affected hunger. D.R. Wilson referred to "personality disturbance" as "probably the main predisposing factor to the obese state."[41] In *Chatelaine*, Sheila Kieran told her readers that a well-known psychiatrist saw the fat man as angry, whereas he thought the fat woman used food as a substitute for comfort and security.[42] The "male change of life" was an "insidious process," and men found "solace" in food addiction.[43] The gendered difference of these explanations were telling, as was the notion that either gender could use obesity as a way of avoiding attention from the opposite sex.[44]

Not all were happy with the way psychology was applied. A 1961 *Chatelaine* article referred to the popularity of psychological causation, but the author, who herself was overweight, was having none of it and rejected the image of those who were obese as somewhat "unbalanced." Neither did all studies see being fat as problematic. A Swedish study found that fat women suffered less from depression and "anxiety neuroses" than their normal or underweight sisters. American studies, too, didn't find the obese individual any more psychologically problematic than anyone else; as a result, obesity was not placed in the *DSM*.[45]

The findings of the Swedish and American studies may have weakened interest in psychological cause, but other reasons added to its decline in the 1970s. Practitioners often rejected psychological theories, especially those of psychiatrists. In *Maclean's*, Dr James Paupst referred to psychiatrists and their way of pontificating:

> As millions continue to overeat, psychiatry ruminates over the symbolic aspects. There are countless theories, including overeating as a sign of repressed hostility reactivating primitive cannibalizing impulses aimed at eating the enemy who is substituted for food; as symptom of yearning for a lost person or situation and orally incorporating the lost person; or as the result of a desire for self-punishment and self-degradation in order to release guilt and to justify rejection by others.[46]

Despite the psychobabble, finding out why someone ate was significant, and often a psychological problem could be a factor. One case was described in the *Canadian Family Physician*:

> Mrs. A: weight 181 lbs. Age 48, height 5' 2 ½". Ideal weight 150 lbs. Mr. W's second wife was not obese until after she joined this family. (The first wife died of a myocardial infarction and was also obese). She gives the impression of being an aggressive, independent woman, but is overpowered by her husband.[47]

Here was a normal weight woman who put on weight after marrying a dominant man, whose former wife had been obese. Many psychological issues could have been raised in such a relationship.

Almost anything could spark a reaction that was psychological. Taking drugs for psychological problems, especially antidepressants, tranquillizers, or antipsychotics, could be a factor in obesity. But was depression the cause or the consequence of obesity? Some health experts saw individuals misreading emotional cues as hunger or others feeling "compulsive hunger" due to experiencing eating as calming. Like those with anorexia nervosa, people who were fat could "possibly have an abnormal perception of their body image." In such an assertion, it was possible to see how the two eating disorders influenced perceptions of one to the other. Indeed, Cappon's 1973 book *Eating, Loving and Dying: A Psychology of Appetites* focused on both, although obesity dominated.[48]

In depicting types of eaters – the nibbler, the voracious eater, the chewer, the "bulk eater," and the faddist – Cappon argued that each type said something about the individuals, why they ate, and why they ate the way in which they did. As a psychiatrist, he emphasized the psychological factors leading to overeating and obesity. However, he did not see obesity only in those terms, but tried to meld the psychological with the physical. He used the concept of the appestat, a "psychological control mechanism, which regulates the amount of food one eats." He compared appestat to a home thermostat with various settings – high, medium, and low – and he maintained each person's appestat could be different from someone else's. Thus, some individuals would simply eat more in order to meet the physical demands of their bodies. In comparing the appestat to a thermostat, he was comparing a biological mechanism to a purely mechanical one. How did one control the biological? In addition, he was creating a hierarchy of appestat settings, seeing a low setting as linked to "brain-centred intellectuals" or people who were creative. Those with high settings were tactile people, "the visceral individual." He almost reverted to a phrenological way of looking at the obese when he mentioned that people who had been obese since adolescence or earlier seldom had "long, tapered fingers."[49]

Only rarely did an alternative perspective appear within the psychological view of obesity. Susie Orbach's 1979 book, *Fat Is a Feminist Issue*, was well known in Canada. Orbach presented a feminist understanding of the experiences of women trying to have slender bodies in a society that was not sympathetic to those who were overweight and the experiences of women who were overweight but feeling that their weight gave them strength and seriousness. For some women, the book encouraged them to accept their bodies. As one Canadian responded concerning her weight: "What makes you think everyone wants to be thin? … I like being big. It gives me a sense of power. It makes people turn around and look at me."[50]

Heredity

If what we eat, and how much, are problems, neither one explains patterns of obesity in the population. While psychology might have answers for some individuals, it doesn't seem to offer answers to the majority. Also, general practitioners, who are at the front line taking care of their patients, are not always sympathetic to or understanding of the psychological or psychiatric world. They are much more comfortable looking to the body. But what does the body tell them? Can our evolution as a species explain obesity? The hardwired theory suggests that our genetic code cannot adapt fast enough to refuse excess food.[51] A more popular genetic cause is family heredity. Statistical studies of parents and children suggest that an individual will have a 1.4 per cent chance of being obese if parents are a normal weight; 8.2 per cent if one parent is obese; and 20.1 per cent if both parents are obese.[52] But how much of family obesity is genetic, and how much is caused by family eating habits?

The idea of heredity as an explanation for obesity is not new, but it was not a factor discussed much in the past. In the 1893 edition of *The Principles and Practice of Medicine*, William Osler recognized heredity as an element in obesity, believing it manifested itself after middle age. By his 1912 edition, he saw heredity as a "marked ... tendency." Thomas McCrae, editor of the 1925 edition of *The Principles and Practice of Medicine*, was more specific, seeing a person's metabolism as hereditary. A 1926 article in the *CMAJ* pointed to race and heredity as significant factors in leading to obesity.[53] If that were true, what could be done about heredity? The assumption was, very little. Indeed, with the eugenics movement becoming stronger throughout the interwar period, race and heredity were increasingly seen as fixed. Weight loss could occur, but maintaining the loss was difficult due to "hereditary nature."[54]

At one level, the hereditary aspect of obesity gave those who were obese, and didn't want to be, some comfort – their fatness was not their fault. Or was it? In a 1931 review of an American article, E.S. Mills told *CMAJ* readers that heredity did not affect appetite, that is, you could not inherit an appetite. What you did inherit was the "constitutional tendency to store fat from whatever food" was eaten. Thus, the individual was to blame for eating too much given his or her propensity to store fat, but the actual storage of the fat was beyond the individual's control. Others saw heredity significant only for prognosis; by 1947, heredity in *The Principles and Practice of Medicine* was only seen as a contribution to obesity, not a cause.[55] No wonder practitioners who listed heredity as a cause didn't discuss how it worked. Before the unravelling of the genetic code, they only had the statistical research on parents and children to back up their claims.

Nevertheless, heredity explained obesity in a way that most lay and medical people could understand. That is why heredity was mentioned, if not dwelled upon, in the popular press. A 1944 article in *Chatelaine* described heredity working through the endocrine (glandular) system (as had the Mills 1931 review article). The author of the *Chatelaine* article understood the difference between inherited metabolism ("the rate at which you burn calories ... controlled by glands") and eating too much, but there was no forgiving people who did not control their food intake to match their metabolism.[56] In the professional literature, what intrigued researchers was how heredity worked. Was it connected to "genes of endocrine glands" or were there "genes for obesity"?[57] But if obese individuals might have liked the idea that their situation was a reflection of their heredity, it didn't mean that fat wasn't dangerous for them.[58]

During the 1950s and 1960s, medical journals increasingly mentioned heredity, more often than not as a factor that had to be considered, but with little explanation of how it functioned. In her 1957 book, *The Importance of Overweight*, Hilde Bruch argued that heredity could be biological or social. The former was "obligatory" obesity, but the latter type only appeared when "environmental" circumstances in life brought to the fore the "inherited endowment." She saw physicians either split between these two types of heredity or not distinguishing between them. She also put forward the idea that in some families the fear of hereditary fatness led them to watch their children's weight constantly, leading to "rebelliousness" on the part of the children, who might eat even more.[59] Cappon didn't consider heredity as a cause in most obese individuals. As for obesity being significant in certain racial/ethnic groups, he tended to see their weight as cultural more than genetic. Other commentators simply dismissed heredity altogether or focused on family eating habits, which could be changed. Yet, proof of heredity in obesity was in the statistics. Or was it? For example, Lucien Dubreuil, in his 1952 article "L'obésité," told his colleagues that if both parents were obese, their children had a 70 per cent of being obese, compared to 40 per cent if only one parent was obese. These statistics were much higher than the 20.1 per cent and 8.2 per cent, respectively, given in current estimates.[60] But did the statistics reflect heredity, or a cultural or social aspect of a family's eating?

The popular literature seemed more accepting of hereditary obesity. In a 1957 issue of *Maclean's*, Byng Whitteker, a CBC announcer, was clear his weight was inherited: "Whenever I am pestered to transform my natural bison shape into something more on the lines of the gazelle, I look at the family album. My father, five-foot-ten, weighed between 235 and 240 pounds and lived heartily for eighty-seven years. My mother was a comfortable 155 or 160 and lived to be eighty-three. I was six-foot-three and 235 pounds by the time I was sixteen." In 1960, Mrs Florence James complained to the readers of *Chatelaine* that the medical profession didn't take hereditary obesity seriously. Doctors were willing to see heredity as a culprit for "everything from low arches to bald heads ... but for something that is as obvious as inherited overweight, they come up with fairy tales. I speak from painful experience."[61] Heredity as a cause permitted families to be more accepting of size; it was just something that most physicians didn't accept.

The genetic factor allowed patients and doctors alike to understand why obesity occurred and why treatment seldom worked. What it didn't explain was the growing rate of obesity. A note in the 1975 *CMAJ* estimated that 60 to 80 per cent of obese patients had a family history of obesity. Other opinions of how many Canadians were obese because of heredity varied from 35 to 65 per cent.[62] Such widely differing statistics couldn't convince many to see heredity as a significant cause of obesity without more research. As Cappon argued, family dynamics could create obesity – after all the family shaped the child. But he remained "skeptical" about heredity as a major factor cause. What would convince him was finding several generations of fatness in the same family.[63]

Studies were trying to understand nature versus nurture by looking at adopted children and their lives to gauge the influence of heredity versus social/family environment. One finding showed that obesity was not determined "only" by heredity, but "family resemblance ... [was] explained virtually only by heredity." Genetics seemed immutable, but those who were optimistic, such as Dr Winick at Columbia University, believed it could be "counteracted" by "environmental factors," especially in children. Researchers also suggested that the hereditary weight of particular ethnic groups was perhaps exaggerated. A look at Canadian school children, for example, revealed that Inuit children's bodies were changing in their weight/height ratios, not through the force of heredity but because of a changing environment in food intake, which was lessening the differences between them and their southern Canadian counterparts.[64]

Genetics covered a wide spectrum of issues. C.H. Hollenberg, Lady Eaton Professor of Medicine at the University of Toronto, summarized the knowledge of heredity in a December 1978 editorial in the *CMAJ*: "All that is known is that genetic factors are important in the causation of the obese state; the genetic determinants that are involved have not been elucidated." As a result, heredity raised all sorts of speculation. Some referred to "genetic abnormalities," suggesting a flaw in the genetic code. Others focused on the urge to eat as something that, as a species, was part of our "propensity to gorge" ourselves, a form of hardwiring.[65] But why did some have that inclination and others not? A 1971 article in *Chatelaine* explained that genetics could account for the propensity to be obese, that is, the tendency towards obesity was inherited, not obesity itself. If the family environment or the wider society did not encourage weight gain, obesity would not result, an argument that had been around for many decades.[66]

Metabolic/Endocrinal Factors

Heredity as a cause of obesity is one that individuals can't overcome, not without seeing their bodies as the enemy. Heredity is an overall explanation, but for obesity it works, in part, through the body's metabolism and the endocrine system. Metabolism is complex, comprising three "components": "resting metabolic rate, metabolism of activity, and energy spent digesting and absorbing food." Of the three, the first uses the most energy to keep the body alive.[67] Rates of metabolism vary, and some argue that those who are overweight/obese have inherited a particularly efficient metabolism, meaning that they can burn their calories with little energy expended.[68] As well, resting metabolic rate is low in obese people, whereas for other people it is higher, which means that thinner bodies are expending more energy even when resting. Of course, as in anything to do with obesity, not everyone accepts the slowness (efficiency) of metabolism in the obese. Some argue the opposite: people who are obese have a fast basal metabolic rate compared to thinner people, and the larger the body, the faster the metabolism.[69] Because the endocrine system controls metabolism, others have put forward the notion of endocrine disruptors.[70]

The issue of metabolism varying from one individual to another had been introduced before the twentieth century and was described in Osler's first edition of *The Principles and Practice of Medicine*. The 1912 edition even placed obesity under "Diseases of Metabolism."[71] McCrae, in his 1925 edition of *The Principles and Practice of Medicine*, noted that low basal metabolism in some patients seemed linked to a "peculiarity" of the thyroid gland, a view that would become quite widespread. Internal secretions from the gonads also played a part in the weight gain of eunuchs and at certain times in women's lives. Both the thyroid and gonads are part of the endocrine system, and thus McCrae was emphasizing the endrocine system's function as a controller of metabolism, as were others.[72] In Canada, Edward Mason and others thought that endogenous obesity (within the body) could be created by some endocrine disturbances.[73]

The idea of a metabolic/endocrine cause was touted more in the 1930s.[74] The fat person did not necessarily eat more food than the non-fat person, but rather processed it at a different rate. The willingness to accept the centrality of a metabolic rate was understandable. It was a physiological explanation that took away blame from the individual who was obese and focused on a reason that made sense to physicians. It presented them with a condition they might be able to respond to by fixing the disturbance or changing the metabolic rate. For those who saw disturbance within the endocrine system as a way to account for the metabolic rate, the thyroid, which McCrae had pointed to, attracted noteworthy attention, although not all were willing to make that connection.[75]

Christie saw the human body as designed to work in balance. If too much food was taken in, the body's metabolism could deal with it, although, he admitted, only to a limited degree. He also argued that the "weight-regulating mechanism" could be damaged through problems in the endocrine system. For example, he acknowledged that when women's ovaries were removed, weight gain followed in 75 per cent of patients, and that 60 per cent of women with amenorrhoea (absence of menstruation) originating from problems in the ovaries gained weight. While he was willing to discuss obesity originating from pregnancy, he believed that most of the weight came when women started nursing and consequently developed an increased appetite and did little exercise. As for men, he recognized "hypogonadal obesity ... after castration or as a result of bilateral atrophy of the testicle." But such cases were not common. Christie also had a racial perception based on "endocrine or cerebral peculiarity," which caused generations of certain families to be obese. For example, he speculated that "Hebrews" had inherited "large appetites and depressed weight-regulating mechanism."[76]

While the metabolic/endocrine cause of obesity was a popular one, it was being challenged. A 1931 article in *Maclean's* by Dr Grant Fleming made clear that the possibility of problems with the "glands of internal secretion" existed, but argued it wasn't a significant cause of obesity: endocrine problems were simply not prevalent enough to account for the majority of those who were obese.[77] The challenges increased in the 1940s.[78] Like Fleming, H.I. Cramer, physician in the Department of Medicine at the Royal Victoria Hospital in Montreal, noted in a 1946 review article that the acceptance of a low metabolic rate as a cause of obesity was "widespread" despite it being "erroneous." As for "endocrine obesity," he dismissed it as a phrase only useful in describing where the excess fat was and how many had it. He tried to account for the persistent belief in endogenous obesity, which more often than not focused on the endocrine system and metabolism, by looking to the standard of the basal metabolism rate (BMR) being used. Some considered a rate between -10 per cent and -25 per cent of the norm as a sign of hypothyroidism (underactive thyroid). But Cramer argued that such a determination was open to criticism for two reasons. First, he pointed out, the accepted normal BMR was placed too high, often based on people who were not relaxed, which distorted the figures. Second, clinical features of myxoedema (dry skin and swelling) must exist to diagnose hypothyroidism, which was not the case for many who were obese. In making his argument, Cramer referred to a 1930 article to prove his point.[79] By doing so, insight into how the scientific or medical process worked emerged. Cramer built on the past, but since so much in the past on this issue was contradictory, not surprisingly he chose studies that supported his argument.

While the endocrine cause of obesity was being negated, no other significant cause took its place. As a result, practitioners tried to hedge their bets. Pointing to the belief in menopause as a cause of obesity in some women, Hugo Rony, an endocrinologist in the Northwestern University School of Medicine, claimed in his 1940 *Obesity and Leanness* that there was little evidence in studies for this theory. However, like Christie had previously, he did see the period during and after pregnancy as a "dynamic phase" for obesity. In doing so, he was putting forward an endocrine hormonal cause. Another text on obesity known to Canadian practitioners observed that some researchers were focusing on damage to the hypothalamus as a way to explain overeating. Given that the hypothalamus links the endocrine system to the nervous system through the pituitary gland, one could argue that the endocrine system was still a focus for researchers, but in a different way. The authors of the text also acknowledged that some aspects of the endocrine system *were* significant in determining the different locations of fat in men and women, which suggested the role of the gonads at some level. Nevertheless, the authors denied any specific cause and effect in relation to obesity. An association between obesity and malfunctioning of the thyroid was also denied except in very rare cases. Yet, thyroid preparations were being used in diet aids to speed up the processing of calories. Indeed, many advertisements for pharmaceuticals used as diet aids made clear to practitioners that "ENDOCRINE OBESITY" existed and emphasized how thyroid extracts could help increase the body's metabolism.[80]

Even though exogenous obesity accounted for most obesity, endogenous obesity would not go away. In 1952, for example, Lucien Dubreuil, assistant-superintendant of the Division of Children's Health for the city of Montreal, argued that the former accounted for 99 per cent of obesity cases. But he still listed endocrine system problems as a cause of obesity, whether they were problems in the pituitary gland, usually found in the young; the thyroid, effecting metabolism; or the sex glands, in males at puberty or in their forties and fifties.[81] Contrary to Rony's opinion about menopause, the reduction in estrogen production during menopause continued to be speculated about as a cause for weight gain. Others still acknowledged weight gain in women at puberty and after pregnancy. Disorders of the hypothalamus, too, were still linked to appetite.[82] The need for a certain amount of calories in order to keep the body functioning suggested that if the metabolic rate was askew, then the body would either lose weight or put on weight. After all, the slowing of the basal metabolism explained, in part, why people tended to put on weight as they aged, especially if they did not exercise much or reduce their food intake.[83]

The mantra of refuting the endocrine theory continued in the 1960s and 1970s.[84] In 1974, University of Toronto professor A. Angel argued: "There is a general tendency to regard obesity as a single disease entity. This view is no longer tenable … [O]besity may arise as a result of: abnormalities at many levels of control including the hypothalamus (control of feeding and satiety); endocrinopathies; abnormal dietary habits, e.g., gorging or cultural traditions of feasting; physical inactivity; and genetic abnormalities." After saying this, he concluded with evidence that "endocrine and metabolic abnormalities in obesity are the result rather than the cause of obesity."[85] Nevertheless, the belief in a metabolic/endocrinal cause didn't disappear. The endocrine system was so varied that the focus could easily shift from one part to another. For example, the thyroid was no longer as interesting as the adrenal gland from the research perspective, but thyroid extract remained one of the ingredients used to treat obesity. Work on the hypothalamus continued, as did work on hormones.[86] While the various editions of *The Principles and Practice of Medicine* from 1912 to 1947 had placed the discussion of obesity under "Diseases of Metabolism," it was placed under "Endocrinology" in 1972. Ironically, the authors of the obesity chapter in the 1972 edition did not place the endocrine system and its hormones high on the list of obesity causation, privileging instead increased caloric consumption and low energy expenditure.[87] Metabolism was still indicated with respect to utilization of calories, and mention was still being made of the elderly and their lowered metabolism.[88] Metabolism also remained part of the obesity discourse through understanding how certain glands worked. Metabolic/endocrinal causes did not lay blame; they described what was, with some believing that metabolism was somewhat genetic and thus individual.[89]

But research seldom looks at the individual. The underlying theory of weight was the energy equation, with its assumption that the amount of energy taken in would and should be expended. Individuals, however, don't live lives according to theory; while stripping individuals down to essential bodies made some sense – it did allow for a finer understanding – eventually the practitioner would have to work with the patient's social, environmental, and genetic baggage. The sense of a body in energy balance was an ideal against which obese bodies were measured. When obese bodies deviated from the ideal, the conclusion drawn by Angel was that they had "in some imperceptible way, lost control of normal homeostatic mechanisms that ordinarily keep the body weight remarkably constant."[90] The language of Angel's statement was telling. The obese person had "lost control" of something over which no person had control. While focusing on the "mechanisms," there was a recognition that these were internal and not volitional, but somehow the language shifted to make it volitional. Also clear was that some people who were obese tended to have a very efficient "utilization of food energy."[91] While in most aspects of life efficiency is a positive attribute, in obesity studies it wasn't – it was problematic and thus an abnormality.

By the end of the period under study, the pursuit of a metabolic cause of obesity had shifted focus to brown fat. As noted in chapter two, Jean Himms-Hagen, professor of biochemistry at the University of Ottawa, explained that "brown fat, a heat-producing tissue, has been fitted together with research on obesity to provide an exciting and challenging new approach to the study of the cause of obesity and could serve as a starting point for the development of new modes of treatment."[92] Underlying that statement is a wonderful summary of the field of obesity studies. It confirmed that scientists and laboratory workers, not practitioners, dominated the field, a development that had been growing for decades. The answer to obesity would not be found in the doctor's office, but in "basic research." The continual optimism in the search for a cause of obesity also shone through, highlighting the ability of those in the field to convince themselves the answer was just around the corner. At the same time, the careful use of the word "could" meant that little was sure in the search for causation, at least not yet.

Lack of Exercise

If differences in metabolism and disorders in the endocrine system helped Canadians to understand why the energy expenditure side of the energy equation was unable to keep an energy balance, there didn't seem to be an easy way to correct those differences – they appeared to be involuntary. Volitional energy expenditure could be pursued through physical activity. Today, we live in a society that doesn't encourage energy expenditure, an environment in which energy expenditure is not naturally as much a part of daily life as it once was. It doesn't take much decline in energy expenditure with food intake either remaining the same or increasing to create a world of heavy people.[93] Not everyone, however, sees the decline in activity as a substantive cause of obesity; nor does everyone see exercise/activity as an easy solution for obesity or think that being obese means lack of physical activity. Michael Gard and Jan Wright in *The Obesity Epidemic* found that what activity means, and how much is enough, is controversial.[94]

Although the energy equation placed energy expenditure as half of the equation, only limited discussion of the role played by physical activity took place in the past. In his 1893 edition of *The Principles and Practice of Medicine*, Osler listed lack of exercise after overeating as the second most important element in obesity causation, but did not expand on the point.[95] And that remained how practitioners perceived it: a factor causing obesity, but not one they saw as a medical issue per se, or one they knew much about. In the 1920s, whenever the relationship between lack of exercise and weight gain was acknowledged, it was usually in terms of older people, although the advice given was to be active but not too active. Middle-aged people over the age of thirty-five were also warned against doing anything too strenuous, such as playing a hard game of badminton. If they indulged in this type of intense physical activity after a hard day of work, it could act as a "slow poison."[96] Exercising and sports were also gendered. For women, walking, golf, swimming, and housework were good for fitness. Men's sports could be competitive and more active than women's.[97]

The popular media was certainly aware of weight gain during winter, in part due to lack of exercise. In all seasons, "authorities" were suggesting that the sedentary life – driving vehicles too much – was a cause of being overweight.[98] When weight loss was required, exercise was mentioned, but generally only in passing. In the 1920s and 1930s, the *Eaton's Catalogue* began to advertise exercise equipment, such as lightweight dumbbells, for men – whether for weight loss or maintaining weight and strength is not known. *Chatelaine* had a tendency to encourage women to see housework as a form of exercise and their home as their "reducing salon." Here, exercise was about appearance, with a concern about weight as part of it. The humour section of *Maclean's* called attention to the limitations of those who were fat – even though they were active, there were limits to what they could do. One cartoon showed two large men playing tennis. Noting a stepladder in front of the net, one explained: "That's for jumping the net to congratulate the winner!" Another version of the cartoon appeared in the 1940s, but instead of a stepladder, there was a gate in the net.[99]

In the 1940s, vigorous exercise was still for youth, and moderate exercise was for the middle-aged.[100] Once an indidivual was fat, however, a vicious circle began: obesity was assumed to lead to a decline in exercise, which, in turn, increased obesity.[101] But it wasn't always seen in such a linear way. As one American text suggested, making any generalization about exercise was fraught: some obese people were active, while some had never been, even as children.[102] It was clear that lack of exercise was not thought to be a significant cause of obesity. When exercise was mentioned in the 1940s, it was with respect to the war and connected to men being fit for military service. Fitness and health were needed for them to rise to their citizenship – fighting for Canada. For women, their health and fitness were necessary for them to take over men's work during the war.

By the 1950s, however, the sedentary life was clearly catching up with North Americans,[103] and the search for fitness came to the fore.

Physical fitness gurus such as Lloyd Percival hectored women through the pages of *Chatelaine* about their lack of fitness, claiming 75 per cent of them were not fit. While he thought women were in bad shape, he observed that men were worse; women had housework and running after their children to keep them physically active, although once past forty they didn't outshine their husbands by much.[104] Lack of activity was one thing, but the lack of fitness was worrisome when added to weight gain.[105] As Deborah McPhail has argued, being unfit and overweight was not the image that Canada wanted to put forward, especially for men during the Cold War era.[106] Young women were entering the workforce more than they had previously (except during the war), and their attractiveness (their slenderness) for some employment was seen as significant – for example, for being a flight attendant.

Fitness became an even bigger issue for Canadians in the 1960s and the 1970s. A "News" section of *The Canadian Nurse* told readers that 50 per cent of Canadians were overweight. Those who were fat did not overeat, the article explained, but 80 per cent of Canadians didn't engage in activity. Russ Kisby, physical director of the Downtown Montreal YMCA, was clear about what was happening: "physical unfitness exhibits itself externally in the form of fat (overweight), flabby muscles, poor posture and in general an unpleasing appearance." Even when Canadians thought they were fit because they played sports, too many of the sports were leisurely ones and not engaged in on an ongoing basis. And it wasn't just southerners in Canada who were unfit and fat. Studies also traced the decline of fitness among the Inuit, especially in the young.[107]

A CBC Radio fitness show, *Sports College*, aired a program on 9 December 1961 entitled "Deliberating Man's Appearance in the Year 2000," in which Percival looked into the future and predicted that men would be less than fit due to "modern-day automation and labour-saving devices," which made them fatter and weaker than they had previously been. In 1968, a CBC TV show, *Newsmagazine*, informed Canadians that they did not exercise enough; coupled with the increased amount of food they were consuming, they were becoming fat. While the focus still tended to be on middle-aged people, middle age was now seen to start in the thirties. *Chatelaine* told its readers that they should maintain the same weight as when they were twenty-five; since they were no longer as active as they had been, they should be cutting back on calories as they aged. Accepting the energy in/energy out equation would mean acknowledging the role of physical activity, especially in a society in which so many appeared to be inactive. Exercise had become a serious business, and it *should* be a daily regimen.[108]

Many Canadians in the 1960s took the advice to heart, perhaps because the early boomers were now in their teens and their numbers brought youth to the centre of attention. Everyone wanted to look young. The 5BX exercise program (and later the 10BX) of the Royal Canadian Air Force became standard fare – too many Canadians were not exercising enough. John B. Armstrong suggested in the *Canadian Journal of Public Health* that lack of interest in exercise was due to the misconception on the part of health experts and the public, who thought "exercise required little caloric expenditure and … that an increase in physical activity is followed axiomatically by an increase in appetite."[109] It seemed some people feared that exercise was not going to help them lose weight, and it might actually put weight on. Trying to offset such beliefs, others noted that a vigorous walk of only half a mile a day could mean a difference of 12 pounds "of fat" a year. Another claimed that twenty-one hours of golf would eliminate 2 pounds. While that didn't seem much for people who were obese, Dr Allison suggested that they also had the work of carrying their own weight around, so they would lose even more weight. As for increasing appetite, it was argued that exercise didn't seem to be a problem if the exertion was only an hour's duration or less.[110]

In the 1970s, the health experts were frustrated about Canadians lives. In 1977, Bert L. Fairbanks wrote an article in the *Canadian Association of Health, Physical Education and Recreation Journal* in which he lamented: "Our 'civilized' world follows the same time proven life pattern that farmers have used for years to fatten their cattle in preparation for market – Pen them up and give them all they can eat." Toronto's W. Harding LeRiche criticized the consumer who wasn't active and didn't seem to care about his health, assuming the government or another agency would find "the solutions for his problems."[111] Such a description of Canadians was a response to certain chronic modern diseases like obesity. Underlying LeRiche's words was the sense of a society in which people did not take responsibility for their health. The world in which Canadians lived did not encourage activity and, indeed, discouraged it. The change in activity didn't have to be much to make a person obese. For example, *Chatelaine* warned that the shift from hand typewriters to electric typewriters meant a 5 pound increase in weight if the typist didn't cut back on her caloric intake.[112] Efforts to be active were needed.

Conclusion

What emerges from the discourse on obesity causation is the frustration physicians and other health experts felt. While at times researchers, nutritionists, physicians, and commentators in the media seemed confident about the causes of obesity, an underlying tone of doubt could often be detected, a worry about not having found a definitive cause. Some commentators were honest – they just didn't know. How could they? There didn't seem to be a causative pattern, a one source fits all. In 1936, Walter R. Campbell summarized the state of obesity studies:

> At present the evidence does not warrant the belief that there is any one qualitative abnormality which predisposes to overweight in all individuals. The specific dynamic response to food has been stated to be abnormally low, and this is probably true in some cases, but is by no means a universal finding. Occasionally one encounters a reduction in the level of basal metabolism. Except in some endocrine disorders, however, this is an unusual factor and the basal metabolism of an obese person may exceed his ideal basal metabolism by larger amounts. The efficiency of muscle work is believed by some to exceed the normal, thus sparing calories. This contention, however, does not go unchallenged. A diminution in muscle activity would undoubtedly lead, when food intake remains the same, to the laying of fat, and may be a potent factor in many cases of obesity; in other words, the patient who is overweight avoids fatigue, becomes lazy, and progressively more economical of muscle activity. Besides the influence of energy conservation, various endocrine influences have been credited with the production of ... obesity, and a lipophilic tendency has been postulated, heredity and constitutional factors have been incriminated, and many other theories have been proposed with more or less evidence to support them. At present we are completely unable to explain the peculiar distribution of fat in certain individuals on a purely energy balance basis, and must look for additional causes in the endocrine system and elsewhere.[113]

This summary is significant. First, Campbell acknowledged that those in the field were looking for one cause. Second, he assessed various theories and pointed out that there were problems with each one. Third, he acknowledged that some theories worked for some cases of obesity, but not for others. Fourth, he admitted the field was a morass and no explanation seemed possible. Fifth, he continued to look to the endocrine system, although he admitted the need to look elsewhere as well. Looking to the endocrine system perhaps reflected his medical training and the desire to find a physiological explanation. It might also have been influenced by all the advances in endocrinology that occurred in the 1930s. Sixth, given the frustration that those working in the field must have been feeling, it was no wonder that many took the easy way out – they focused on food intake and lack of exercise, both of which put the blame on the individual. The dissatisfaction with the causal explanations offered in the early decades continued for the rest of the years covered by this study.[114]

It is difficult to figure out causation for obesity. Overeating was the favoured cause, and most of the debate revolved around what led to it. As they do today, experts in the past often gave a list of various factors: heredity, learned behaviour, lack of exercise, emotional issues, difficulty sensing when full, metabolism, thyroid problems, and others. At times, the list could be quite specific, with each cause seemingly a problem in and of itself. In the 1980 edition of *The Principles and Practice of Medicine*, the authors of the obesity chapter admitted their quandary. While over decades more understanding of eating and obesity had emerged, "the normal physiological controls of body weight are incompletely understood."[115] There were so many theories – psychological, biological, cultural, and social – that it was next to impossible to get an overview. It still is this way. No single cause for obesity has been agreed upon, and multiple causes are still being proposed. Indeed, the "multifactorial" nature of obesity is where the consensus lay in the past and remains in the present. For a practitioner dealing with individual cases, the long list of causes would make effective treatment difficult. Some, however, took the list as meaning that there was no real causation.[116] This study of perceived causation indicates that the factors seemed endless and complex. But for most people it was simple – eating too much and not exercising enough. Little has changed.

4 Treatment: "Stubbornly Resistant"

"A stout lady was told by her doctor, 'You have too much around your hips and the weight has retreated to your rear ... effecting [sic] your posture. You have to reduce!' Looking at the doctor's large protruding stomach she commented, 'Seems to me I'd rather pull it than push it.'"[1]

With so many perceived causes of obesity, it is not surprising that treatments are multivarious. Even as new treatments emerge, older ones don't necessarily disappear. Determining a treatment is fraught since there is no proof that a cause, if removed, would eliminate obesity – that is, sustained obesity might be a different issue from the onset of obesity.[2] And treatment, no matter what form it takes, has consequences. This chapter examines two treatments used for weight loss: exercise and dieting. The first addresses the energy expenditure side of the energy equation; the second addresses energy intake. The two are more often than not put together as a mantra for losing weight: exercise more, eat less. Both have a long history, but exercise, while often mentioned in the obesity literature, has been overwhelmed by the focus on dieting. There were two aspects to increasing energy expenditure in the past. The first comprises exercises, sports, and any movement of the body that an individual initiates voluntarily. The second consists of the involuntary movements resulting from the use of products, which range from soap to machines. Choosing the best diet is a complex decision and an issue for debate. What diet will help in weight loss, and what diet will Canadians stay on? Diets were many and varied. To understand the elements and types, diets have been broken into four sections: medical diets – diets that physicians felt would help their patients lose weight in a safe way; fad diets – diets that Canadians got from friends, families, media, doctors, or others who thought that their "new" diet was the best for losing weight; product diets – diets that grew out of consumer culture; and unsafe diets. No matter what the diet, dieting has a history of failure; consequently, adjuncts to dieting were introduced to make dieting both easier and presumably more effective. Psychological counselling and support from professionals or other dieters was one of those adjuncts. Canadians needed to understand why they ate the way they did and to learn ways to avoid doing so. Joining a support group was positive for many women, a psychological mainstay that has maintained its popularity to the present day.

Exercise

A biological problem underlies the assumption that exercise is necessary to increase energy expenditure and offset energy intake. When the body loses weight, it tends to reduce energy expenditure since signals go out warning that the body could be in a starvation mode. When this occurs, the body is oriented towards gaining weight or at least maintaining weight, not towards losing it.[3] Some suggest that this signalling also happens with exercise. If exercise uses up energy, the body stimulates appetite so that energy is maintained. Nonetheless, the commitment to physical activity as part of the treatment for obesity is strong. And, as with obesity, pundits see "inactivity" as a "global pandemic." A 2011 federal report on obesity suggests that one million Canadians could avoid obesity by simply doing fifteen minutes of extra physical activity per day, advice that Dr Sharma, scientic director of the Canadian Obesity Network, deemed "simplistic."[4] Nevertheless, being active is something that many Canadians believe will help them maintain a stable weight or lose weight.

Effective or Ineffective Exercise

Although William Osler in his 1893 text listed the lack of exercise as a second cause of obesity, he didn't discuss exercise as a treatment to any degree. In his 1912 edition, he noted that exercise could be helpful, especially for children and for women who gained weight during pregnancy or menopause; otherwise, he didn't see exercise as a significant treatment.[5] Little changed over the decades. In the 1920s and 1930s, exercise and sports were part of the new regime for women and

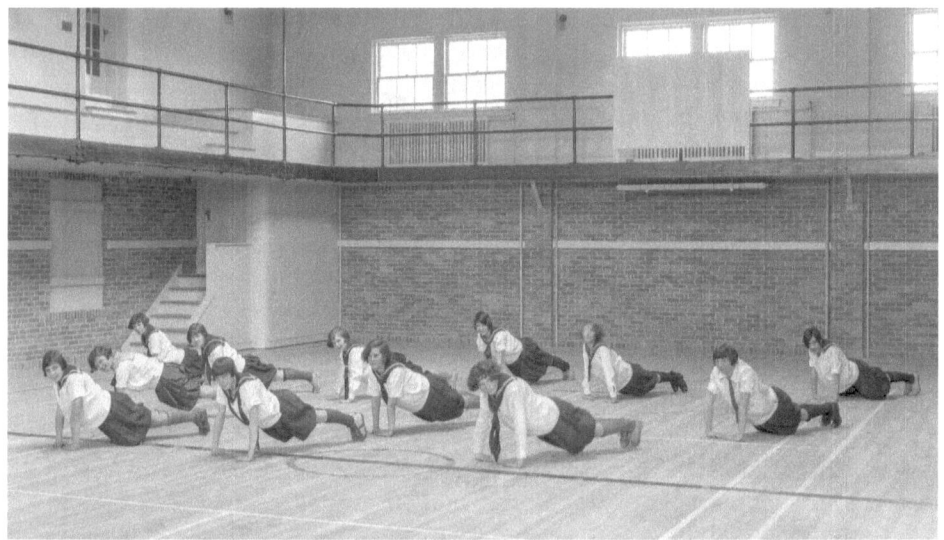

Fitness was equated with good health, and being fit was considered a defence against getting fat. Some Canadians were fit because of their work, but others had to exercise. These young ladies were exercising at the Young Women's Christian Association (YWCA) gymnasium, Edmonton, Alberta, in 1926. Source: Photographer: McDermid Studio; ND-3–3114e, Glenbow Museum.

seen as good for all, but there were limits. In the 1921 *L'Union Médicale du Canada*, Maurice Boigny, chief physician of l'École de gymnastique de Joinville, France, suggested vigorous activity was not healthy for adults after thirty-five or forty years of age. The rather broad age range was meant to take into account an individual's constitution.[6] Neither was exercise deemed an effective weight-loss treatment for those who were obese, with some physicians arguing that strenuous activity for people "already exhausted by the task of carrying too much fat" was not beneficial. Exercise, however, was considered helpful to make sure that weight loss didn't weaken a dieter.[7] In his 1938 book on obesity, Dr W.F. Christie was more optimistic. He noted that for some individuals exercise resulted in weight gain in the form of muscle replacing fat, but that eventually exercise did reduce weight. Some of the medical beliefs mentioned made their way into the popular press, sending the message that exercise was not a good weight-loss treatment, in part because it allegedly increased appetite. But exercise was positive for firming up the body while dieting.[8]

Little changed during the 1940s and 1950s. Some physicians who were interested in weight loss did not see exercise as a stand-alone solution – it didn't use up much energy, could stimulate appetite, and "strenuous" exercise might aggravate the health problems that too often came with obesity, especially for older Canadians.[9] The September 1950 issue of the *Canadian Medical Association Journal* (*CMAJ*) reported an American specialist's estimate that an individual would have to walk thirty-six miles to lose one pound of weight. No wonder exercise did not loom large in obesity treatment. Those who supported exercise for both weight control and weight loss tended to be physical education experts. Medical practitioners were not against exercise, but found it was difficult to get patients to engage in physical activity. As a comment in the humour page of *The Canadian Doctor* noted, every patient wanted to be able to get rid of fat through "mental concentration. Wishful shrinking in other words."[10] A more serious article by Morton Hunt in *Maclean's* entitled "Exercise is the Bunk – Relax" concluded that exercise was "a black fraud." It didn't help lose weight and didn't even prolong life. Sidney Katz agreed, pointing out that to lose one ounce a person had to climb eighty stairs. Josephine Lowman, the guru of dieting for husbands, saw in exercise a danger to men who had not done any for many years. If they wanted to exercise, it should be to shape their bodies and for no other reason.[11]

Fitness, however, became hugely popular in the 1960s, as evidenced by the 5BX and 10BX plans for men and women. The 1970s saw the pervasive presence of ParticipACTION, a national organization to get Canadians engaged in physical activity. But its founding also reflected the perceived need to make headway in Cold War sports. The goal was not necessarily weight loss but health. Marc Lalonde, the minister of health and welfare, saw fitness as "health promotion"; and Canadians became more interested in fitness and sports when the 1976 Olympics were held in Montreal, Quebec.[12] *Chatelaine*'s readers were told about the Slim Jym device, designed to shape the body and help them lose inches within the "privacy" of their homes. Spas offered "treadmills, roller machines, bicycles, pulleys and weights."[13] Most of these approaches targeted body attractiveness as the goal, although losing weight was part of improving appearance and an added bonus. Those who saw themselves as both active and overweight were frustrated by any emphasis on exercise for weight loss when it seemed obvious to them that some people just put on weight no matter what they ate or did.[14]

The medical and health literature didn't emphasize exercise as a "treatment" per se for obesity, other than as an adjunct to dieting.[15] Exercise could help a dieter lose some weight to add to the weight loss achieved by dieting; exercise could also be a weight maintenance strategy. All Dr D.R. Wilson of Edmonton could say about exercise for weight loss was that "it limits the patient's access to food for part of the day." Dr Firstbrook, School of Hygiene, University of Toronto, even suggested that the health benefits of exercise had been exaggerated. However, not all the health experts were negative. Sandy Keir from Fitness and Amateur Sport reminded readers in the *Canadian Journal of Public Health* that the Nutrition Study of Canada survey had determined that the caloric intake of overweight and average weight people did not differ greatly. The difference in weight, then, was most likely caused by the former's lack of activity. Exercise certainly could be preventative, if not a weight-loss method. In explaining diet failures, Bert L. Fairbanks, professor of kinesiology at the University of Lethbridge, looked to the possibility of exercise offsetting low energy expenditure. Supporters of exercise were also trying to overcome the long-lasting notion that exercise led to increased eating.[16]

Passive "Exercises" for Reducing

As a way of encouraging physical stimulation for patients who were overly fat, some practitioners in the 1920s recommended hydrotherapy, massage, or electricity treatment. Each implied a class of people who could afford such treatments. Underlying these treatments was a belief that getting inactive obese people to be active was difficult.[17] Indeed, companies used the lack of effort as their products' attraction. The Renulife Violet Ray was advertised as an undemanding treatment that could be used at home. Appealing to credulous women was Osmos, "the famous Swedish Reducing Foam Bath." The advertisements assured readers that Osmos, unlike most other products, actually worked because it was a scientific "innovation." Osmos represented a partnership between beauty and health specialists, and was "prescribed" by both. Nothing needed to be done but bathing, the punch line asserted – the pounds would apparently flow down your bathtub's drain. The Little Corporal Belt was promoted in *Maclean's*. Wearing the belt would allegedly take four to six inches off the waist and do away with the "unsightly, uncomfortable bulge of fatty tissue over the abdomen" without "fasting, hot baths, or back-breaking exercises." There was also the electric roller to break tissue down on certain spots on the body. The Beasley Reducing Corset would make women both look and be slimmer through its "gentle massaging."[18] The lack of specific information was part of the allure of all these products.

The easy exercise sales pitch appealed to middle-class Canadians. In 1945, Gordon Sinclair, a radio personality and reporter, described one example – the weight reduction machine. All you had to do was stand in the machine and electricity "would do the rest." He quite liked it – "a barber's head rub extended to the whole body." Eaton's offered its steam baths to "help whittle those extra pounds if you are on a weight-reducing campaign." The Relax-A-Cisor, too, could be used at home to decrease the size of stomach and hips; like all such devices, it apparently did so with little effort. Unlike dieting, this machine didn't leave the user with sagging skin, and both sexes could use it. In 1958 alone, 500,000 Canadians used such machines in salons, and 25,000 purchased them.[19]

For those who were unable to lose weight, there were items that hid the weight they carried. For example, the Spencer Body and Breast Supports, advertised in *The Canadian Nurse*, was one such product. Others were closer to medical items, such as the Camp Support girdle, advertised in *The Canadian Doctor* in 1948. The accompanying images depicted an older, overweight woman, the first showing her with a "pendulous abdomen." The text was lengthy and warned about the collapse of the body's balance, unhinged by the "pendulous abdomen" and forcing the woman's centre of gravity forward. The result was "strain on muscles of back and feet ... round shoulders and increased cervical and lumbar curves ... the diaphragm and abdominal viscera ... on a lower plane than normally; [and] eventually respiratory and circulatory symptoms appear." The image of the body of such a person needing support was not a pretty one. This type of image was used again in 1957. One advertisement depicted an older man who wore the "girdle" over his undershirt, with the photo showing various straps surrounding his girth. The result claimed was a formidable and firm girth that hid any sense of jiggling or overhanging fat. The role of the girdle was "to balance the flesh of obesity," which the picture represented.[20]

116 Fighting Fat

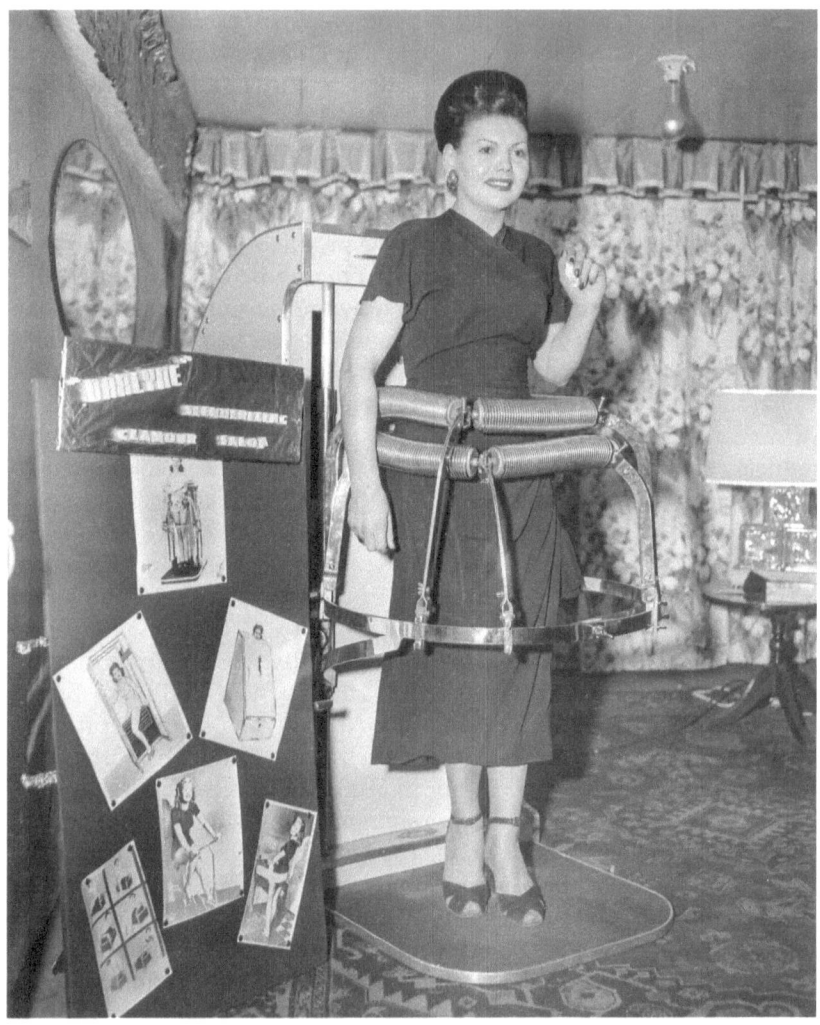

In the 1950s, passive exercise became popular, appealing to people who wanted or needed to lose weight but did not like exercise. This photograph, taken at the Pacific National Exhibition (PNE) in 1950, shows the Darlene Slenderizing Glamour Salon Device, a product that claimed to help people lose weight easily. Source: Photographer, Art Ray; AM281-S8-: CVA 180–1636; © COV, City of Vancouver Archives.

Easy-to-work exercise equipment and other devices for weight control and fitness abounded in the 1960s and 1970s: the Exercycle (Automatic Exerciser), "spa-inspired shapers," and the automatic massage belt.[21] If weight decreased, however, it was a bonus. If you didn't have time to engage in exercise, a weightlifting champion's advertisement offered a "weightlifter's physique" with only 70 seconds a day of effort using the "i-sometric-isotonic" method based on muscle contractions.[22] An article in *Chatelaine* mentioned the staplepuncture, a form of acupuncture for those who were overweight. A surgical staple (1/8 inch long) was placed in a particular part of the ear lobe, which, according to acupuncturists, was an appetite control spot. Dr Elie Cass, head of the Acupuncture Foundation of Canada in Toronto, used small metal pellets taped to the lobe, since the staples could result in infection. As well, he suggested that his patients follow a "sensible" diet.[23] Apparently he claimed good results, but the diet, if followed, would by itself lead to weight loss.

Even though Canadians were interested in the Olympics, too many didn't participate in sports or exercise themselves. One cartoon in *Canadian Doctor* summed up the situation. A fat man was shown sitting on a tennis court. When asked why, he replied: "My doctor told me to spend three hours a week on the tennis court." In 1977, John Robertson wrote a sports column article in *Maclean's* entitled "You Know the 60-Year-Old Swede Who's Fitter Than a 30-Year-Old Canadian? To Hell with Him." The only new discovery to emerge from studies of fat indicated that cold temperatures resulted in "appetite suppression, vigorous activity ... and fat mobilization." Even though some experts were working with overweight people and having them exercise in a cold environment, it was hardly practical for most. Dr Abraham I. Friedman's advice might have been more attractive: he wrote *How Sex Can Keep You Slim*.[24]

Exercise as treatment for obesity didn't seem to be effective. First, physicians throughout the decades didn't see proof of weight loss as a result. They didn't reject exercise – exercise was positive for fitness, a sign of health. But for patients who were obese, exercise alone didn't work. Second, practitioners knew little about exercise; other than being concerned about vigorous exercise at certain ages, they seldom suggested a specific exercise regime. Exercise was general advice without specific guidance for patients who were overweight. It was advice that those who were fat would have to work out on their own. But would they? In the early decades, Canadians didn't seem to be interested in exercise. Indeed, passive activity was the goal. Even with the rise of Canadians' concern about the sedentary life more people were living, few accepted that exercise would make them attractive, thin, or happy.

Dieting

Unlike exercise, dieting as a treatment for obesity has held sway throughout the twentieth century and beyond. It is a control device and a repudiation of former eating habits.[25] Yet, for most people, dieting is not a permanent solution; those who diet, more often than not, regain their weight. As a result, dieters live in a liminal space between the weight they don't want to be and the weight they hope to achieve. Dieting is also complex and encompasses various stages – first, the catalyst that "triggers" interest in dieting; second, being on the diet; and finally, quitting the diet – each with its own demands. Too often the body at the end of a successful diet is not what the dieter wants. "[T]he post-weight loss state is nothing like the biology of someone who has never lost weight," pointed out Dr Arya Sharma of the Obesity Network. "Simply stated, someone who was 150 lbs and has lost 20 lbs cannot hope to maintain that weight loss by simply eating the same amount of food or doing the same amount of exercise as someone who is 'naturally'… 130 lbs."[26]

Medical Diets

Dieting reflects culture in its motives, goals, and methods. At the turn of the nineteenth century, the term "diet" came to apply to weight-loss programs rather than being only an eating plan to treat illnesses. As such, it was largely directed at men rather than at women, whose obesity was understood more in terms of fluids connected to puberty, pregnancy, and menopause.[27] As for dieting, Osler's 1893 text advised a diet of low carbohydrates and low fat, a diet that is still popular today.[28] Most medical diets are concerned with nutrition – not just having the nutrients you need, but also keeping to the calorie intake suited to your age, gender, and working energy. While it may sound easy to find such a diet, keeping to it is not, especially as a family, where each member – mother, father, children of various ages, and maybe grandparents – has his or her own food preferences. Some might need to eat more to put on weight and others might need to lose weight. Having someone on a diet can upset a family's meals, depending who is on the diet and why. It certainly can make cooking more complicated.

Historians agree that the 1920s was the decade in which slenderness in women and leanness in men emerged as the dominant image of a modern, young, and healthy body. The result was the desire for many to lose weight, not just those who were fat. Dieting for the obese was the main treatment – as were "fasting" and "special" diets.[29] In one of the first articles on the treatment of obesity in the *CMAJ*, Dr Edward H. Mason argued that "it is wise to 'reduce'" those who are obese. Note the language: it was the physician's task to "reduce" the patient, not the patient's responsibility. The subjectivity of the patient in this case disappears.[30] For extreme obesity, the 1925 edition of *The Principles and Practice of Medicine*, edited by Thomas McCrae, advised a diet consisting of 1,200 calories a day. Protein was not to be decreased below 90 grams per day, and sugar (a carbohydrate) and sweets were forbidden, but saccharin (a calorie-free sweetener) could be used. In 1924, the Canadian government had limited the use of saccharin in foods to people "suffering from disease" and "preferably under medical direction," both of which could apply to obese patients. It was curious that McCrae was willing to suggest certain dieting food days such as milk days, when the only food was milk, or "green vegetable days," accompanied by some bouillon.[31] Another diet supported in *The Canadian Nurse* was a fruit or liquid diet of 500 to 600 calories for three days to give a good start to weight loss, followed by a regular diet.[32] But what was a regular diet? As noted in chapter one, medical experts were not always up to date on nutrition. But they worried that Canadians might become enthralled by "freakish and temporary diets" instead of maintaining "habitual moderation" in their diet along with a balance of proteins, vitamins, and minerals. In 1936, Dr Walter R. Cambell pointed out that there was no sense in putting patients on a diet they couldn't or wouldn't stay on. He also rejected institutional dieting (in a hospital) for most patients; the "coerced" patient brought "little credit to his physician."[33]

Various magazine articles, as well, described how dieting worked. A successful diet needed to be preceded by thoughtful planning: Would your diet conform to scientific eating? What were you expecting from dieting? If you were successful in losing weight, were you prepared for unforeseen consequences, such as constipation or wrinkles about the eyes? While fasting was popular, articles warned Canadians against extreme dieting and starvation methods.[34]

The medical view of dieting changed very little during the 1940s and 1950s. The kind of foods to be avoided in a diet remained fats and carbohydrates.[35] In 1946, H.I. Cramer, Department of Medicine, Royal Victoria Hospital, Montreal, wrote a literature review on dieting for his colleagues. He reiterated to his readers that dieting was "the principal way" to achieve weight loss. But he was not impressed by the 400- to 600-calorie diets on which some practitioners placed patients, unless they did so with patients who were hospitalized and for whom a quick reduction in weight was needed, for example, those who were obese and had cardiac problems. Not all physicians agreed with Cramer on the limited use of hospitalization. Since most people had difficulty dieting for any length of time, being in a hospital was the only sure way of guaranteeing weight loss for "the majority of overweights." But how many could afford to go to a hospital or could leave their work or family to be in a hospital? And after being in the hospital, could such patients keep the weight off? The diet Cramer supported was for people who were living their usual life and who reduced their caloric intake to 1,000 to 1,200 calories, that is, a moderate diet, which Cramer believed had more chance of success than any extreme diet.[36] Some physicians saw calories underlying dieting: weight loss was the same whether you were on a high-fat, low-carbohydrate diet or a high-carbohydrate, low-fat diet. Not all agreed – for many, fat was the problem.[37] And that view lasted for some time.

Studies of dieting examined what kind of diet would be more feasible for patients to stay on and more successful for losing weight. In 1956, the Faculty of Food Sciences at the University of Toronto surveyed seventy-eight women divided into six groups who had been on a twenty-four week diet. The average weight loss was only 23 to 31 per cent of the excess weight that needed to be lost, and most of that loss occurred in the first half of the study. The study concluded that weight came off when enthusiasm for dieting was high.[38] Keeping on a diet was not easy. In an article entitled "I'm Reducing," Gordon Sinclair warned readers not to expect quick results, but to be prepared for at least forty days of work. James Bannerman, critic and broadcaster, described his diet as full of hunger, and commented that during his diet he felt compelled to keep checking his weight. The entire process had been "torment," although he admitted he was sleeping better as a result, didn't snore, and was eating like a man rather than a horse.[39]

Despite the problems of dieting, physicians in the 1960s continued to advise dieting as the treatment for obese patients to follow. Many ways of losing weight were tried. While cutting back on calories was the obvious way to lose weight, some suggested that the key was how an individual ate: it was better to eat five small meals a day rather than three larger ones, adding up to the same number of calories.[40] Similarly, the 1976 edition of *The Principles and Practice of Medicine*, noting studies that showed animals ate many small meals a day, suggested humans do the same to help them lose weight (or prevent overweight from developing). But wouldn't more meals be difficult for those in the workforce? Other studies among human subjects came to the opposite conclusion: more meals were not the way to lose weight.[41] While some were still interested in starvation (fasting) dieting, an editorial in the *Canadian Family Physician* reported that more weight was lost with a restricted diet than with a starvation one.[42] The whole process of dieting was fraught. Summarizing the situation, Wilfred Leith, a physician at McGill University and the Royal Victoria Hospital, Montreal, noted that it was "difficult for most patients seen in clinical practice to follow a low caloric diet." One estimate was that 25 per cent of patients advised to lose weight never tried to do so; 25 per cent made the attempt for a month; 25 per cent for three months; and only 25 per cent kept to a diet for a year or more.[43] Despite this recognition, physicians tried to find some way to ensure patients would stay on their diet rather than question whether they should have been put on a diet in the first place. Such questions would bring into doubt the whole underlying assumption of obesity treatment – the need to get the weight down.

The challenge for physicians was both keeping their patients on the diet and determining what the goal of the diet should be. Few people actually managed to lose the amount of weight they wanted to lose. So what was reasonable? Advice given in the December 1964 *CMAJ* suggested that physicians had to be prepared to put their patients on a "long-range" plan. The diet had to be simple or else the patient would not follow it; it also had to be varied to avoid monotony. The dieter needed to understand that being overweight was a "lifelong problem" and was not going to disappear quickly. As well, dieting meant a significant change in dietary habits and not simply cutting out carbohydrates and using sweeteners in coffee. Some experts considered eating to be an addiction and being overweight a symptom that could never be cured, only managed.[44]

Practitioners, however, couldn't control the dieting process. Even if they did for some time, as in a hospital setting, sooner or later patients had to leave and be on their own.[45] At the end of the 1970s, both the

Corporation professionnelle des dietistes au Québec and the Departement de nutrition de l'Université de Montréal concluded that nutritional education and proper eating habits were key to solving the problem of obesity,[46] ignoring the decades of nutrition education that had already been offered to Canadians. Studies on individuals who were obese kept being reported and seemed more refined, but were not of much use to general practitioners. Auréa Cormier, professor at l'Université de Moncton, looked at how weight loss correlated "with certain physical, biochemical and psychological data." He found that it didn't matter if group or individual dietary instruction occurred. Men tended to lose more weight than women, and weight loss was faster for those "moderately overweight than when only slightly overweight." Others were studying the "mechanisms of appetite."[47] Referring to the work done by American Ancel Keys in the 1940s on semi-starved men and the effect on their basal metabolic rate (BMR), Fairbanks described how, at the beginning of a diet (say 1,000 calories a day), the body responded by lowering the BMR to protect its energy source. In long bouts of dieting or severe dieting, the BMR could decrease by 50 per cent as the body went into survival mode so that the energy needed for basic survival was protected.[48] While fascinating and informative, little of this research helped people who wanted to lose weight through dieting or their physicians who prescribed the weight loss.

"Fad" Diets

Not all diets were balanced in nutrients. Indeed, Canadians were bombarded by advertisements and articles to lose weight and offered easy diets to do so. In the October 1929 issue of *The Canadian Magazine*, Virginia Lea referred to the Mayo Brothers' "18-day diet," noting that "prominent ... doctors," both French and American, had experimented with the diet for five years. Lea also mentioned that a Hollywood actress had gone to the Mayo Brothers' clinic, went on the diet, and then "told a friend who told a friend." "Prominent" doctors and a "Hollywood" actress were a significant duo to make a diet popular. The fact that doctors had worked with the diet for five years added to the perceived seriousness, safety, and efficacy of the diet. Individuals would readily believe in a diet if they heard someone else had tried it and found it helpful. Nevertheless, Lea's history of the 18-day diet appeared to be an amalgamation of rumours. The diet itself revolved around eating grapefruit at every meal and taking in only 600 calories a day. A year later, Lea regaled her readers with another diet that a doctor had encouraged a woman who was 40 pounds overweight to follow: a cup of coffee (no milk, no sugar) for both breakfast and lunch, and then whatever she wanted for her dinner.[49] Another diet put forth in *The Canadian Magazine* recommended a spinach fast for five days – the point of it was not to eat starch.[50] One of the extreme diets that physicians commented on in the 1930s was the diet advocated by American William Howard Hay. Reprinting a blurb about it from the *Journal of the American Medical Association (JAMA)*, the *CMAJ* let its readers know that the Hay diet prohibited eating starches and sugars with protein and acid fruits. The *JAMA* reviewer rejected such a peculiar diet, referring to American pride to do so: "Americans have been eating meat [protein] and potatoes [starches] and drinking milk [carbohydrates and protein], and have, as a result, produced some extraordinarily healthful and powerful human beings." The moral – eschew "freak diets."[51]

Dieting has become part of our culture. In 1941, dieting humour in *The Canadian Doctor* featured an anecdote of a little girl who was asked what she would do when she grew up and became a big girl. She answered: "Reduce." "Dietary racketeers" were luring Canadians into various dieting fads. Even the 1947 edition of *The Principles and Practice of Medicine* was still pushing its milk days and green vegetable days.[52] In 1955, A. Corinne Trerice, director of nutrition at the Bakery Foods Foundation of Canada, responded to the society around her by noting: "It is the FASHION to be thin!" The consequence was all sorts of "food faddists" and followers who had forgotten that the basic way to lose weight was to cut back on food consumption while maintaining its quality and variety. But eating was pleasurable, and being on a diet, even a nutritional one, was not. Noting factors working against good eating habits, Trerice listed superstitions, cultural traditions, family traditions, social pressure, laziness, lack of knowledge, and misleading advertisements.[53] Not listed was that diet fads were seen as modern, something to talk about. Indavertently placing diet fads in the "misleading advertisements" category, Mrs B. from Edmonton wrote a letter to the nutrition division of the federal government explaining her problem and frustration. She wanted to lose 12 pounds, and she claimed that the "Canadian Food Rules" didn't seem to allow for it. She wasn't under a doctor's supervision, but she was on the "orange-juice-knox-gelatine diet (4 oranges & 2 envelopes daily plus 1 grapefruit at night)." The diet had not helped, and she had already taken forty-four envelopes out of the fifty-four that the diet recommended. She then asked if the people in Ottawa "kn[ew] anything about the STAUFFER Home Reducing Plan, where you lie on a 'Magic Couch' and are *supposed* to loose [sic] weight effortlessly?" She ended her letter with a request: "Any diet List or recommendation will be appreciated. I'm not a faddist."[54] Why she did not see the "orange-juice-knox-gelatine diet" as a fad diet wasn't clear. At least she did not believe in the "Magic Couch." In an article in *Maclean's*, Sidney Katz worried about the enticement of the easy and fad diets such as the ones mentioned by Mrs B. These diets tended not to be balanced nutritionally; according to Katz, while 1,000 calories was "fine for a housewife who stays home and has little to do … it can be dangerous for a man who has to do a full day's work." The gendered nature of his advice was breathtaking, as if women at home didn't work and all men were employed at physical labour rather than many spending their days at office jobs where they sat on an office chair.[55]

Despite the failure of most diets, their popularity increased throughout the 1960s and 1970s. Healthy and stable diets were not popular; the quick fix that diet fads offered was preferred. In *Chatelaine*, E.W. McHenry noted, as others had, that the popular diets often lacked nutrition. He admitted that a high-fat diet worked for some individuals, but largely because such a diet was "unpalatable" and so food consumption declined. Another article in *Chatelaine* told readers about a British study comparing a high-carbohydrate diet, a high-protein diet, and a high-fat diet. Over three weeks of dieting, no difference in weight loss between the three groups was found. The conclusion was not new – it was all about calories, not where they came from.[56]

Chatelaine constantly put forward diets to its readers. Diets were something that its readers expected to see and liked to read: a "new snack diet"; "The Thinking Woman's Diet"; and its own "Diet Cook Book." *Chatelaine* even described the diet that Queen Elizabeth II followed.[57] In *Maclean's*, Eric Hutton regaled his readers with a list of diets he had tried: "the banana and buttermilk diet; the violent-exercise-and-starvation theory; the Maritime all-potato diet; the high-fat protein diet; the 900-calorie package that drug companies and dairies now offer; and a memorable routine of eating an undressed head of lettuce to start every meal, followed by anything else I wanted – which wasn't much." All were fad diets. Bob Blackburn referred to variations on the low-carbohydrate diet or what he and others liked to refer to as the DMD, the drinking man's diet, and he assured his readers that it worked. Then there was the "drab-food" diet.[58] Canadians were willing to try almost any kind of diet.

Treatment: "Stubbornly Resistant" 125

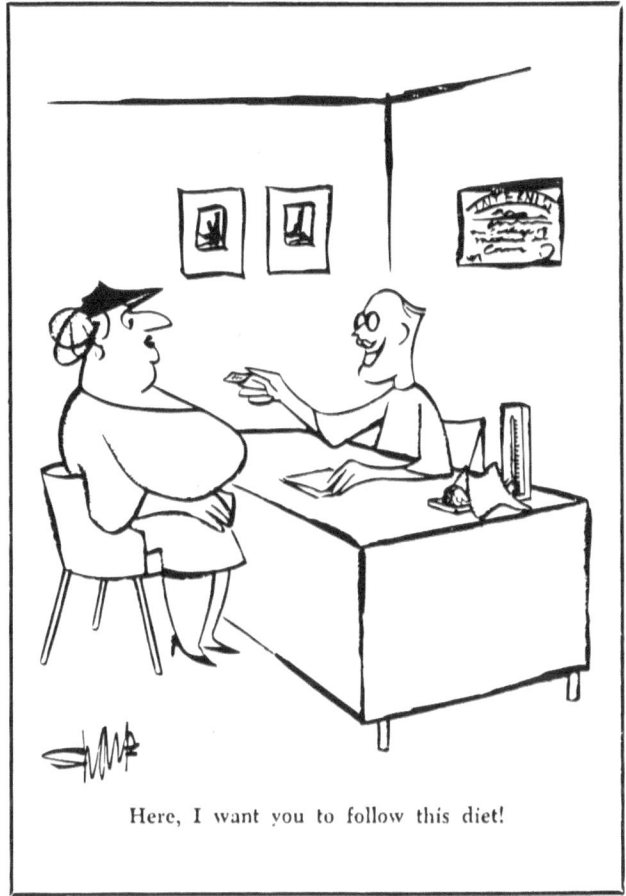

Here, I want you to follow this diet!

Dieting was a major treatment for weight loss. Physicians, families, friends, groups, and magazines came up with diets for others, and those who wanted to lose weight could also create their own diet. In this 1961 cartoon, a doctor is giving a diet written on a very small piece of paper to his large patient. Obviously, the diet would not have much food for the patient to eat. Dieting was something that most Canadians didn't like. Republished, with permission, from *CanMed Assoc J* 85, no. 3 (15 July 1961): 22. © Canadian Medical Association 1961. This work is protected by copyright and the making of this copy was with the permission of the *Canadian Medical Association Journal* (www.cmaj.ca) and Access Copyright. Any altering of its content or further copying in any form whatsoever is strictly prohibited unless otherwise permitted by law.

The Pennington diet created by American Alfred Pennington had a certain amount of caché in Canada. Like many diets before, it was based on low-carbohydrate intake, high in protein and fat, and rejected any focus on calories. The dieters could eat all they wanted, which sounded remarkable. Dr Leith, McGill University and the Royal Victoria Hospital, thought the Pennington diet showed some promise since it allowed dieters to feel their hunger was being satisfied at the same time as they were losing weight. Yet, the diet had problems. Leith looked at some of the claims for the diet – for example, the theory that there was a "fat-mobilizing hormone … present in the urine of patients on this type of diet" – but found no confirmation except in biased sources. In his own trial of the diet on his patients, Leith found that eight of forty-eight quickly lost interest in the diet after a month. They complained about the "monotony of the diet, its constipating effect, the absence of taste and its failure to satisfy their desire for sweets."[59] No wonder Pennington could tell his dieters that they could eat all they wanted – who would want to? Liquid protein diets were also popular. As early as 1966, *Chatelaine* published an article entitled "LP (Liquid Program) Diet" by Barbara Croft, which explained Dr Gold's liquid diet. Gold was "a fellow of both the Royal Canadian and the American Colleges of Physicians, associate physician at Montreal General Hospital, and consultant at Queen Mary Veterans' Hospital, Montreal," and his diet was extreme; for the first two weeks, the dieter could not eat more than 500 calories a day. After Croft's critical article, women wrote to *Chatelaine*. The magazine published three of their letters in which they praised the diet and were specific about how it had helped them lose weight.[60]

The 1970s saw the popularity of the Atkins diet. Robert Atkins argued that calories did not matter, as had Pennington and others before him. Indeed, there are historical precedents for his diet going back to the mid-nineteenth century. Atkins believed that if a dieter eliminated carbohydrates (including sugars), the body would burn off its fat. At the same time, the dieter could eat all the proteins and fats she or he wanted.[61] It sounded like the Pennington diet. A consumer reporter in the *Weekend Magazine* said of the Atkins diet: "Like pornography, it owed its basic appeal to its naughtiness." Another called the diet "quackery."[62] There was little evidence that the weight loss through the Atkins diet was permanent. But then, the same could be said for most diets. Nevertheless, many have followed the Atkins diet, right up to the present day.

Product Diets

Diets revolved around food, but some were part of product marketing that claimed to make dieting easier. Like the advertisements for food that used nutrients to sell products, advertisements also used low calories – low fat – to sell dieting products. For example, in 1924 an advertisement for Nujol salad dressing claimed it would offset the problem of fattening salad dressing. An advertisement for Bovril ensured readers that by using Bovril in their drinks (water or milk), they would receive the nourishment they needed, and they could cut back on fattening food without fear of endangering their health. The Quaker Oats Company advertised Tillson's low-calorie "*natural* bran" as a substitute for food with high calories. In 1932, an advertisement claimed that half a teaspoon of Kruschen Salts in a glass of hot water taken in the morning before breakfast for thirty days would "get rid of pounds of unwanted weight." Of course, the advertisement suggested that to improve the results of the salts, the consumer needed to eliminate "fatty" meat and pastry, and cut back on potatoes, butter, cream, and sugar. There was no way that someone following that food advice would not lose weight, with Kruschen Salts taking the credit. Standard Brands advertised the value of bread for "safe dieting." One of its advertisements was gendered, stating it would help women lose weight but promising men it would give them increased energy, as represented by visuals of two hockey players.[63] It all seemed so easy.

By the 1950s, other products were available. An advertisement in *Chatelaine* for Vita-Thin, an early liquid meal, featured Trudy Jensen of 18 Sunnylea Ave. E, Toronto, Ontario. In her endorsement, Jensen talked about the many people unable to keep to their diet "safely and enjoyably." She, too, had looked for a different way to diet. After searching drug stores "by the dozen," she had finally found Vita-Thin.[64] Liquid meals appealed to women. They were easy: wives or mothers could make breakfast and lunch, meals for their family, without having to make a different dieting meal for themselves except for Vita-Thin. Dinner would be a normal meal for everyone. First person narratives such as Jensen's were used to convince readers of the efficacy, honesty, and easiness of the method being touted.

While saccharin pills were designed for people with diabetes who had to eschew sugar, dieters found saccharin useful, as did people during the war when sugar was rationed. Its use, however, was such that Pensions and National Health warned Canadians that saccharin was "not a food [but] ... a chemical substance without nutritive properties. It should be used in moderation."[65] Similar products were increasingly available, and advertisements for them could be found in the medical journals and popular magazines. D-Zerta advertisements assured doctors that desserts using D-Zerta "CAN'T HARM your *low-carbohydrate patients!*" Significant ingredients in D-Zerta were "saccharin and cyclamate sodium." A news item about Sucaryl (a trade name for sodium cyclamate) noted that it did not have the bitter taste of saccharin and did not break down with heat. A prescription was not needed, but physicians were warned that no more than eight pills a day should be taken, and care was necessary if used by those with kidney problems, given the sodium salts in Sucaryl.[66] Nevertheless, in 1959, L.S. White claimed in the journal *Health* that cyclamates could be "safely consumed by both children and adults on low-calorie or low-sodium diets." But would patients use cyclamates as a substitute for sugar? Or would they use these sweeteners to increase their food intake, believing that with artificial sweeteners they were keeping to a diet, even when eating sweet food? And how safe were sweeteners? In 1969, cyclamates were banned in the United States, based on a study that linked cyclamates with cancer in rats. In October 1969, Ottawa created a staggered deadline to completely ban sodium cyclamates by 1 June 1970.[67] By 1978, Canada allowed certain uses for cyclamates, such as tabletop sweeteners, after more studies suggested the substance was not carcinogenic.[68]

Safety

The federal government's concern about cyclamates was a sign of the danger that diet products posed to dieters. But the safety of dieting had long been a worry. Mason's and Campbell's articles in the 1920s and 1930s had warned that not everyone was a good candidate for reducing: children, adolescents, and the elderly were not good candidates, and neither were those who were anaemic or "suffering from chronic infections." In 1933, E. Fowler, Department of Metabolism, Montreal General Hospital, warned that dieting was too often sponsored by "cultists and quacks." For example, promises such as "Take Off the Fat Where It Shows" were made for products containing thyroxin, which could result in the development of myocarditis. The "bran fad" was fine for constipation, but it could aggravate already existing problems such as ulcers in a weak digestive tract. As for the 18-day diet that allowed only 500 to 600 calories a day, Fowler thought it was too "drastic."

In his 1946 review, Cramer also rejected the cycle of fasting, seeing it as both impractical and dangerous. The cycle began with a five-day fast, followed by a limited and insufficient caloric total, followed by another fast.[69]

The 1950s were more detailed about safety. For the young healthy adult, a "radical" decrease in calories was possible. For older people, especially those with atherosclerosis, the recommendation was to decrease fat intake slowly and retain a reasonable caloric intake in order to lose only 3 to 4 pounds a month. Henry W. Brosin in a reprint from the *JAMA* cautioned colleagues about middle-aged citizens who were "adjusted to a set of habit patterns which are in a delicate state of balance ... [A]ny change may cause a serious upset leading to severe irritability or depression or, in rare cases, suicide."[70] In 1957, L. Bradley Pett from the Department of National Health and Welfare warned about the problem of yo-yo dieting, seeing it as "especially bad for coronary arteries." Elizabeth Chant Robertson, too, understood the inherent danger of many diets and warned her readers against semi-starvation diets accompanied by vitamin and mineral tablets. The assumption underlying dieting was that standalone nutrients would offset the nutritional lack in the diets. But, as Chant Robertson noted, pills did not contain all the necessary "food factors" found in nature.[71]

Dr Stillman was an American whose diet was very popular in Canada in the late 1960s and seemed to anticipate Atkins in many ways. He promoted a whole protein regime with low caloric intake. Designed to be a "quick weight loss diet," it was incredibly unbalanced in that no fruits or vegetables were included. It also "caused severe dehydration through a combination of low-carbohydrates and a copious intake of water, with no plan for rebalancing the salt lost through excessive urination."[72] Such diets may have helped weight loss, but the weight would not stay off once the dieter resumed a healthier way of eating, which the dieter would eventually have to do.

A winter 1977–78 article in *Health* looked at the American experience with liquid protein diets. For the healthy or overweight, these diets probably wouldn't cause harm if the dieter had one good meal a day. But the reality was alarming: in the United States, twenty-six people – some sources reported as high as forty – had died after being on a liquid protein diet for between two and eight months. Although there was no proven cause and effect relationship, the deaths did raise concern at the time,[73] especially since such products were easily available. Canadians, too, were at risk. Kaspars Dzeguze in *Maclean's* described the case of Janine MacDonald. She was washing dishes with her mother at her mother's home when she became lightheaded, somewhat faint, and lost consciousness. She had had a similar episode before. She was taken to Joseph Brant Hospital in Burlington, Ontario, where Dr Edward Kwong saw her in the emergency room and noted she was near starvation. Janine died. She was only twenty-five years old. The autopsy showed myocarditis (inflammation of the heart); at the inquest into her death, it was revealed that she had been near starvation, subsisting on a diet of tea, coffee, water, and eight tablespoons of liquid protein. As Dzeguze made clear, the consumer needed to be aware. Indeed, he informed his readers that Health and Welfare Canada had made a list of "diets not recommended," among them "Dr. Atkins' Diet Revolution, the Mayo Clinic Diet, the Calories Don't Count Diet and the Drinking Man's Diet," along with what Dzeguze considered women's favourite diets revolving around grapefruit and bananas.[74] Dieting was bad for the body, and it could cause malnutrition if needed nutrients were not being consumed.

Reducing had become a "fetish," and one that could result in "irritability, poor concentration, anxiety, depression, apathy, lability of mood, fatigue and social isolation." Dieting attracted charlatans and quacks, who offered a hopeful audience the ease of one diet over another. Crash diets, usually focused on low sugar content, at times resulted in "mental confusion, dizziness and fainting." Low-carbohydrate diets could affect the working of the kidneys and the liver.[75] Dieters often wanted to have a diet that was easy and up to date; when one diet didn't work for them, a new one could always be found. The exasperation of physicians was palpable. In 1975, Dr Charles H. Hollenberg, Sir John and Lady Eaton Professor of Medicine at the University of Toronto, commented that in medical practice, obesity led to frustration in both doctors and patients. At the Canadian Dietetic Association meeting in 1977, Dr Winick, professor of nutrition and pediatrics at Columbia University, was questioned about whether it might be best for some obese individuals not to lose weight. As noted in chapter two, he admitted that if the individual had normal blood pressure and normal glucose levels, "the obese person may be healthy."[76] This statement was extraordinary for the time. Of course, since it was the physician who kept track of whether aspects of the body became abnormal or not, it was questionable how many would allow patients who were obese to continue carrying their current weight without suggesting a diet.

Dieting as a way of controlling weight spanned the whole period from the 1920s to 1980. At the end of the 1970s, Dr Marliss, Division of Endocrinology, University of Toronto, queried why people seemed so attracted by fad diets. Like others, he was aware of the social pressures on people to be thin and recognized that dieting was not only the prerogative of the obese but also of the many others who saw themselves as overweight.[77] His analysis reflected a society in which the easy solution was the one wanted and advertisements had become a major source of information for people, even on health issues. The constant failure of so many dieting methods had taken people to the point that they would try anything.

Psychology

Dieters, physicians, and nutritionists were all frustrated by the difficulty of losing weight. Why did many dieters not understand the rules of nutrition? Why did they look to fad diets? Why could they not stay on diets? Why did they eat the way they did in the first place? Why did they eventually regain the weight they had lost and more? Something else was at work, and the rise of psychology at mid-century seemed to offer some insight. If a psychological problem was causing obesity, perhaps lessening that problem would also make dieting easier. On the other hand, if obesity was causing a psychological problem, losing weight might ameliorate the psychological trouble. Today we live in a time when the psychological often dominates. For example, behaviour therapy is a strong "adjunct" to both dieting and exercise. It includes "self-monitoring, stress management, stimulus control, problem-solving, contingency management, cognitive restructuring, and social support."[78] Psychological treatment for obesity came relatively late compared to dieting; as an adjunct to dieting, it strengthens control over the body through counselling, self-surveillance, and awareness of behaviour. All three were and are used in self-help groups.

Medical Approaches to Psychology

In common parlance, a psychological treatment of obesity in the early decades simply referred to the relationship between the patient and the physician, and the kind of influence the latter had over the former. If the patient's problem was weight, the doctor needed to find something of importance to that individual – health, being attractive, being able to play sports – to help modify the patient's eating habits and keep her or him on a reducing diet until weight had decreased. As noted, Mason gave the practitioner the responsibility to "reduce" the patient. Campbell, in his 1936 article "Obesity and Its Treatment," agreed and went further: if the patient didn't have a motive to lose weight, the doctor would be obliged to "invent" one. The patient's weight loss would be a success for the practitioner and the patient. In the 1947 *Manitoba Medical Review*, Dr A. Keenberg, too, suggested to his colleagues to look for a patient's motive to lose weight. For example, he explained that "most patients ... are women who worry about their appearance. Advantage should be taken of their vanity to make them eat for the benefit of their health."[79]

Psychological treatment seldom meant psychoanalysis in Canada because of the difficulty in finding therapists, the expense of paying for them, and the time such therapy took. Neither were there many trained psychiatrists in Canada. Only in 1942 did psychiatry become a recognized specialty in Canada with its own certification and exams. In 1951, a Canadian Psychiatric Association was formed, a sign of increasing interest in psychiatry within the profession and among medical students studying it.[80] But the association didn't really overcome the problems of getting patients to undergo psychoanalysis. Nevertheless, in the 1950s, more discussion of psychotherapy took place in the medical literature. As a treatment for obesity, psychotherapy was assumed to be useful to help the patient stay on a diet, that is, it could be an adjunct to dieting. Daniel Cappon, associate professor of psychiatry at the University of Toronto, however, saw psychotherapy as more than an adjunct, arguing that the problem of many obese individuals was that they did not have a realistic body image of themselves and weight loss would not occur until they did. Obese people also had to understand the psychosocial factors that had led to their obesity. If not, the result could be "dieting depression."[81]

More common than psychotherapy in the formal sense was physician awareness of the psychological stress of being obese. Placing an overweight person on a diet needed to be accompanied by "large doses of emotional support and analysis, guidance or reassurance." Even the use of weight charts and various laboratory tests could give the patient a sense of being supported. Group therapy was mentioned in the literature, as well as learning the "psychological factors" and "psychological conditioning" of overeating. In view of the role of food and eating in society, the Faculty of Food Sciences, University of Toronto, began a project in 1956, in part to get psychologists to create a test to predict a client's success with weight loss. While the results would be more of an aid for the psychologist or physician treating patients than for the patients themselves, the project suggested a desire to find a template for treatment, for example, a way to look at patient issues and determine what treatment would be best.[82]

While psychotherapy as an adjunct treatment to make dieting more effective continued to be mentioned in passing in the 1960s,[83] psychology was becoming a significant part of dieting treatment. Pharmaceutical advertisements often referred to the psychological issues accompanying obesity and acknowledged the need to address them. For example, a 1965 advertisement for the appetite suppressants Biphetamine and Ionamin noted that "for long-term success, the patient needs re-education in his eating habits and activity, plus removal of underlying psychological causes."[84] Both recommendations were difficult to manage, but it was easier for the advertisement to instruct physicians on what to do than for physicians to do it. Many who supported pharmaceutical diet aids believed that drugs would help the person lose weight; as result, the negative psychological aspects of obesity would disappear, that is, the psychological problems were not those of the person, but of obesity. While some physicians were hopeful, others were more pessimistic. For patients whose psychological problems caused their obesity, no weight loss would occur without psychological treatment to help them understand what underlay their obesity. The emphasis would be on talk therapy, that is, the psychological uplift of having a good practitioner who believed in the treatment.[85]

Could sympathetic care get to the root cause of obesity? A study of eighty-six general practitioners in the late 1950s and 1960s in Ontario and Nova Scotia revealed that few physicians had a good grasp of emotional or psychological problems based on any professional qualifications. Also, most of the physicians in the study admitted they disliked dealing with such issues, even though they were not able to escape doing so. Neither did they have a high opinion of psychiatry or psychology.[86] Perhaps these findings explain why experiments in electroshock as an avoidance treatment (as with sexual deviants) were tried by Dr Richard I. Hector at the Toronto General Hospital. Given his perception through tests that obese patients were "tense, insecure, demanding, suspicious and emotionally immature" as well as "self-sufficient, resourceful and creative," he might have hoped that electroshock would be a "quick fix." A more "gentle" therapy was hypnosis. In explaining how hypnosis worked, Dr F.W. Hanley described getting the patient to define his or her goal and motivation. Once that was done, the next step was teaching the patient to "enter a hypnotic trance," which took one or two sessions. At that point, the physician could begin making positive suggestions: for example, "the patient is told that he will derive a great deal of pleasure from eating ... and that when he swallows the first mouthful he will begin to feel satisfied and full." In describing the patient, Hanley used the male pronoun, but all his patients under hypnosis were women. Hypnosis continued to be used into the 1970s.[87] Electroshock and hypnosis were in the hands of the physician or the psychologist, not the patient. The treatments were tried, but they were not popular. Most general practitioners didn't have the equipment for electroshock or the time to give several appointments for hypnosis. Undergoing electroshock or even the easier hypnosis seemed radical to patients; even if they could find a doctor to administer the treatment, most Canadians didn't have the time or the financial resources to pay for such sessions.

In the 1970s, the psyche and its relationship to obesity was increasingly understood to be complex. As a result, there was little consensus on whether psychological/psychiatric problems were the cause or effect of obesity or both. Daniel Cappon even pointed out that some therapists were not competent to analyse patients. Even if the therapist was competent, a good analyst still needed the support of a patient willing to probe into the cause of his or her overeating. Indeed, Cappon estimated that the patient would have to spend at least eighteen months in weekly meetings with the therapist. Clearly, such treatment could not deal with the number of people who were obese. Neither could group therapy, which for Cappon meant no more than six people working together. No wonder Cappon, in his book, imagined a future in which he saw the possibility of electrodes being implanted into the brain to control appetite. In his fictional future, some centralized control centre would run the electrodes.[88]

Before an annual meeting of dietitians, Ottawa's Dr Kenneth Breitman argued that an obese individual being treated needed to have self-awareness, perhaps not a surprising conclusion from a psychologist. He claimed that obesity had no organic causes, so dieting would probably not be successful until the external stimuli for eating were addressed. Certainly, social pressures were present in the 1970s, with an emphasis on maintaining a slender or lean body.[89] While most physicians focused on organic causes of obesity, they had long used a psychological perspective: they "counselled" their patients on what to eat, how to perhaps cut down on their eating, queried their reasons for eating, provided support, and believed in the beneficial psychological effects of daily trips to the doctor as part of treatment. Optimistic physicians thought that the psychological problems of their patients who were obese were a consequence of the obesity.[90] Remove the obesity and the problems would lessen. This trajectory appeared straightforward and certainly easier than dealing with deeper psychological problems. But, given the difficulty people had in keeping weight off, the steps to psychological wellness were fraught. Whether the psychological issues were cause or consequence, dealing with someone who had psychological problems created complications for traditional obesity treatment.

The psychological method that garnered most attention in the 1970s was behaviour modification. Even in the 1960s, the popular literature often reflected the general medical approach of belief in mind over matter. In 1963, Sidney Katz explained behaviour therapy to his *Maclean's* readers, pointing out how it differed from psychotherapy, which concentrated on neuroses locked in the mind. Behaviour therapy did not worry about the origins of the neuroses, but sought to change the habits contributing to a problem so patients would feel better. *Chatelaine*, in its dieters' series, often included psychological tricks that people used to keep themselves on their diet. For example, one young woman asked her sister to mention the name of a certain young man whenever she felt tempted to eat too much, the assumption being that she would be more attractive to the young man if she kept to her diet and lost weight. The tricks were easy and a way to modify behaviour. Similarly, group therapy employing the addiction model for alcohol to food addicts provided another psychological treatment. Once again, the goal was a different behaviour. Dr Gordon Bell, who had long worked with alcoholics, turned his gaze to those who had trouble limiting what they ate. He saw his treatment as a combination of psychology and physical tests, both in an effort to find out why the person couldn't stop eating. Similar to treatment for alcoholics, group therapy was part of Bell's program with those who were obese.[91]

In the 1970s, according to one article, there were twenty different behaviour therapies available; they varied, depending on their target audience. Drs Barbara A. Davis and Daniel A.K. Roncari, both of the Toronto Western Hospital and the University of Toronto Department of Medicine, deconstructed the eating process into three stages: the stimuli for eating, the eating itself, and what happened following eating.

But since individuals were so variable, they found it was difficult to generalize. Nevertheless, behaviour therapy seemed to result in more weight loss compared to other "traditional measures of active therapy," although it hadn't been confirmed through long-term and follow-up studies.[92] Whatever its form, behaviour modification was popular, perhaps because the methods were easy to understand and gave control to those trying to lose weight. Many physicians believed behaviour therapy was the one treatment that worked. In 1972, *Chatelaine* informed its readers about one woman, Mrs G., a middle-aged housewife who, after years of dieting off and on, managed to lose weight and keep it off without pills, dieting, or exercising. She had joined a group run by Dr Ernest G. Poser, director of the behaviour therapy unit at Douglas Hospital in a Montreal suburb. Underlying Poser's experimental group was a list of behaviour instructions for the women in the group to follow in their everyday lives to keep them aware of what they were eating.[93] Behaviour modification theory assumed that people who ate more than others responded to external cues about food more than others, and the program was designed to help those who were overweight avoid the cues. By the end of the 1970s, however, some studies indicated that people who were obese didn't respond to cues any more than other people. Even so, many of the suggestions coming out of behaviour therapy seemed to help.[94]

Self-Help Groups

Many Canadians didn't find diets easy to follow, and they each had their own reasons why diets didn't work for them: fat ran in the family or all the food they ate turned into fat. One cartoon showed two fat women at a restaurant table, with one woman explaining to her friend that the first day of a diet was the hardest. Then she continued on to say: "By the second day I'm not on it any more."[95] What would make dieting easier for her and other Canadians? Some of the behaviour modification strategies were appreciated mostly by women and worked with the support of other women.

Group support became significant in the 1960s with the expansion of self-help groups. Taking Off Pounds Sensibly (TOPS) had existed in North America since 1948 and was very popular. Like many self-help groups, TOPS did not have strict rules or diets; instead, it offered members (mostly women) tricks to help them lose weight. For example, dieters could eat off a small plate, add a drop of yellow vegetable colouring to skim milk to make it look creamier, reduce oil in salad dressings, eat slowly, and keep snacks like raw carrots and celery always available. By 1967, TOPS had 265 chapters in Canada and 5,000 members. Weight Watchers entered Canada in 1967. Canadian Calorie Counters also started in 1967, beginning in Dundas, Ontario, as a centennial project; its members followed a diet informed by Canada's Food Guide. Overeaters Anonymous (OA), which began in Los Angeles in 1960 and based its program on that of Alcohol Anonymous, came to Canada as well.[96]

Self-help organizations seemed to offer people the support they needed. Because they didn't have medical professionals to lead the group, volunteer self-help groups had been overlooked in the obesity literature. Their expansion, however, meant that by the 1970s they could no longer be ignored. In addition, after decades of failure in treating obesity, many physicians were relieved to have a group to recommend to their patients. One of the earliest mentions of such an organization in the medical journals was a 1972 letter to the editor of the *CMAJ* by Dr Beverley A. Burgess, a physician from Stoney Creek, Ontario, who wrote:

> Weight Watchers offer a program that is a new way of life, not a diet. No calorie-counting is done although the program amounts to 950 to 1050 calories per day. Cardiovascular experts might argue with four to seven eggs per week and we hear a few complaints about so many fish meals per week but we also hear the incredible news that members are never hungry. They feel well on this diet and have none of the crankiness, anxiety or dizzy spells of previous low-calorie meals.[97]

Here was a program that seemed to work. It was a program that empowered those who were fat to take control without resorting to other aids, and it did so in a supportive and group environment. Weight Watchers offered a different kind of behaviour modification with some therapy.

Smaller groups also existed. New Image in Toronto, like others, used support, sympathy, and behaviour modification in order to assist its "clients" to lose weight. New Image was a profit-making "club" in that it would put you on a fasting diet for $295. The Centre for Human Metamorphosis was located in Toronto as well, and guaranteed weight loss of 4 to 5 kilograms. Of course, whether the weight could be kept off was another issue. Sarah Henry, who wrote about self-help groups for the *CMAJ* readership, lost weight at the centre, but it gradually came back. At least a dozen weight groups existed in Montreal for the francophone population, with names such as "Rayons d'espoir," "Vie nouvelle," "Maturité," and "Entregent." With so many groups forming, concerns about the business of weight loss emerged. L'Office de la protection du consommateur du Québec visited twenty-two health clinics/offices in the Montreal region and couldn't recommend any of them. As for obesity clinics, only one merited a recommendation.[98]

All the organizations were based on women helping women. Women attracted to self-help groups were often those who had tried everything to lose weight with little success. Of all the TOPS chapters in Canada, only one was a men's chapter. As one commentator noted, the lack of men was "not because there are not enough overweight men in Canada, but because they will not admit it." Few men would admit they were fat and needed help. Harvey L. joined OA. Self-described as a compulsive overeater, he reported that OA was helpful, and he had learned from the group that he wasn't alone. As he commented, he benefited from "the relief of knowing that it's not my fault I am the way I am."[99] Some groups accepted teenagers as members, and some Weight Watchers groups tried to cater to teenagers through a weekly group only for them.[100]

Of all the self-help organizations, Weight Watchers received the most press. In the journal *Health*, advertisements and articles connected to Weight Watchers were prolific. One of the first articles introduced Adelaide Daniels, the woman who played the starring role in Canadian Weight Watchers, having founded groups in all the provinces east of Manitoba with the exception of Quebec. She herself had lost 102 pounds in the mid-1960s, and so knew how being overweight felt and how difficult it was to lose weight. That she had managed to keep the weight off offered hope to those who were overweight. Weight Watchers' "Canadian Family Meal Plan" was easy to follow but nutritious, low in calories, and apparently appetizing. The organization insisted on a weekly visit from their members, where they found an accepting and challenging environment, and also offered a telephone helpline, group support, and motivation. Its literature, however, tended to focus on the negative aspect of being overweight, touting how "wonderful it is to rejoin the slim world."[101] It wasn't until the end of the 1970s that fatness activists emerged in Canada, and their groups were small compared to Weight Watchers and other groups.

Weight Watchers made a point of aligning itself with professionals in the health field, another reason why many practitioners were positive about it. One of its advertisements associated the organization with a

"Behavior Modification method ... designed ... by ... Dr. Richard B. Stuart." Stuart, a psychologist at the University of Michigan's School of Social Work, was a leader in the field beginning in the late 1960s. He educated his mostly women patients to understand how to control the eating stimuli, for example, removing tempting foods from the house. Unlike health experts, he didn't blame the individual for lack of willpower.[102] Weight Watchers also introduced a "Personal Exercise Plan," developed for them by "a leading cardiologist."[103]

So involved were Daniels and her husband in weight loss that they created Adelaide Daniels Enterprises, which endorsed the Counterweight "calorie-reduced" foods. In January 1977, Weight Watchers altered their menu plan to incorporate some formerly "forbidden foods." This new menu meant that their members could now eat unflavoured yogurt, soft cheeses such as Camembert and Brie, shellfish, and commercial diet foods, as well as cut down on the number of fish meals and add more legumes and vegetables. By 1981, an even newer menu plan was introduced, which included "wine, peanut butter, popcorn, and home-baked bread." Weight Watchers also created a national association, the Canadian Association of Organizations for Weight Watchers, to bring together and encourage commonality among the various weight organizations and as a holding organization for research data using Canadian statistics. Professionals involved in obesity studies and practice could join as well.[104]

The popularity of weight-loss organizations was testimony to their psychological appeal. But even with the help of these organizations, when the results of all the psychological treatments were assessed, there was little permanent success. Some practitioners, however, were not so quick to reject the psychological needs of patients. The whole issue of self-acceptance was important, especially for youth, and psychological support, whether through counselling or other means, was beneficial.[105] It would, at the very least, make the patient feel that he or she was not alone. That reassurance was what the group organizations offered best. The appeal of group organizations was many-sided: the regular attendance at meetings with friends; a sympathetic group with whom to discuss weight issues; the insight into how others managed to lose weight; and even the payments to maintain membership, which served to remind a member of her commitment. However, while some considered weight-loss groups to be positive in the short term, not everyone did. In a 1980 debate in the Saskatchewan Legislature, concern was expressed that some weight-loss groups were encouraging their clients to lose too much weight too quickly, harming their health.[106]

In many respects, psychological approaches to obesity treatment were a fallback position, something to try because exercise and dieting didn't work in a sustained way. While behaviour modification worked better than other approaches, even its success was not significant. Neither did many psychological methods address the psychological needs of patients after losing weight. For example, one woman described to readers of the *Globe and Mail* that after having lost weight, she was unable to recognize herself in a mirror among several women. It was only for a "split second," but it was as if she had lost her identity.[107]

Conclusion

Underlying dieting and its adjuncts was an acceptance of the power of the mind over the body. People had long tried to figure out what prodded them to eat the food they did. What was new was involving the insights of psychiatry and psychology. With respect to obesity, the treatment was rather watered down. Few people could afford psychotherapy and the time needed for it. There were not enough analysts in Canada, even if Canadians had the money or time to work with them. Psychology was more acceptable. The use of behaviour modification in the treatment of eating disorders appealed to those who wanted a practical response to their own weight problem and to practitioners who were searching for a treatment to offer their patients to help them lose weight. Success, however, was limited. Dieting, even with the light of psychology shining on it, didn't seem to lessen the dim prospect for people who wanted to lose weight and keep it off. Exercise wasn't an adjunct to dieting but rather a weak partner. Health experts were determined, however, that there were other methods that would offer a solution. Two methods are the focus for the next chapter. The first, the use of appetite suppressants, is, like psychology and psychiatry, an adjunct to dieting. The second, surgery, is an admission of dieting's failure.

5 "Dietary Drugland" and Surgery

"The very large number of new drugs currently on the market and introduced each year, and the extensive advertising which supports their sale has made it extremely difficult for the practising physician to learn and remember their characteristics."[1]

Appetite suppressants are adjuncts to dieting, and their use is a reaction to the failure of dieting on its own. They are also a reflection of the gradual proliferation and power of pharmaceutical companies. While the use of appetite suppressants to treat obesity is not central to the rise of pharmaceuticals, it is a model of how drugs were integrated into medicine and how pharmaceutical companies became partners with practitioners. The early histories of medicine didn't see a substantive role for pharmaceutical companies in how medicine was practised, but in the late twentieth century, histories of medical drugs became significant.[2] Within that literature, however, there are only a few histories of obesity drugs.[3] Yet, drugs have long been an aid to losing weight, either facilitating the ability to keep to a diet or altering the metabolic rate to permit energy to be expended more quickly. Doctors also saw pharmaceuticals as a means to suppress psychological problems – problems that could be the cause of obesity or the result of it – allowing doctors to treat patients who appeared and acted normally, that is, patients who could keep to a diet.

Similar to the use of appetite suppressant drugs, surgery came about because of the failure of dieting, even with appetite suppressants. As a treatment for obesity, surgery is relatively new and radical; yet, as part of the history of surgery in medicine, rather than the history of obesity, the surgical treatment of obesity is not as radical as it seems. Despite its increasing popularity in the present, surgery is not a treatment of choice for the majority of Canadians who are deemed obese. Over the period from 1920 to 1980, Canadian practitioners were very hesitant to propose surgery as a remedy for obesity.

Drugs

The history of drug treatment for obesity in Canada begins with the legislative framework for approving drugs and regulating pharmaceutical companies' marketing of their products. Over time, the number of products increased, but this chapter can only mention some of the drug types and relate their acceptance and, for some, their decline. Practitioners were concerned about both the efficacy and safety of obesity pharmaceuticals, as well as which drug to prescribe to a patient. In making that decision, the gender of the patient played a significant role in both the medical literature and, to a greater degree, in the advertisements for appetite suppressants.[4] The latter became a venue for the education of practitioners, albeit a biased one. The advertisements were sophisticated, appealing to their readers, providing an understanding of the actions of drugs, and attracting doctors by addressing their patients' problems. By doing so, a partnership between physicians and pharmaceutical companies was created.[5]

The Legislative Context

The pharmaceutical industry in Canada was, and is, a lucrative business. Sales of prescribed drugs increased by 1,141 per cent from 1960 to 1982. In the early twenty-first century, profits in the pharmaceutical industry were "double those in all manufacturing industries."[6] To keep practitioners up to date on what drugs are available, pharmaceutical companies advertise their drugs in medical journals. They also have salespersons visiting the doctors to sell their products. In the past, the salespersons were called "detail" men. For Canada, the ownership of the companies complicated the pharmaceutical landscape. A 1960 study determined that "of 40 companies responsible for producing 90% of all the ethical drugs sold in Canada only 4 were Canadian controlled."[7] The situation has not improved. Of the foreign-controlled companies, the American ones have been significant, in part, because of their proximity and numbers. Consequently, an understanding of the historical context of medicinal drugs in both the United States and Canada is necessary.

Two types of drugs, patent medicines and ethical medicines, were sold in nineteenth century America. Patent drugs were marketed with "expansive therapeutic claims" and did not reveal their ingredients, whereas ethical drugs were standardized products, generally marketed to pharmacies and later practitioners, and voluntarily followed the American Medical Association Code of Ethics.[8] Most ethical drugs in the first half of the twentieth century did not need a prescription; as a result, sales representatives focused their efforts on getting pharmacies to carry their products.[9]

In 1906, the US Pure Food and Drugs Act required drug content labels as a protection against dangerous ingredients, followed six years later by an amendment to stop the marketing of drugs that fraudulently claimed therapeutic benefits. In 1938, the US Federal Food, Drug, and Cosmetics Act allowed the Food and Drug Administration (FDA) to inspect pharmaceutical factories and to insist on proof of safety before marketing drugs. Ten years later, the US Supreme Court ruled "that the FDA had the power to define and restrict the sale of prescription-only drugs." In 1951, an amendment restricted drug products that would be unsafe without expert oversight; their sale was limited to physicians, veterinarians, or dentists. In 1962, a significant shift came with the Kefauver-Harris Drug Amendments that required drug companies to "demonstrate efficacy prior to new-drug approval," including a retrospective study of drugs introduced from 1938 onward. The 1962 amendments also placed the safety and efficacy of drugs under the jursidiction of the FDA. The FDA then insisted that companies get its approval for testing procedures "*before* proceeding with clinical studies of an investigational new drug."[10] The power of the US federal government to oversee drugs was strengthening.

The 1962 legislation also transferred oversight of prescription drug advertising to the FDA from the Federal Trade Commission.[11] For most of the first half of the century, advertising of ethical drugs had been limited, and publicity was achieved by persuading pharmacies to stock brand names. This was done through detail men and other means. Once prescription regulations were extended, the individual practitioner became the target of advertisements. Physicians in the United States, however, were increasingly antagonistic towards drug companies advertising to the public, seeing it as an infringement on their control over their patients. As a result, advertisements for brand drugs began to emphasize the doctor-patient relationship to keep doctors on side.[12] Also to appease doctors, the companies increased their advertisements in the medical journals, thus providing revenue needed to maintain the journals. For example, between 1949 and 1953, advertising revenue for the *Journal of the American Medical Association* (*JAMA*) increased 50 per cent.[13] From 1962, advertisements directed to the medical profession had to have a summary of drug side effects, contraindications, warnings, and the benefits and risks of the drug. All of the advertising, in whatever form, was part of educating physicians, and by doing so encouraged them to use brand name drugs. Between 1951 and 1961 alone, 4,562 new prescription drugs came on the market, and with those drugs came competition.[14] Despite the growing influence of the FDA, the alliance between the drug industries and the medical profession in the 1960s often undermined the FDA's effectiveness.[15]

The Canadian legislative context reveals some parallels with developments in the United Sates. In Canada, laws were introduced in the late nineteenth century to prevent adulterated food and drugs from reaching the market.[16] In 1920, the Food and Drugs Act replaced the adulteration legislation and empowered, through the federal minister, inspectors to test food samples to make sure they conformed to quality standards. False labelling was also a focus. Not until 1927, however, were drugs included in the act, although the legislation governed patent medicine.[17] In 1934, an amendment to the Food and Drugs Act prohibited the sale of products "represented by label or advertisement to the general public as a treatment for any of the conditions specified in Schedule A of the Act." Obesity was listed. Prior to 1939, the sale of drugs in Canada had been controlled by provincial pharmacy legislation. In 1939, however, the federal government became an active participant when the Food and Drugs Act established the authority to regulate sales of drugs that could be harmful to health. In 1941, the sale of "amphetamine, benzedrine ... Ortho-dinitrophenol ... Thyroid," and thyroxin as an ingredient to anyone except a licensed physician or dentist was prohibited.[18] All these drugs were used in obesity treatment.

In 1942, a Drug Advisory Committee was created to advise the Department of Pensions and National Health on drugs. It later became the Canadian Drug Advisory Committee and was composed of various stakeholders: the medical profession, pharmacists (both academic and practising), and pharmaceutical companies. It was a powerful committee since it determined which drugs would go into Schedule F (prescription drugs). In 1951, regulations over the sale of new drugs required that "a new drug submission must be filled prior to marketing the drug to support the safety of the drug." In the early 1960s, drug companies had to submit efficacy data before being allowed to market products, a requirement designed in response to the tragic consequences of the use of thalidomide. Yet, the regulation was not applied retroactively to drugs that were already on the market, and companies were not even obliged to report to Canadian authorities adverse reactions of a drug outside Canada or those documented with the parent company. In the 1970s, there was a "review of protocols for clinical trials ... and the development of guidelines for New Drug Submissions." The review found problems in some of the protocols, such as a weakness concerning patient consent, for which the Health Protection Branch had not set standards.[19]

From 1966 to the early 1970s, drug marketing was guided by the principles and marketing practice code of the Pharmaceutical Manufacturers Association of Canada (PMAC), a voluntary organization of pharmaceutical companies. Due to government concern about marketing practices, federal and provincial ministers wanted more regulation over the industry. The industry's response was to create the Pharmaceutical Advertising Advisory Board (PAAB) in 1975, with representatives from the generic drug sector, the patented (having a patent) drug industry, physicians, pharmacists, and the Health Protection Branch. But neither the code nor any PAAB decision was binding, and the PAAB remained a voluntary body. Until the 1990s, the only PAAB code covering images or other nontextual content of advertisements was that companies not imitate one another's advertisements.[20] As in the United States, drug advertisements in Canadian medical journals helped the publications stay afloat. Drug companies also lobbied to connect with the public. While they were not allowed to advertise directly to the public, some placed articles about specific drugs (using ghostwriters) in magazines such as *Canadian Home Journal* and *Chatelaine*.[21]

Types of Drugs

At the turn of the twentieth century, the use of pharmaceuticals for obesity was based on organotherapy (use of endocrine organs or extracts from them). Thyroid was the organ that was most used.[22] One of the more popular products in the 1920s was Marmola tablets, with dried thyroid as an ingredient. A Marmola advertisement in *The Chatelaine* told readers that losing weight was easy: Marmola was able to "increase the factor which turns food into fuel and energy rather than into fat." All that was needed was to take four tablets a day – exercise or dieting was not required. Referring to the belief in endocrine obesity, another advertisement reminded Canadians that losing weight through dieting wouldn't work because science had determined that the problem of weight was due to a "deficient gland," but Marmola could help "combat" it.[23]

In the 1929 *Canadian Medical Association Journal* (*CMAJ*), an advertisement for Iodesin from the Anglo-French Drug Company listed among Iodesin's contents the following: hepatic extract, pituitary extract, orchitic extract, ovarian extract, thyroid (deprived of lipoids – fat-like substances), and suprarenal extract. Iodesin (or Iodobesin as it was also called) with its cocktail of extracts was one of the main drugs on the market that focused on endocrine obesity.[24] The assumption was that using thyroid extract would increase the basal metabolism rate (BMR), no matter whether the rate was abnormal or not, causing a rise in energy expenditure.[25] G. Harvey Agnew, assistant physician at Toronto Western Hospital, didn't go that far, but was optimistic that people who were obese and had a "minus" BMR would benefit from the extract. Others feared an "uncontrolled employment of thyroid extract" for weight-loss purposes. What "uncontrolled" meant was unclear, but it most likely referred to the drug's application beyond endogenous obesity,[26] that is, the use of the extract to increase the BMR even if it was normal.

In the 1930s, practitioners began to recognize that thyroid treatment was not a straightforward solution for obesity – low metabolic rates were not all thyroid in origin, and not all patients with hypothyroidism (an underactive thyroid) were obese. Despite challenges to the use of thyroid extract for obesity treatment, the practice continued. For example, the 1938 edition of *The Principles and Practice of Medicine* approved thyroid use and mentioned the benefits for menopausal women as well as for those with a low BMR. In his 1936 review of obesity and treatment, Walter R. Campbell, Toronto General Hospital, argued against the condemnation of thyroid use, and blamed its problems on "the laity" through their purchase of patent medicines, many of which contained thyroid, such as the Marmola tablets. In the hands of professionals, however, and with "safeguards," he insisted, thyroid's potential had not been disproved.[27] Whether its potential had been proven was left unsaid.

In the 1940s and 1950s, as practitioners were focusing more on the causes of obesity outside the body – not enough exercise, eating too much – they seldom discussed thyroid extract as a treatment. It didn't mean, however, that they were not prescribing drugs with thyroid extract. Even new drugs in the 1940s used thyroid extracts. For example, Clarkotabs had thyroid powder along with amphetamine, as did Probese. Nevertheless, L. Bradley Pett, Department of National Health and Welfare, rejected the endocrine origin of obesity except for a small number of people and argued that "indiscriminate use of thyroid preparations often suppressed what little function there was, and led to real obesity," hardly a message physicians using thyroid extracts wanted to hear. That experts like Pett and others felt the need to keep reminding their colleagues about the lack of substance behind the thyroid origin of obesity revealed how tenacious the belief was.[28]

As a result of the debates over the origin of obesity, the market was becoming competitive, and older drugs had to compete with newer ones. In the 1940s, amphetamine entered the Canadian field and became a major drug for obesity treatment. One of its brands, Dexedrine, took the opportunity in advertisements to critique the weaknesses of thyroid-based drugs as a way of losing weight.[29]

Amphetamine was synthesized late in the nineteenth century and used in the decongestant Benzedrine (benzedrine sulphate) in the 1930s. It was also used for weight loss, and Canadian physicians would have been aware of the latter use since some of the major medical texts recognized its application.[30] During World War II, amphetamines were also pressed into service by the military in Germany, Britain, and the United States to overcome sleep deprivation (although the practice did not last in Germany because of amphetamine's addictive characteristic). On the home front, Canadian officials acknowledged that many drug users in British Columbia were getting Benzedrine inhalers and using the amphetamine in them with morphine to create a "twist on the cocaine-opiate 'speedball.'"[31]

In 1946, two Edmonton physicians, Leonora Hawirko and P.H. Sprague, described how they came to use amphetamine for obesity treatment. A "rather obese" patient had been given benzedrine for narcolepsy and found that she had lost 5 pounds in ten days, something she had never been able to do. To compare drugs, Hawirko and Sprague proceeded to give benzedrine sulphate as an "appetite depressing drug" to some patients, but most were given d-amphetamine. Of the original 162 patients (mostly women), 72 remained on the diet and treatment for more than two months, and it was only those 72 who were reported on. One woman in the study was only 9 pounds overweight. Over the life of the treatment, care was taken to ensure vitamin deficiency did not occur from the low caloric diet that the patients were on. As well, an intravenous of salyrgan, "an aqueous solution containing about .37 mg ... of metallic mercury, to act as a diuretic," was given to a minority of the patients who were very obese to offset any kidney problems. Hawirko and Sprague were optimistic about the use of salyrgan as an "adjunct" to obesity treatment since it eliminated water retention and thus encouraged loss of weight. When weight loss reached a plateau, they increased the amount of amphetamine given to the patients. The average weight loss of those in the study was about 5.5 pounds per month; of those individuals who stayed the course for over two months, six were failures in that they lost less than 20 per cent of the pounds they were overweight. Five of the patients became pregnant. The physicians went to the expert literature to support their results: d-amphetamine reduced appetite by "diminishing hunger contractions," stimulated the urge to be active, and lessened water retention. Turning to the findings of other studies on benzedrine, they found that the drug was reported to result in much more weight loss than "diet alone, with or without thyroid," and could improve "the state of mind," and thus reduce the desire to eat as a result of depression or "dissatisfaction with life." Hawirko and Sprague concluded, however, that d-amphetamine had all the advantages of benzedrine without its side effects of "insomnia, irritability, edginess and tenseness." They also warned readers that medical supervision was needed when using such drugs, since patients could get carried away and overuse them.[32]

Hawirko and Sprague's article is an entry into obesity treatment of the time. The article presented a scientific experiment conducted with the participation of 162 obese individuals. The authors were clear about what they wanted to do: find out how well d-amphetamine worked as an appetite suppressant, suggesting that this was a question that would interest their readers. Their description stressed the care taken when placing people on a significant diet – the body was vulnerable without access to its normal amount of food and nutrients. The study also showed a willingness to experiment on the individual – when a patient stopped losing weight, the physicians increased the drug dosage. Fewer than half of the original people in the study stayed with the treatment. It didn't seem to matter that they were given a drug; they could not stay on either the drug or the diet. Thus, the dropout rate was high, which constituted a warning to other physicians not to expect too much. When the weight loss was examined, it really wasn't that much – for the whole group an average of 5.5 pounds per month. Of the seventy-two subjects who stayed with the study, the physicians considered that six were failures because they didn't lose enough poundage. Seeing their weight loss as a failure suggested that the goal was more than just weight loss, but rather achieving a specific weight loss. While weight loss was the measurement of success, so was pregnancy for women. Obesity could weaken the ability to conceive; for women, their ability to conceive in the world of 1940s Canada was a reflection of their womanhood and their citizenship. The mention of the woman who was overweight by 9 pounds calls into question the definition of obesity. We have already seen that obesity's measurement was quite varied. Last, the physicians essentially were endorsing one particular product over another one.

Just as amphetamines lessened the use of thyroid, new drugs on the market tried to weaken the dominance of amphetamines. Challenges to amphetamines encouraged some of the companies producing amphetamines to expand their flexibility and to increase emphasis on safety, which was necessary as amphetamines were getting publicity as addictive street drugs.[33] By the late 1950s, Dexedrine Spansule Capsules came out with a new lower-strength version of the drug; physicians could now prescribe the new 5 mg capsules, or keep to the 10 or 15 mg ones.[34] If physicians were concerned about the effects of the amphetamine-based drugs, they now had a range of strengths from which to choose.

Dexedrine continued to be available in the 1960s and was advertised, not only for appetite control, but also for depression, alcoholism, and narcolepsy. Its advertisements assured physicians that the drug was "widely accepted" and "superbly documented." Dexedrine not only curbed the appetite but also "encourage[d] mental and physical activity," a comment on the life of the obese before dieting. By 1962, the advertisements could assure their readers that Canadian physicians had had over fifteen years of experience with the product.[35]

New drugs were always being introduced by various brands. In 1957, Dr Antonio Martel from Quebec City wrote an article on Preludin (phenmetrazine) in which he criticized the side effects – "tachycardia [rapid heart rate], nervousness, insomnia, hyptertension, dizziness, nausea and perspiration" – of many of the amphetamine-based drugs used as appetite suppressants. He supported what he saw as a much better product, which had been available for about a year. He had undertaken a study of 118 patients to assess Preludin. According to him, many of his patients were happy with it; it had allowed them to develop an acceptance of their diet and, after a bit of time, continue the diet without the drug. He admitted that amphetamine derivatives suppressed appetite "and created a state of satiety in the course of the meal." But with Preludin, he wrote, "we have observed that patients lose their appetite even before starting the meal." He acknowledged that Preludin did not seem to be very effective in women after menopause. However, he did so in a way that didn't blame the drug but rather women's bodies or the treatment of them with estrogens, which he told colleagues would undermine any kind of therapy for obesity.[36] Indeed, Martel's article reads like a paid endorsement for Preludin. Increasingly, Preludin advertisements referred to "older anorexiants," placing Preludin into a new generation of "modern" treatments, as did Martel's article and others endorsing the drug.[37] Newer variations on phenmetrazine kept being developed. For example, a 14 March 1964 advertisement in the *CMAJ* told physicians: "Prelutal, by adding the proven tranquilizing action of promazine to the predictable anorexiant effect of Preludin, assures maximum patient cooperation."[38]

One of the newer obesity treatments in the 1960s, and among the most controversial, was the use of human chorionic gonadotropin (HCG), a hormone "secreted by the placenta, or afterbirth." According to Lawrence Galton in his "Here's Health" column in *Chatelaine*, HCG was safe and worked through daily injections. However, Galton was not always to be trusted, since he was often employed as a ghost writer for pharmaceutical companies.[39] A year later, another article in *Chatelaine* described a treatment that used HCG injections for twenty-three to forty days along with a 500-calorie diet, which had been pioneered by Dr Albert T.W. Simeons, a British endocrinologist working in a Rome hospital. The theory behind HCG was that three types of fat were found in the body: the first type was necessary for the functioning of the organs; a second was fat used for energy and "emergency food"; and the third was "locked-in" fat, which the body, for whatever reason, seemed unable to lose. HCG "release[d]" the latter fat so that eating a limited calorie diet could then eliminate it. The article noted, however, that the American Medical Association had no evidence that HCG worked as an obesity treatment. Another English physician also noted that saline solution worked as well as HCG for his patients, and posited that it was the 500-calorie diet that caused weight loss, not the HCG.[40]

The use of HCG continued to be contested, and Canadian physicians in general did not approve of it. Readers of the *Canadian Family Physician* in 1975 were informed that the Royal College of Physicians and Surgeons of Canada had looked into the practice of four physicians who together had billed the Ontario Health Insurance Plan (OHIP) for $400,000 in one year. Their practice was to provide HCG in small daily doses to their patients. The result of the investigation was that "the Ontario Medical Association and OHIP ruled that in future physicians may not charge OHIP for any injection used to treat obesity. The ruling also stipulated that physicians may not treat a patient for obesity more than once every two weeks." HCG had been a moneymaker for physicians, but its popularity was at an end. Ayerst Laboratories, which marketed HCG under the name APL in Canada, cut back on the amount they were bringing into the country; apparently its researchers confirmed that it wasn't useful for obesity treatment.[41]

Obesity drugs were becoming more specialized, and brands used this specialization to advertise their new drugs. For example, New Tenuate (diethlproprion), according to its own publicity, was designed for the "cardiac/hypertensive obese." There were also drugs for the obese diabetic, or for "faulty fat metabolism."[42] Combinations of drugs continued to appear in different products. One such was Bamadex (meprobamate with d-amphetamine sulphate). According to its advertisement, the d-amphetamine limited the appetite and improved the mood of the individual, while the meprobamate "ease[d] the tension of dieting." Desbutal Gradumet combined Desoxyn (methamphetamine hydrochloride, an appetite suppressant and mood enhancer) with Nembutal (a barbituate and hypnotic for calming). Among others were Eskatrol Spansule (dextroamphetamine sulphate and prochlorperazine, an antipsychotic), Ambar #2 Extentabs (methamphetamine hydrochloride and phenobarbital), and Probesil (phenmetrazine and amobarbital).[43] There seemed to be an endless combination of drugs, which led to "new" drugs that didn't really differ much from others already on the market. Given the numerous brands, it was difficult for physicians to keep track of them.

Treatment Considerations

The increasing popularity of pharmaceuticals for weight loss was based on dieting and the difficulty people had in staying on a diet. While practitioners attempted to assess the value of drugs for treating obesity, consensus about a drug's effectiveness was not always reached. The debate over endocrine obesity in the 1940s resulted in the use of thyroid extract. Some practitioners worried that increasing the BMR artificially could harm those whose bodies were already stressed by their weight, while others supported its use, even to treat obesity that wasn't endocrine in origin.[44] As the number of drugs in the pharmaceutical market increased, efficacy became more difficult to determine.

The 1960s opened with W. Harding le Riche, professor of public health at the School of Hygiene, University of Toronto, belittling the dependence on drugs for treating obesity. He noted that most drugs sooner or later ceased to curb the patient's overeating, and the physician needed to change medication over time. The drugs alone could not do the work; it was more important to put the individual on a low-calorie diet.[45] In 1961, Wilfred Leith of the Royal Victoria Hospital, Montreal, accepted that appetite suppressants such as amphetamine, phenmetrazine hydrocholoride, and "bulk substitutes" were "of some value," a rather lukewarm endorsement. Edmonton's Dr D.R. Wilson wrote "Drugs for Obesity," an article commissioned by the editorial subcommittee of the Canadian Medical Association Committee on Pharmacy. In the article, he recognized the usefulness of the "appetite-depressing" drugs, especially when the dieter's weight had reached a plateau. He concluded, however, that all the amphetamine-based products were basically the same, and phenmetrazine (Preludin) was "pharmacologically similar to the amphetamines" and didn't seem any better. As for the sedatives and tranquilizers often added to the appetite-suppressing drug, he didn't see they had any place in weight loss but rather were there to counteract the amphetamines being used.[46] His survey was hardly a rousing support of drug therapy. The involved process of deciding "what dosage should be given" and determining safety in the face of side effects added to his concerns about giving patients drugs.[47]

Most of the advertisements in the medical journals addressing obesity were for pharmaceutical aids to dieting. The specifics of the dieting didn't matter, as long as it was low calorie. It was the drug that mattered. Indeed, the advertisements tended to leave readers thinking that losing weight was going to be straightforward. Probese advertisements in the 1950s used a male silhouette in four figures going from the right side of the page to the left. On the right, the figure had an obese profile; the profile of the other figures gradually became thinner until the last one at the end showed a very long-legged male climbing up a stylized ladder.[48] One could interpret the last figure as an action silhouette, climbing for success. A 1963 advertisement for Dexedrine showed a friendly doctor and a well-dressed, overweight woman patient sharing a laugh together. The advertisement was subdued, and the woman was treated like any other patient who had legitimate needs – needs that would be met by the "encouragement" of her physician and the "help" of Dexedrine. Dexedrine would not only control her appetite for the full day, but would also overcome the "lethargy" that was a problem with many overweight patients. By doing so, the drug would give the woman her life back.[49] Indeed, many advertisements employed before and after images, that is, pictures taken before dieting and after dieting, when weight had been lost with pharmaceutical help.[50] The difficulty of dieting wasn't conceded in these advertisements.

Drug efficacy, in part, was based on trust. For example, some drugs advertisements suggested it was best if a person could lose weight with diet alone. Two reasons for the apparent willingness to play down the drug's value come to mind. First, seeming to advocate for the individual rather than the drug company put an altruistic face on a company's advice with little harm to sales – the odds of an individual keeping to a diet were slim (so to speak), so it was quite likely the drug would be tried as an adjunct. Second, such references were a response to the criticisms emerging about the side effects of specific types of diet aids, particularly amphetamine-based ones. By endorsing diet only, pharmaceutical companies appeared responsible to practitioners. After all, it was the practitioner who decided what drug was best for a patient – the practitioner was the conduit between the drug (product) and the consumer. An advertisement for Biphetamine-T, however, took a different tack. It advocated a number of different treatments going on at the same time: exercise, diet education, learning about calories, counselling, and "adjunctive medication" such as anorextic agents.[51] Through such advertisements, companies were beginning to admit the limitations of their products, for example, the period for which pharmaceuticals could actually work.[52]

In the late 1960s and the early 1970s, the acceptance of drug therapy for any number of medical problems, including obesity, continued to expand, but the concern about recreational drugs did create some problems. In the 5 December 1970 issue of the *CMAJ*, an advertisement for Dexedrine and Dexamyl, in the form of a letter, noted:

> In recent months, the indiscriminate use of amphetamines, barbiturates and other medically useful drugs has been the subject of numerous articles in the medical literature and the popular press. Most of these reports have dealt with the non-medical misuse of drugs, and the emphasis has often been sensational. As pioneers in the development of amphetamine drug products for medical use, we at SK&F [Smith Kline & French] feel

this is a good time to restate both the advantages and limitations of "Dexedrine" and "Dexamyl" in the area of their widest medical usefulness – the treatment of obesity.

The statement attempts to ward off criticism of the medical use of amphetamines resulting from the reaction against the recreational use of drugs. The advertisement went on to explain that dextroamphetamine sulphate reduced "hunger and lethargy" brought on by lowering the caloric intake when dieting. In an effort to show it was the patient who mattered and not the drug sale, the advertisement acknowledged that "many patients can restrict their caloric intake without the help of anorectic medication, and this should be encouraged." As the SK&F letter implied, at most the appetite suppressant was a crutch, and just as a crutch could not cure a broken leg, medication could not "cure" obesity. Neither could the failures of dieting be blamed on the medication; too many patients looked for "easy cures" through medication, and they were unwilling to give up pleasurable activities, like overeating.[53]

The claims of drug companies continued to decline over time, as if companies were trying to avoid exaggerating what their products could deliver. Ponderal (fenfluramine hydrochloride) advertisements emphasized that drugs were only "short-term" aids to help those who were obese lose weight through dieting. Pre-Sate (chlorphentermine hydrochloride) advertisements focused on what overweight persons needed to do. Losing weight depended on a "program," not just taking a pill. Individuals needed to determine why they ate the way they did and figure out how to stop; set themselves realistic goals, which meant not going on "crash diets"; educate themselves about food and proper diet; become more active; and learn to eat less (and the right food) and do so on a permanent basis.[54] Despite these qualifications expressed by the drug companies and the general assessment that drugs were only helpful over a short time,[55] anti-obesity drugs continued to thrive.

Part of efficacy is safety. Only rarely did the popular press in the 1920s warn Canadians about safety concerns with the use of drugs for obesity. In the 1930s, however, concern was expressed, perhaps because of the drugs being used. The Metropolitan Life Insurance Company warned Canadians that they needed to be very careful in taking "reducing" concoctions and to see a doctor first to assure the safety of taking any drug. Dr John W.S. McCullough, through his writings in *Chatelaine*, also warned readers that drugs of any kind for losing weight needed to be overseen by a physician. The advice to be careful could also apply to physicians who were not always able to keep up with new drugs on the market, both for obesity or otherwise.[56]

The medical journals, however, did try to keep practitioners up to date. A reprint in the 1935 *CMAJ* informed readers about dinitrophenol, an organic compound. "When taken in adequate dosage, the increased metabolic activity burns extra fat and carbohydrate without appreciably affecting the protein." However, the efficacy of its use was debated. L.-Henry Gariépy put forward in a review that dinitrophenol wasn't as good as thyroid extract. There was also a sense that dinitrophenol was dangerous and should be accessible only by prescription and only if and when other weight-loss methods had failed. The 1938 edition of *The Principles and Practice of Medicine* agreed about the dangers of dinitrophenal – it increased the metabolism too much. The edition noted, however, that there was a related drug, dinitrocresol, which "may" be less problematic. And "may" was the operative word. Four years before, the *CMAJ* had reviewed a British article on obesity and told readers that the author considered Dekrysil (dinitro-o-cresol) dangerous, with poisonous consequences when given in doses slightly above their therapeutic value.[57]

Early in the 1940s, there was a suggestion in the medical literature that patients wanted a quick fix, a pill that represented medical care, rather than taking responsibility to eat less and exercise more. In a 1948 article in *Maclean's*, journalist and author Pierre Berton warned Canadians about the danger of drugs by telling the story of a Winnipeg housewife who had asked her physician for thyroid tablets to help her lose weight. The pills interfered with her sleep, and thus she was given sleeping pills. As a result, she began to "hoard" pills that she managed to get from a number of physicians and became addicted. No wonder companies such as the Metropolitan Life Insurance Company continued to warn Canadians not to take "reducing drugs" without a doctor's advice.[58]

Many Canadians were taking pills for health problems. Pills were a $30 million per year big business in Canada,[59] and diet pills were part of the business. Canadians learned about diet pills from their friends and popular literature; the information and the desire to be slim encouraged many to ask their physicians for prescriptions, an easy fix that became increasingly popular for both patient and physician. But there were warnings. In 1951, the Metropolitan Life Insurance Company told

Chatelaine readers about the danger of diet pills, pointing to the possibility of damaging the heart's ability to work efficiently and "other serious conditions." With the last phrase, the warning left the reader to imagine the worst.[60] Sidney Katz in *Maclean's* was very clear: drugs were not a good diet method and could be fatal. Only a doctor could and should prescribe drugs, and then only to help a person get started on a diet. *Chatelaine*, however, in an article on Preludin, seemed to be endorsing it as a safe way to control weight gain in pregnant women. *Canadian Home Journal* also appeared to endorse Preludin in one of its articles, and Levenor in another. All three articles were authored by Galton, the pharmaceutical ghostwriter.[61] Whom could Canadians trust?

Over time, pharmaceutical advertisements provided more detail about their products. Listing side effects and warnings in small print became much more elaborate in the 1960s because research on the side effects of various drugs such as amphetamines was increasingly being published in the medical journals. Also, American legislation demanded such information in drug advertisements; given that many of the companies selling drugs in Canada were American, the lists and warnings became the norm. Criticism of amphetamines persisted as an advertising tactic for non-amphetamine drugs.[62] In 1962, one article listed potential side effects of amphetamine as "restlessness, excitement, depression, irritability, exhaustion, headache, dizziness, halitosis, dryness of mouth, burning of the throat, heartburn, nausea, vomiting ... diarrhea"; another article noted psychosis. Some countries were even contemplating prohibiting prescriptions for amphetamines.[63]

Side effects were more detailed when the advertisement was for a pharmaceutical product that addressed obesity or excess weight in someone who was in a vulnerable category. At that point, the details could read like a medical article.[64] Some advertisements were cleverly designed and placed the list of potential side effects on a page adjoining the main advertisement. Others, like those for Prelutal (phenmetrazine hydrochloride), blamed the patient for experiencing side effects, referring to the "problem obese" who did not seem to respond to "routine therapy" in a satisfactory way.[65] Of course, the side effects and warnings could only be based on the knowledge at hand and made public. Such warnings, however, put doctors on notice that their patients must use the drugs with responsibility and that they, as physicians, needed to be aware of their patients' general health and not just their obesity. These warnings protected manufacturers from any liability if the drugs were used by contraindicated patients and made the detailed advertisements seem open and honest.

As for the popular press, it didn't make much mention of drug treatment, in part because the drug companies couldn't advertise in those publications. In a September 1960 issue of *Maclean's*, Sidney Katz interviewed Dr Gordon Bell, a drug authority who was concerned about the number of drugs people were consuming when the effect of their use was not always known. Bell was so worried about amphetamine use that he put himself on Dexedrine to see what the side effects were. He was energized by it, but when he stopped after only ten days, he seemed to experience withdrawal symptoms – lethargy, depression, and impaired mental capabilities. His question was, what happens to a patient who takes the drug for months? Doctors didn't always understand the addictive aspects of new drugs coming onto the market,[66] or even of the old ones.

In December 1971, the Canadian Medical Association (CMA) queried the Food and Drug Directorate about why two anorexiants, diethylpropion and methylphenidate, had not been placed into Schedule G (which was concerned "with the abuse or misuse of other stimulants") of the Food and Drugs Act along with phenmetrazine (used in Preludin and Probese) and phendimetrazine. In a statement in the January 1972 issue of the *CMAJ*, Dr A.B. Morrison, assistant deputy minister, Food and Drugs, replied by saying how pleased he was that the CMA approved of the action against phenmetrazine and phendimetrazine. While at this point the same action was not directed at the two drugs the CMA had mentioned, it might very well have to occur.[67] In the 20 May 1972 issue of the *CMAJ*, under Special Report, Dr D.A. Geekie, CMA director of communication, announced: "[A]s of September 1 the use of amphetamines, phenmetrazine and phendimentrazine as anorectics for weight reduction purposes will be prohibited."[68] It was one of the few notable incidences of the Canadian government actually restricting drugs that had already been on the market.[69]

But the federal government was not always able to protect Canadians. A new drug product, Pondimin (fenfluramine hydrochloride), was introduced as a "new non-stimulating" treatment. Yet, in the 1972 *Canadian Family Physician*, Anne B. Kenshole warned that fenfluramine didn't have a track record so its efficacy and safety could not be assumed. She was right. In the 1990s, a scandal in the United States emerged over fenfluramine – popularly called Fen-Phen, a combination of fenfluramine with phentermine – due to accusations that it caused heart valve disease, pulmonary hypertension, and cardiac fibrosis effects. Pondimin was eventually taken off the market.[70] In 1997, the two drugs were still registered in Canada, but with the Therapeutic Products Directorate in Canada advising doctors not to put the two together. Yet the Directorate knew of physicians who provided both drugs in combination.[71]

The world of drugs was a quagmire for doctors, but more so for patients. Sometimes individuals who asked for treatment for obesity were unclear what the doctor was prescribing. In the December 1973 issue of *Chatelaine*, Sheila Kieran, in an exposé of three diet physicians, told readers about her experience of going to Dr X, who explained to her that the body could only burn fat in the bloodstream chemically, not in the tissues of the body. During weight loss, there was the actual burning of the fat, but also the "mobilization and transportation of fat." The latter was the most significant, according to the physician, since it allowed him to be able to transport fat from various parts of the body to others. Kieran reflected that the idea that anyone could move fat from different parts of the body would "be grimly amusing to the thousands of women who, while dieting, watch their faces melt into hard lines while their spare tire of flabby arms seem cemented into place." To keep his pill working, the physician assured Kieran that if she went off the diet, it would stop its effect for three to five days, and weight gain would occur, a concept Kieran found intriguing: a pill that punished! That the physician was a charlatan was confirmed by an independent lab assessment of Dr X's "medicine." Nor was Dr X the only one whose practice seemed problematic. Dr Y had a reputation among his colleagues for following questionable practices. Even the OHIP would not pay for the needles Dr Y used in his HCG weight-loss program. Kieran deemed Dr Y's booklet outlining his program "bizarre." First, patients were told to gorge for three days, during which they were also to drink quarts of liquid. On the fourth day, a near abstinence from eating began, along with six weeks of injections. The third physician Kieran discussed was Dr Z, whom she had seen in the past to help her lose weight, which he did with the aid of amphetamines. She eventually quit both the doctor and the diet pills. When she saw him again, she was pleasantly surprised that he was no longer an advocate of appetite suppressants and, indeed, warned his patients against them. She concluded the article by telling her readers that there was a new type of drug available if they felt they wanted it. "But, after my adventures in Dietary Drugland, you won't get it from me."[72]

Gender and Treatment

As a patient, Kieran was educated about drugs for obesity; as a reporter and a patient, she tried to inform readers about obesity and drug treatments. Seldom was a patient's perspective put forth in the medical literature, but patients were very present in the drug advertisements. Depicted as respectable, middle-aged, middle-class, heterosexual, and white individuals who were fat, patients portrayed in the advertisements were people who needed to lose weight and who could afford to see a physician and to pay for prescription drugs. Given that women dominated most of the studies of obesity in the period under examination, the expectation is that they would dominate the visuals of the advertisements. Looking at the advertisements in the *CMAJ*, women did dominate, but perhaps not to the degree anticipated.[73]

Gendered perceptions, however, prevailed in all the cultural and social aspects associated with being a woman or a man. For example, an advertisement for Marmola in *The Chatelaine* in 1928 appealed to men, letting them know that fat was a "blight" on them for it meant "less health and vigor," as opposed to the "loss of youth and beauty" for fat women.[74] Advertisers in the medical journals did not create the gendered social perspective per se, but applied an existing one to a specific situation (obesity) and audience (physicians). In the drug advertisements, men were usually depicted as being at work or away from home and family during their workday, whereas women, not surprisingly, were depicted at home, performing chores for the family and themselves, or in a doctor's office as a patient. Women were represented as less active than men and often shown snacking throughout the day, whereas men working outside the home could not take time off to eat snacks or would be criticized if they did. Instead, advertisements often described men as night eaters, eating after they returned home from the office. Although the advertisements did not direct physicians to see emotional eaters as female, the medical literature already did through the belief in the emotional/psychological element of women's obesity. Ironically, some of the advertisements using the businessman image did reflect emotional personalities, but ones seen as characteristic of men's working persona – assertive or somewhat aggressive – necessary for them to get ahead in their work.

A Dexedrine advertisement in the 1953 *CMAJ* showed a photograph of an obese man, dressed in shirt, tie, suit, and overcoat, putting his hat on a coat rack and gazing straight at the reader. By his demeanour, it was clear that taking Dexedrine would not interfere with the man's work (he was obviously a businessman) or his masculinity, an important message at the time.[75] Photographs were powerful tools for selling products – the advertisement with a photograph of a patient was believable for a physician. A second Dexedrine advertisement used a photograph of a woman, showing a middle-aged housewife (recognized by the apron she wore) sitting, reading a book, and eating a rather large cookie with others piled on a table within reach. The dress under the apron signalled a middle-class woman. In this case, the message implied was that weight was the result of eating (which the photograph of the man did not make explicit) and that eating did not have to be egregious to be harmful.[76] The busy businessman was not blamed for his own obesity, at least not overtly, but the housewife was. According to Heather Molyneaux in her study of these advertising images, the man was presented as in control, whereas the woman was not.[77] An advertisement in 1961 depicted two significantly overweight people, a woman and a man. The woman, who was reading a romance book or magazine, was referred to as a "sedentary overeater," whereas the man, shown at a business meeting in an assertive position, was called an "active overeater." The gendered aspect of the advertisement was obvious, with the product Biphetamine being for the woman and Ionamin for the man.[78] Another Ionamin advertisement, subtly criticizing the use of amphetamines, stated: "Well-adjusted people who talk business at mealtime are as subject to overeating as the neurotic for whom food is an emotional substitute. Yet the anorexiant suitable for the latter – often amphetamine – may be excessively stimulating to the busy executive." The visual showed the restaurant table after the customers had left. The dishes were dirty, and on the tablecloth were scribbled financial figures, indicating that what had just taken place had not been a social occasion but a business lunch. The text made clear that the executive's eating was not neurotic in origin but rather linked to his busyness, and Ionamin would be best for the executive.[79] He was overweight or obese as a result of focusing on business, and not on himself and what he was eating.

These advertisements were typical in their gendered portrayal of women and men. While their need to lose weight was common, the cause of their weight was visually different. Women were often portrayed as more emotionally needy than men, at times looking anxious. The advertisements also depicted women's lives as lacking. Some advertisements talked about the depression that women experienced because they could not fit into fashionable clothes due to their weight.[80] Underlying such advertisements was a view of women's problems as somewhat trivial. They also reflected a medical literature that depicted women as culturally dependent and, as such, susceptible to moods. The "psychological weakness" of women played into the way some drugs were used. Physicians prescribed amphetamines to treat some psychiatric problems as well as to aid dieting. Indeed, the two came together when the obesity literature looked at the psychological issues behind overeating.[81]

Most advertisements were serious, but at times fat patients were ridiculed to make a point. One of the earliest cartoon drawings was an advertisement for Probese in the 1949 *The Canadian Doctor*. In the upper left-hand corner, a large woman wearing a dress and heels was standing on a tall public weight machine. The machine was breaking under the woman's weight, indicated by the machine leaning backwards straining and its inner workings disintegrating. In the lower right-hand corner was a larger representative drawing of a curvaceous young nude kneeling on the floor with her head tilted to one side and her hands behind her head so that her breasts were lifted up and visible. The fat woman and her situation was a cartoon figure to amuse the onlooker. The nude was the drawing of a very sexualized and idealized woman. The message to the practitioners who saw it was clear – an obese woman was a source of mirth; if she lost weight she would become a desirable woman.[82] But the prospect was a lie, since most women could not look like the ideal woman. Because most practitioners of the time were men, the depiction of women was intended to appeal to them. As the number of women physicians increased, advertisements adjusted to the new readership. Idealized female nude drawings, for example, did not appear much beyond the 1950s.

A series of advertisements for Ionamin and Biphetamine in the 1960s were gendered cartoons. One of the first was a drawing of a rather abstract, but clearly obese man whose body went from a pointed head to the large base of a triangle somewhere above his knees. Wrapped in a flowered towel labelled "hers," he was standing on a scale trying to see his weight. Unable to see over his protruding abdomen, he resorted to looking through a periscope with a 90-degree turn in order to do so. The cartoon is humorous because it is ludicrous. His shape is ridiculous and unreal. He is a man, but not a man – for what

162   Fighting Fat

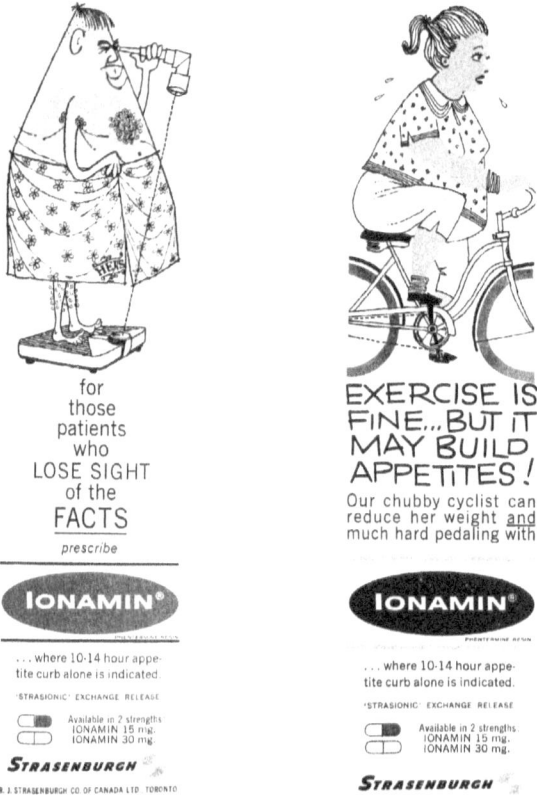

Ionamin advertisements often used cartoons that made fat men look ludicrous. While most of the fat men in the cartoons were funny, the man wearing a towel in this 1963 cartoon (left) isn't. He looks unhappy, anxious, and somewhat annoyed. He has lost "sight of the facts," and needs help curbing his appetite. The fat woman riding on a bicycle in another 1963 Ionamin cartoon (right) is quite different from the man with the towel. She is attractive: she is dressed in nice clothes; she has a bracelet on her right wrist; and even while riding her bicycle, she is wearing make-up (lipstick). She is trying to lose weight through exercise, but the advertisement informs physicians that exercise "may build appetites." Clearly, this woman may need help to control that increased appetite. Source: (left) Ionamin advertisement, *CMAJ* 88, no. 26 (29 June 1963): 26; (right) Ionamin advertisement, *CMAJ* 89, no. 10 (7 September 1963): 22. Used with permission under a non-exclusive licence issued by the Copyright Board of Canada in cooperation with Canadian Artists Representation Copyright Collective.

kind of man would put a flowered towel labelled "hers" around his girth? The implication was that undressed men who were obese were slightly effeminate; the man beneath the business suit was vulnerable to ridicule. Another advertisement depicted a trampoline expert bouncing on the trampoline so that his body floated upwards – not surprising since he is shaped like a balloon. The advertisement suggested he had lost control, and he needed to come "back from orbit" and to lose weight.[83] There were at least sixteen cartoons in the series, only three of which portrayed women, perhaps a reflection of some kind of chivalry. The first was somewhat risqué. It showed a rather shapely, but clearly overweight woman trying to get the bottom part of a two-piece bathing suit over her hips. But with the right drug, she would be able to get into her suit for another season. What comes to mind when looking at the drawing are the woman's curves. Unlike the men, her body is clearly that of a woman (not a stylized blimp), and she is a rather sweet-looking woman (as were the cartoon women in the other two advertisements).[84] In these advertisements, the manufacturer, R.J. Strasenburgh, crosses over the line to make fun of the people its products were supposed to help. But from the perspective of gender, the advertisements ridiculed the men, whereas the women might have generated a gentle smile.

Most of the cartoon advertisements illustrated men and women before they saw a physician. They had "allowed" their weight to get the better of them. The blimp-sized bodies drawn were clearly aspects of out-of-contol individuals. Dexedrine, for example, used the visual of a balloon with a stretched-out face (unclear what sex) in one of its advertisements. A very thin string attached to the inflated balloon suggested a tenuous grip on "normalcy." The image conveyed the message that very little could keep such people grounded, safe, secure, or under control. Yet, being in control was necessary, especially for those who had co-morbid conditions such as hypertension along with their obesity. If they were not in control, their blood pressure could increase, placing their health in danger.[85]

Partnership between Medicine and Pharmaceuticals

Despite the negative view that saw people who were obese as failures and out of control, many of the advertisements made the return to control seem relatively painless. The advertisements also assured physicians that the product marketed was safe and based on science.

The presence of all three of these factors signified that drug treatments would be successful. Control over eating was necessary in order to take weight off. Advertisements in the 1940s for Probese A, B, or C assured physicians that amphetamine would "lessen appetite ... and increase the will to diet."[86] As a result, a patient would remain calm throughout the dieting phase, and practitioners wanted to see patient control. One of the few depictions of men in a non-business setting in the 1950s was an advertisement in which the picture delivered the message. It showed a dapper youngish man, not particularly overweight, dressed in hat, chequered jacket, shirt and tie underneath, and a very fashionable scarf thrown over his right shoulder. He was standing behind a supermarket buggy full of food and in his left hand he held out a cake. Looking straight at the reader with his right hand by his mouth, he seemed to be asking if should he buy the cake or put it away. Only at the bottom of the page was the message confirmed: "Successful appetite control begins in the supermarket." If the man could resist the temptation to buy the cake, he would be on the road to lasting weight reduction. Only then does the reader discover the advertisement was for Dexedrine Spansule, which would curb appetite at meals and in the supermarket. The advertisement was subtle: the visual dominated with the message a doctor wanted to see – a patient who thought before he bought food, a patient who had self-control.[87] From the doctor's point of view, having a patient who was in control would make life easier for both doctor and patient, and their relationship would be much more pleasant.

The drawings and photographs of real "fat" people were not as negative as the cartoons. A 1961 Tenuate Dospan advertisement suggested that people who were overweight had many things in common, including the need to be on its drug. The visual depicted a painting class with people identified as students (all older) and teacher; the figures were all labelled according to their health problems: very overweight, gravid (pregnant) overweight, a little overweight, hypertensive overweight, diabetic overweight, and cardiac overweight. Underlying all the advertisements, however, was the need for these people to change, to lose weight, and to keep it off. The whole thrust of patient weight loss was to have them be like others. Preludin appealed to this underlying message in a drawing of a swimming pool surrounded by enlongated silhouettes of slender people, both men and women. In the foreground was the back view of an overweight woman who looked like she didn't fit into

"Dietary Drugland" and Surgery 165

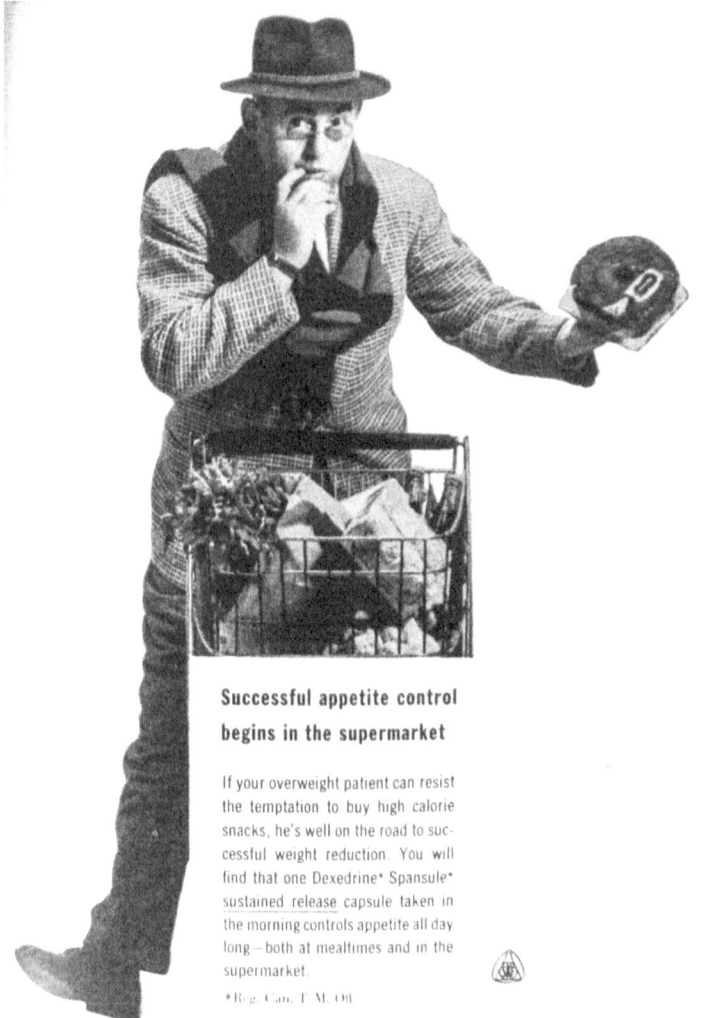

The photograph here shows a man who is not very fat but needs to "resist the temptation to buy high calorie snacks." He is the type of patient that doctors liked: he is overweight but not obese; he is thinking about buying the cake but resisting; and his clothes convey middle class. This 1957 advertisement suggested to doctors that Dexedrine could help such a patient. Source: Dexedrine advertisement, *CMAJ* 76, no. 10 (15 May 1957): 915; © Paladin Labs Inc.

the picture. The text – "when overweight becomes more obvious" – makes the situation very clear. Being obvious was not what you wanted to be.[88]

Given the lack of information at a doctor's disposal about the various drug treatments available and the powerful nature of appetite suppressants, safety was a key enticement to get physicians to consider prescribing a specific drug. In the late 1940s, a Dexedrine advertisement assured readers of the drug's general safety, quoting from a recent *JAMA* article stating that "prolonged" use in studies resulted in "no evidence of toxicity … [and] no evidence of deleterious effects of the drug." Little specific information was provided, but by quoting a highly regarded source, the advertisement reassured physicians that they were dealing with a safe and reputable drug.[89] Physicians were interested in safety, and advertisements used vulnerable groups to depict the safety of their products. For example, Dexedrine advertisements in the 1950s and 1960s assured their medical readers that the drug was so safe a woman could take Dexedrine throughout her pregnancy. Other vulnerable groups were overweight people with co-morbidities such as diabetes, hypertension, or heart disease, especially men in executive positions. The latter were considered to be more at risk for coronary disease when they put on weight than other men or women.[90]

References to science also gave practitioners a sense of safety. A Dexamyl advertisement in 1953 with a visual depicting a sad-looking, overweight older woman had a text that asked: "How many clinical problems do you see in this patient? … You see that she is somewhat exophthalmic [protrusion of the eye]. You see also that she is overweight. Perhaps less apparent is an even more common clinical problem: mental and emotional distress." Dexamyl contained "*two* mood-ameliorating components: 1. 'Dexedrine' Sulphate – the antidepressant of choice – to lift the patient's mood and provide a sense of well-being. 2. Amobarbital (Lilly) – the sedative that elevates mood – to relieve nervousness, anxiety, and inner tension."[91] This particular advertisement was popular and appeared frequently. But what was it saying? It appeared to promise that with the help of drugs the woman could become happy. She was experiencing emotional and mental problems – whether they were the cause of her obesity or the result was unclear – but for the advertisement it didn't really matter. What she needed were mood-altering drugs, one to overcome her depression and another to keep her calm. In the drugged state, she would be able to lose weight. The advertisement

"Dietary Drugland" and Surgery 167

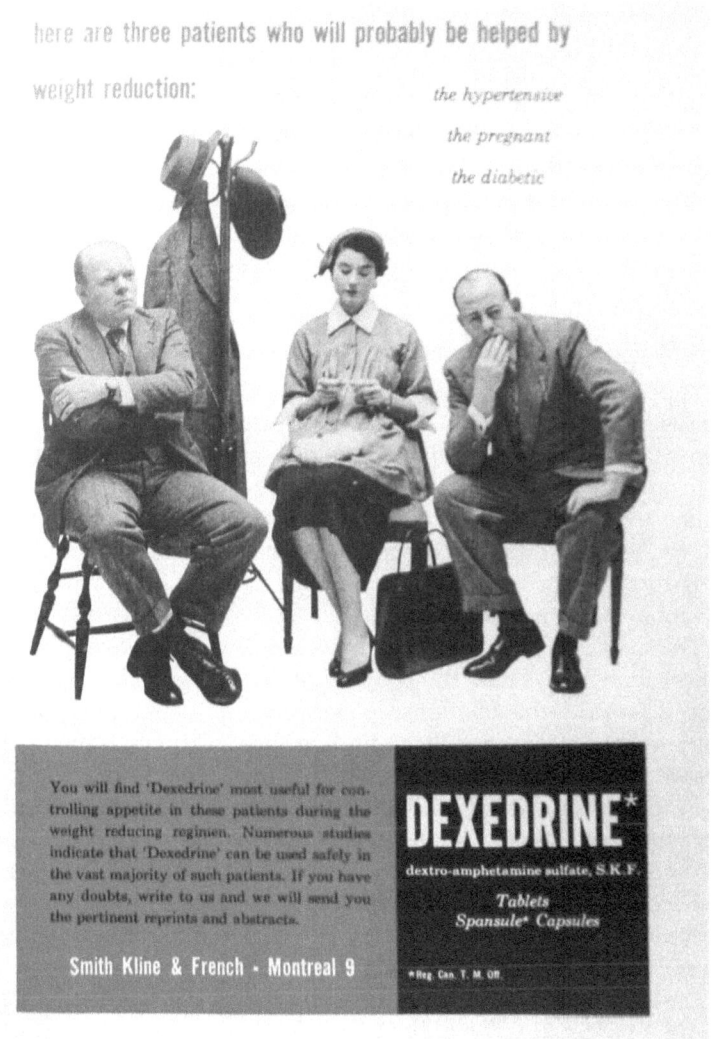

Over time, pharmaceutical companies tried to make drugs that targeted many different types of patients. This 1956 Dexedrine advertisement features three people who need to control their appetite. None of them are obese, but if they became overweight, their conditions – hypertension, pregnancy, and diabetes – could result in complications. Source: Dexedrine advertisement, *CMAJ* 75, no. 7 (1 October 1956): 617; © Paladin Labs Inc.

claimed that modern science through drugs would be able to help her reach her goal.

A series of cartoons advertising Probese and Dexobese (dextroamphetamine) were headed by the caption "Famous because ..." One cartoon depicted a very skinny and hairy man, intended to be Archimedes, sitting in an overflowing bathtub. No connection was drawn between Archimedes and obesity, but placing a famous classical scientist in the advertisement implied the scientific credibility of obesity treatment with Probese or Dexobese. A Dexedrine advertisement emphasized in its text that the Dexedrine Spansule capsule would last the whole day. The capsule was full of "tiny coated pellets" that would "disintegrate at pre-determined intervals" releasing the "active ingredient," a formulation appealing to the wonders of science through the words "active ingredient" and to the technological innovation that came up with time-release pills. It was modern![92] The advertisement also showed a willingness to appeal to and adjust for the patient's needs or perceived needs. Adjudets even added multivitamins to its lozenges with amphetamine, as did Probese VM, and Revicaps (d-amphetamines and vitamins).[93] All these additions and adjustments were designed to make prescribing drugs more attractive for practitioners.

Patients may have trusted practitioners, but how were physicians to wend their way through so many advertisements and competing claims? Certainly the relationship between the drug companies and physicians was closer than Canadians realized. Although medical students were taught the basics of pharmacology, once in practice physicians faced the challenges of keeping abreast of new pharmaceuticals and their applications. They relied not only on detail men but also on the drug advertisements as a way of keeping up with new drugs. The pharmaceutical companies were more than willing and financially able to become a partner in this education.[94] From interviews with physicians conducting therapeutic trials on new drugs, it was clear that they depended on the drug companies for information about the drugs. According to Joel Lexchin in his 1984 book *The Real Pushers: A Cultural Analysis of the Canadian Drug Industry*, some articles in support of a specific drug were drafted by a physician, but finished by professional writers in the pay of the pharmaceutical companies.[95]

Looking at the role of pharmaceuticals in the treatment of obesity, it is clear that physicians had a partner in pharmaceutical companies, but not a disinterested one. Certainly, the advertisements for pharmaceutical aids tried to enter into a dialogue with physicians. Advertisements

"Dietary Drugland" and Surgery 169

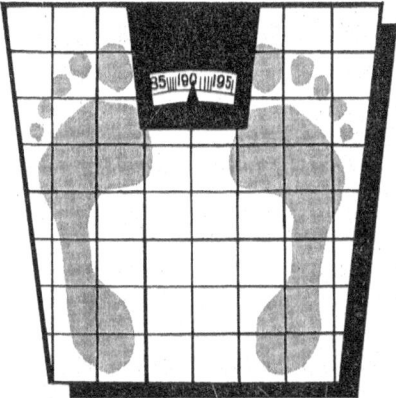

This 1962 Probese advertisement shows how the pharmaceutical companies worked. Readers would see listed four types of Probese that doctors could use for different patients. A note in the advertisement informs doctors about two other versions of Probese they could choose for patients if amphetamine therapy was contraindicated. According to the advertisement, Probese would be safe for any member of a "real" family. Source: Probese advertisement, *CMAJ* 86, no. 19 (12 May 1962): 20. Used with permission under a non-exclusive licence issued by the Copyright Board of Canada in cooperation with Canadian Artists Representation Copyright Collective.

could be comforting, commiserating with physicians about patients who did not seem able to lose weight and were obstreperous as a result. Underlying some of the increasing detail given in the advertisements was the assumption that the physician understood all the references. The advertisement scripts were designed to make physicians, even those in a general practice, feel part of the experimental aspect of medicine. The scripts issued an appeal to knowledge shared among a select group of people, physicians among them, whether they understood the details or not. Essentially these advertisements were a primer on specific drug use. They attempted to be the mediator between the research people (in the employ of the pharmaceutical companies) and the practitioners, making the physician and the pharmaceutical company partners in the fight against overeating. But it was an unequal relationship, since the source of information was often one sided. What the physicians were encouraged to do was choose from among the different types of products companies offered (based on the type of obesity the patient had), determine the dosage, keep track of how the patient was doing, and decide when a new prescription was needed. Pharmaceutical companies focused physicians' attention on drugs and offered physicians some expectation that the situation was not hopeless. Yet, looking at the data from the 1970s, it was clear that the promise of appetite suppressants was limited. They only helped for a short time. Surgery, on the other hand, offered a permanent treatment.

Surgery

Surgery was, and is, the most extreme treatment for obesity; by the 1970s, it was just beginning to be performed in Canada. For that reason, there is no ongoing narrative about surgery for the period under study as exists for dieting and other treatments. Surgery is recommended only when a persons's weight affects the ability to function and places his or her life at risk. Two types of surgery are available: intestinal malabsorption and gastric restriction. Gastric banding, which is less invasive, is now available for those with a 30 BMI if they have co-morbidities. But, as with most obesity treatment, banding has its critics.[96] No matter the surgical method, there is a gender dimension; the vast majority of surgeries – 80 per cent – are done on women.[97]

While obesity surgery was seldom performed in Canada until the 1970s, there were a few articles about using surgery. An article in the 1925 *L'Union Médicale du Canada* (*UMC*) by Dr Aimé-Paul Heineck from

Chicago raved about surgery for removing fat from the abdomen. He saw it as quite safe with permanent results. Similarly, a physician from Sault Ste Marie, Ontario, while taking a tumour from a thirty-five-year-old woman, also removed fat tissue at his patient's request. Other doctors were negative. In his extensive article on "Obesity and Its Treatment," Walter Campbell expressed his dislike of surgery as a treatment for obesity, although he understood its attraction if another surgery was being performed. On its own, however, surgery was simply too risky a procedure, and not enough fat was removed to make a significant difference.[98] In the 1960s and 1970s, the jejunoileal bypass (bypassing most of the small intestine) was popular in the United States, and Canadians were apprised of it through magazines such as *Chatelaine* and physicians through the American and their own medical journals.[99] Cosmetic surgery, in part to correct "flabby" stomachs and thighs, was described in the 1966 *Chatelaine*, and some of it focused on obesity treatment.[100]

While liposuction was a popular surgical treatment in Europe during the 1970s,[101] the situation in Canada concerning this treatment is unclear, since throughout most of the decade Canadian professional literature on surgery for obesity was limited and generally negative. The discourse on surgery was a response to something most Canadian practitioners knew little about. Obesity had long been a concern of general practitioners; however, while they were willing to steer some of their patients towards the self-help groups or to prescribe appetite suppressants, general practitioners were reluctant to advise patients to look to surgery as a cure. Surgery was simply too full of the unknown. In 1973, P.A. Salmon, Faculty of Medicine at the University of Alberta, discussed shunt surgery (jejunoileal bypass) and its consequences in a paper presented at the annual Ontario Medical Association meeting. He reported on 148 cases in which weight loss was significant, with little weight regained. However, "morbidity" was included in the report of adverse reactions: "infections, 19%; wound dehiscence [wound opening], 8%; and evisceration, 3%. Pulmonary complications, fatty infiltration of the liver, diarrhoea, and electrolyte disturbances occurred" as well.[102] Nevertheless, surgery was becoming more popular. By the end of the 1970s, the Toronto General Hospital was using bariatric surgery (weight-loss surgery) to help obese patients.[103]

There was unease about bariatric surgery within the profession. In a 1975 issue of *CMAJ*, an unattributed author claimed surgery for obesity to be "unphysiologic, even if it occasionally works." In 564 cases, "collected" morbidity was significant, and mortality was high at 6 per cent.

The author could only conclude that surgery "must be the last resort when the patient otherwise faces incapacity or death." Two years later, Dr R.C. Bowen and L. Shepel, both of the Department of Psychiatry, University of Saskatchewan, described the case of a thirty-three-year-old woman who was experiencing "cognitive changes, depression, arthralgia [joint pain], and dermatitis" five years after surgery (a jejunoileal shunt). Suspecting vitamin and mineral deficiencies, Bowen and Shepel instituted a regimen of nutrient replacement, and most problems lessened or disappeared.[104] Not enough care had been taken to oversee long-term effects after the surgery.[105] In the 1980 edition of *The Principles and Practice of Medicine*, the authors on obesity mentioned the new "gastric bypass," but noted that there was a 19 per cent mortality rate in patients over fifty years of age.[106] In the same year, Maurice Verdy in the *UMC* wrote an article entitled "L'obésité: la maladie nutritionelle la plus importante de notre société" [Obesity: the most important nutritional illness in our society]. Verdy noted that the long-term benefit of bariatric surgery of any kind was still unclear.[107] Nevertheless, surgery has continued in large part because other treatment modalities have not had any significant results.

Conclusion

In looking at obesity treatments – exercise and dieting with its adjuncts of psychology, self-help groups, and appetite suppressants – the prospect of success from 1920 to 1980 was dim, hence the hope for surgery. In 1958, Paul Dumas, in an article in *UMC*, was clear about what medicine offered: "Le traitement de l'obésité demeure donc encore un traitement symptômatique, à base de régime et de médicaments palliatifs, il est une source de frustration pour plusiers malades et il demeure inopérant dans un petit nombre de cas" [Treatment for obesity still remains just a treatment of symptoms, essentially comprising diet and medications that are palliative in nature, and is a source of frustration for many patients and completely ineffective in a small number of cases]. In 1978, Louise A. Demers-Desrosiers, writing in the same journal, concluded that the majority of those who were obese would have to accept that eating would need to be regulated for the rest of their lives. Some saw obesity as "an insolvable problem," no matter what the treatment. Others in the present day acknowledge that we still know so little about obesity that most treatment is doomed to failure.[108]

A 1972 cartoon of a doctor talking to his patient reflected the desperation felt by practitioners who were willing to try almost anything to help their patients lose weight. The caption read: "Have you tried worrying a lot?" Despite the frustration, a team global approach was put forward in hopes that if no one treatment worked sufficiently, perhaps several treatments together would.[109] It was a narrative of different treatments tried and not succeeding, but nevertheless remaining part of the treatment list. Obesity was baffling for practitioners; the causes seemed to be obvious, but treatments weren't. A survey of Nova Scotian practitioners conducted in the late twentieth century asked doctors what they did when faced with an obese patient. Only 39 per cent tried to treat obese patients; 34 per cent referred them to others; 16.5 per cent recommended their patients seek treatment, but didn't give them any specific referrals; and 11 per cent did nothing. Most did not rely on drugs. In the present day, some experts see obesity as a "chronic" disease in which "patients are struggling against their own body's coordinated effort to stop them from losing weight." Other voices wish to "transform fat-phobic culture" instead. As Michael Gard and Jan Wright have suggested, perhaps it would be best to "'get over' body weight altogether." Treatments for obesity have not worked well, and they "affect people socially and psychologically," which is seldom recognized in much of the scientific literature on obesity.[110]

6 Infant, Child, and Teen Obesity

"A perfect baby does not have the outlines of his muscles obliterated by wads and cushions of fat."[1]

Up to now, the chapters on obesity have focused on adults. This chapter concentrates on infants, children, and teens. Views on the causes and treatments of obesity in children and teens are somewhat similar to those for adult obesity, except that these vulnerable populations don't have adult agency – control and responsibility. As children grow, their ability to exert their wants becomes stronger, but they are still largely under the care of mothers, fathers, and educators. Teens are under the same care, but compared to children, teens spend more time away from adults and assert more control over what they do and eat. Even then, they have the pressures of youth culture, at times as strict as any parent. The situation for infants is different: they are the most vulnerable Canadians, and they have little agency. Although the discussion about infants and obesity over the period under study is limited, it is more extensive than most historians acknowledge.

Infant Obesity

Today, the rates of obesity and its causes extend to infants. Theories based on the experience of the foetus in utero abound: studies suggest that poor nutrition in a pregnant woman can result in fat being stored in the foetus; other researchers have found that a diabetic woman may affect her foetus in a similar way; and older mothers-to-be have been linked to heavier children as a result of exposure in

Infant, Child, and Teen Obesity 175

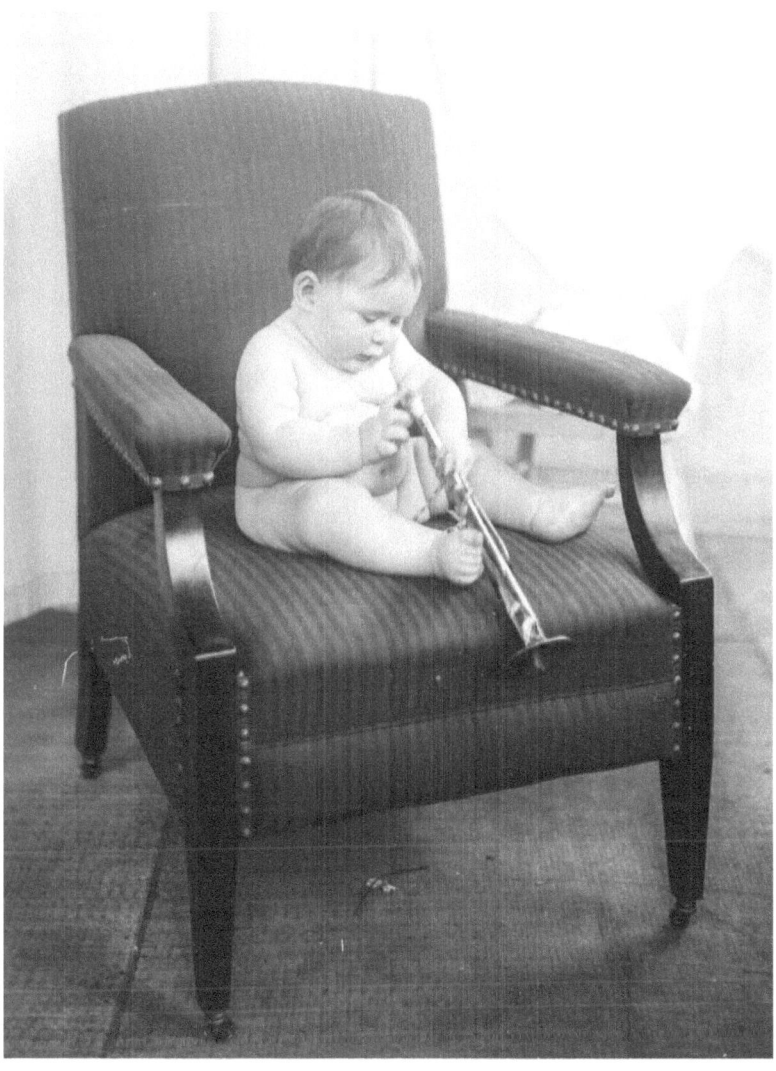

In the early twentieth century, parents wanted their babies to be fat because they thought fat babies were healthy babies. Baby contests showcasing fat "healthy" babies were popular. This baby won first place in the "Better Babies Contest" at the Pacific National Exhibition (PNE) in Vancouver, c. 1920. Source: Photographer, Stuart Thomson, 1913 or 1920; AM1535-: CVA 99–1297, City of Vancouver Archives.

176 Fighting Fat

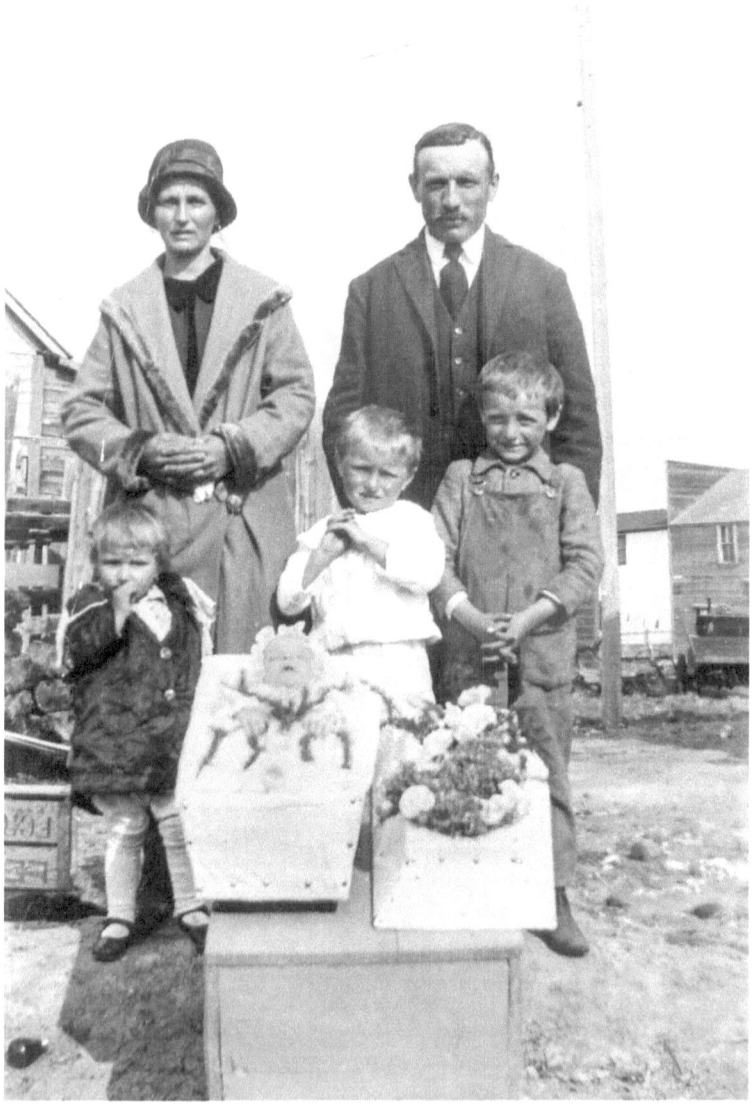

Mortality was high for infants and young children in Canada during the 1920s, and many parents feared their children might die. A thin baby or a thin young child was not thought to be healthy. This haunting photograph from that period shows a family with their baby in a home-made coffin. Source: NA-3596–153, Glenbow Museum.

utero to polychlorinated biphenyls (PCBs). Some studies suggest that obese mothers often give birth to infants with low metabolic rates, and such babies are overweight by age one. Other studies see the birth of both low- and high-weight infants as risk factors for future obesity. An infant's sleep and feeding habits can also be considered factors contributing to obesity.[2] All of these theories reflect concern for infants' health, but also for their future weight.

In the past (as in the present day), the health of the foetus and infant was linked to the pregnant woman and her health. If the mother was healthy, her infant would have a better chance of being born healthy. Nutrition was key; malnourishment, the enemy. While being underweight was a sign of malnutrition, concern also existed about women putting on too much weight during pregnancy. After birth, the worry was infant mortality. Infant mortality rates had long been high in Canada, and the loss of life during World War I and the influenza epidemic that followed made infants' health even more of a concern. In 1919, the federal government created a Division of Child Welfare within the Department of Health. The Depression of the 1930s raised fear that too many families couldn't care for their infants. Only towards the end of the 1940s was there optimism that infants' health would be more secure in the future. Keeping infants thriving was necessary, and debates on how best to do it were contentious. Health experts considered breast milk the best food for newborn babies, but the length of time babies should be fed only breast milk was disputed. How long mothers would be able and willing to breastfeed was also debated, especially when companies were promoting bottle feeding and infant formulas. Underlying the various ways of feeding infants was the image of a healthy, chubby infant. Only gradually did physicians question that image and look at the problems of a fat baby. Even then, the chubby baby image remained iconic, both for many parents and for the baby formula and food advertisements.

Maternal and Infant Weight

In the 1920s, popular literature was suggesting to women that they should not gain too much weight during their pregnancy – it was "dangerous" for both the mother and the foetus. Eating well was even more significant. But not all women could afford nutritious food. The nutritional study of 100 low-income Toronto families in the 1930s found that pregnant women consumed on average only 70 per cent of needed protein, and nursing mothers only 57 per cent. Alan Brown and Elizabeth Chant Robertson, in their popular 1948 book *The Normal Child*, emphasized the need for better nutrition for pregnant women and warned readers that overconsumption of sugar could result in the pregnant woman putting on too much weight. Their advice was that women should gain only 20 pounds during pregnancy. Others, however, accepted a weight gain somewhere between 25 and 30 pounds.[3]

The lack of consensus over weight gain during pregnancy continued. The foetus shouldn't be too big, especially for women with diabetes or women who were obese and might be prone to gestational diabetes. As late as 1970, an article in *The Canadian Nurse* recommended a pregnant woman gain no more than 16 to 20 pounds; others preferred 20 to 25 pounds. If the pregnant woman couldn't control her weight gain, appetite suppressants could help, although some feared that such drugs might harm the foetus, lowering its birth weight and even causing perinatal death.[4] While doctors had long tried to limit their patients' weight gain during pregnancy, in the 1970s they also worried that too many women were not putting on enough weight. The emphasis on being slender for women could prompt some pregnant women to have a negative reaction to their weight gain. Women who were too thin (20 per cent under the ideal weight for height) were considered at risk, as were their babies.[5] The result could be the birth of underweight infants, whose doctors and mothers would want to see them gain more weight than they needed. Today "so many factors influence the connection between mother and child" that some authors argue that "mother's nutrition during pregnancy" may not cause the child's obesity.[6]

Because of the concern about weak babies and infant mortality in the past, it was not surprising that the image of a healthy infant was a smiling, chubby baby throughout most of the nineteenth century and much of the twentieth.[7] At the 1929 Canadian National Exhibition (CNE) baby show, Master Donald Baldock, a "sturdy" one-year-old, was the grand winner from among 600 children; the sturdiness of Donald was what Canadians parents were assumed to want for their own children. Marketers used images of fat babies to sell their products, letting mothers know the importance of keeping track of their infants' weight gain. Virol, a malt extract, blatantly appealed to parents' (and specifically, mothers') fears. Its 1930 advertisement showed a baby boy, both before and after taking Virol. In the first image, the baby was emaciated with ribs protruding and stick-like arms. After taking Virol, he was plump and healthy. At fourteen, he was no longer plump, but an active young man.⁸ Infant formulas, too, were becoming more popular, and advertisements for them abounded in the popular press. One Carnation Milk advertisement told *Chatelaine* readers that providing an alternative to mother's milk would give baby boys a "husky" start.⁹ Surely a "husky" boy was the goal of any parent.

In a 1954 advertisement for Heinz, the visual showed a weight scale and a naked baby lying across it looking huge and fat. In bold type, the baby was declared a "Heavyweight Champ." He was touted as "one of the thousands of healthy husky youngsters who thrived on Heinz products right from the start." Added proof was that Heinz babies "overwhelmingly" were the prize winners in Canada's baby shows. In such an advertisement, weight was depicted as desireable, and there seemed to be no weight limit. Why would there be a limit when pounds were deemed "precious"? Chubbiness signified that the infant was getting enough food (the assumption being that the food was nutritionally good), and a sturdy weight would thus pave the way for a healthy childhood and adulthood. Fat, after all, was a reserve that would be needed to fight off disease, and steady weight gain was associated with normal growth and health well into the 1960s.¹⁰

Infant Feeding and Fat

The key to raising a healthy infant was proper feeding. But how to feed an infant was contentious. The debate over breastfeeding versus bottle feeding emerged in the late nineteenth century and has carried through to the present day. In 1929, Dr M.J. Carney from Halifax, Nova Scotia, noted that the "amount of literature at present on the artificial feeding of infants is colossal, and … is to my way of thinking only equated by its contradictions." Dr A. Chandler, director of the Montreal Welfare Association, blamed baby welfare clinics for the decline of breastfeeding. Too often, the clinics weighed the infants as part of assessing their health. When mothers who breastfed their infants compared their infants to those who were given cow's milk or infant formula, they noted that their babies were not putting on the same kind of weight. As a result, many decided to wean their infants and resort to artificial feeding. As one immigrant mother at a Victorian Order of Nurses (VON) clinic declared, the nurse wanted "to see how much my baby make fat." The "baby-scale" had become the ruling tool to assess an infant's health.¹¹ The issue of breastfeeding versus bottle feeding continued well into the 1970s.¹²

Sooner or later, neither breastfeeding nor bottle feeding is enough for a growing infant and weaning the infant to solid food is necessary for optimum nutrition. But when to wean was disputed over the early decades.[13] The private sector encouraged early weaning of babies by offering baby foods to make weaning easier. Swift's Strained Meats used its advertisements in popular magazines to remind readers of the need to start babies eating meat early. A 1944 advertisement in *Chatelaine* for Swift Canadian bacon showed the visual of a fat baby being given bacon to eat as a way to sell its product. Baby food had become big business. In 1955, one company alone offered forty-seven types of strained food for infants and thirty-one types of ground food for older babies. For the Canadian canning industry, baby food represented up to 25,000 tons of their business, a significant branch of the industry.[14]

Despite the adoption of a fat infant as the image of a healthy infant, some health experts queried how fat an infant could be and still be healthy. Alton Goldbloom, in his 1928 edition of *The Care of the Child*, referred to infant overeating, although he didn't see this as a problem and certainly didn't connect it with future obesity, as others did later in the century. He did suggest, however, that a baby weighing 19 pounds at six months would be "definitely overweight," and a 32 pound infant at one year would be "abnormal." He connected such weight to mothers who wanted to see a weight gain of half a pound per week in their infants. Alan Brown included a section on "Fat Babies" in his 1923 edition of *The Normal Child*. He, too, didn't approve of babies putting on weight rapidly, and blamed mothers' belief that fat babies and health were synonymous. The *Chatelaine* Baby Clinic in 1933 pointed out to its readers that fat babies could have health problems such as rickets, bone deformities, and digestive problems. Nevertheless, the magazine understood the competition between mothers for the fattest infant[15] – winning would be a sign of their successful mothering. The fat infant remained the goal.

Increasingly in the health professions, a fat baby wasn't necessarily seen to be a healthy baby. A study of infants in the Swan Valley area of Manitoba, based on 1,225 baby records from 1946 to 1950, showed the weight gain of different feeding groups. Babies who were breast-fed doubled their weight by three to six months and tripled it by nine to twelve months. Babies fed cow's milk did the same. But babies fed Carnation Milk put on weight significantly faster, to the point that some girl babies weighed up to 30 pounds by age one. In 1952, L.L. Kulczcki, an official from the Manitoba Department of Public Health, deemed this high weight gain "an example of over-feeding, which cannot be regarded as a beneficial gain of weight." Mothers were blamed.[16]

Overfeeding of infants was seen as a problem within the growing obesity rate in the country as a whole. Dr L.B. Pett, head of the Nutrition Division of the Department of National Health and Welfare, considered the overweight status of many Canadians to be the result of an era accepting large, fat babies as healthy. Pett understood that a healthy infant/child had a certain look and that for many decades the look had been a chubby one. But his concern about obesity in the wider population signalled a different way of looking at fat babies – "big babies are often nutritional problems." W.A. Cochrane, Department of Paediatrics, Faculty of Medicine, Dalhousie University and Children's Hospital, commented on how mothers were "bombarded" by advertisers telling them that big babies were healthy babies. Not content to blame the advertisers or the mothers who believed them, Cochrane also chastised his own colleagues for encouraging mothers to feed their infants solid food much too early, leading to infant obesity. While the old standard of weight gain had been for an infant to double his or her birth weight by six months and triple it by a year, too many infants now doubled their weight by three to four months.[17]

Three signs of the concern over infant obesity existed in the 1960s. First was the debate: breastfeeding versus formula feeding. In the eyes of many, artificial feeding tended to encourage overfeeding because the mother often felt obliged to make sure the infant drank everything from the bottle. With breastfeeding, surveillance of the infant was not as focused – the mother couldn't "measure" how much breast milk her infant was taking. Second was the assignment of a measurement for infant obesity – 15 per cent overweight. And third was the response of the food companies, which came forward to provide physicians with a solution to infant obesity. Products such as Mil-ko, a form of skimmed milk with a low calorie level, began promoting their value for infants, including those who were too fat. Heinz came out with its new "cottage cheese with pineapple" for infants. Since the cottage cheese had skim milk in it, the product met physicians' demand for a low-fat diet for the youngest of their patients, including those with obesity.[18] How this product would help when it was an "addition" to infant meals was unclear.

In the 1970s, Dr Donald Hill, assistant professor of paediatrics at the University of Toronto, informed his listeners at a symposium on infant obesity that the earliest time obesity could be diagnosed was six months, arguing that if the weight gain at six months was over 5.4 kilograms, the baby was obese. The fat cell theory considered obesity a result of overfeeding in infancy. "According to this hypothesis, the number of our fat cells is established by the way we are fed as infants." But you didn't need to resort to the "fat cell" theory as a cause. Nutritionist Dr David Yeung, who was studying 403 babies in the Montreal–Toronto region, determined that the Canadian Dietary Standards for newborn infants up to a month were appropriate, but the standards for those from three to eleven months of age were too generous by 10 to 20 per cent.[19]

The literature on infant obesity indicated that it had become a significant problem. But if the problem was recognized, how were health experts to address it? In a 1975 letter to the editor of the *Canadian Medical Association Journal* (*CMAJ*), Dr T. Hancock from Chipman, New Brunswick, was adamant that Canada should "stop the sale of milk formulas except on prescription until their safety can be established." Others, too, were concerned about the link between infant obesity and bottle feeding.[20] Not surprisingly, some health experts contested Hancock's assumption.[21] Others speculated that weaning a baby at too early an age was the reason for infant obesity. Some suggested six weeks to two months was too early, yet the national median was six weeks to two months. Marketers were encouraging an even earlier introduction for their products. Early weaning was becoming the norm. Pushing the discussion further was "double feeding" – bottle feeding and giving the infant solid food at the same time, and praising the infant for eating it all. As Anthony W. Myres, Health and Welfare, Nutrition Education and Advisory Division, argued: "In this way, the infant's own physiological signals concerning satiety may become suppressed and a habit of overeating may be established."[22]

At the end of the decade, Myres and Yeung published their article "Obesity in Infants: Significance, Aetiology, and Prevention" in the *Canadian Journal of Public Health* (*CJPH*). They began with a summary of opinion:

> In recent years both the public and professionals have become anxious about obese infants. This concern has stemmed from such widely known hypotheses as: a) infancy is a critical period for fat-cell development; b) bottle feeding and early weaning are causes of overfeeding leading to obesity; and c) infantile obesity is the first step in a pattern of lifelong obesity. These hypotheses have been controversial ... However, new evidence and further arguments both supporting and contradicting these hypotheses are being presented.

Three points emerged from this summary. First, one of the authors (Yeung) was an employee of a company that made baby food, and yet he was going to address the issue of early weaning and the consumption of baby foods at an early age. Second, the perception was created that infant obesity had become a concern, not only among "professionals," but with the public as well. Third, people looked to the history of obese individuals for the source/cause of obesity and in some cases found it in infancy.

The rest of the article addressed the complexity of infant obesity. For example, the authors distinguished between being overweight and being obese. The latter was a measurement of fat, the former may not have been. They acknowledged a "strong" connection between infant obesity and adult obesity, but suggested that a similar connection between infant obesity and child obesity was less clear, even though the Canadian Paediatric Society Nutrition Committee saw a connection between infant and adolescent obesity. Myres and Yeung recognized infancy as a time when fat cells could form and increase in size, but it was not the only time. In any event, the significance of an increased number of such cells was uncertain. The two authors called for more research. The best course of action in infant obesity was not to treat it, but to prevent it. Going back to an earlier debate on what to feed infants, the authors noted that bottle feeding increased the possibility of the baby eating more than needed. Added to that was an earlier introduction of solid foods resulting in overnutrition, although the authors admitted that there was no consensus from the experts on the subject. The way around the feeding issue was not to blame the milk source or the type of food eaten, but the amount. And the amount was determined not by the infant but by the mother. Eating improperly or too much was considered a learned behaviour.[23]

Infants needed to be monitored, but even those who were obese should not lose weight. Instead, control of future weight gain was the key.[24] Some studies indicated that infants at four to nine months of age did not really differ in food intake whether they were overweight or "normal" weight. Indeed, some infants who were fat did not eat as much as those who weren't. A skim milk diet wouldn't work – studies had indicated that skim milk could result in depletion of the fat needed to ward off disease and illness. Two per cent milk wasn't good either, since it contained too much sodium, potassium, calcium, phosphorus, and protein. Treatment amounted to controlling the feeding method – breastfeeding versus formula feeding – but both methods were contested, complicating the scene. And sooner or later, breastfeeding and formula had to be supplemented by solid food. Low-fat food was not the solution since it could result in babies wanting to eat more and also denied them fatty acids, which were key to their growth.[25] The problem of infant obesity had been recognized, but what to do about it had not been determined. Would the narrative of obesity in children and teenagers be any different?

Child and Teen Obesity

A 2009–11 Canadian Health Measures survey reported that 19.8 per cent of Canadian youth aged five to seventeen were overweight and 11.7 per cent were obese. The children of the poor were at risk, especially those in "multi-ethnic, urban neighbourhoods" and Indigenous children. Rates for being overweight or obese among First Nations children were 55 per cent on reserves and 41 per cent off the reserves.[26] As with adults, obesity rates in children and teens are based on contested measurements. Two different measurement methods were used in the survey, the skinfold thickness and the body mass index (BMI). While this choice might seem straightforward, a 2011 article noted that three different BMI standards were used in Canada for children: one put forth by the US Center for Disease Control and Prevention, another from the International Obesity Task Force, and a third from the World Health Organization. Each organization's standard gives rise to different statistics. The BMI for children as a measurement of fat, as with adults, varies with age, ethnicity, and sex, but is also specific to children's maturation patterns.[27]

Obesity in children and teens revolves around health issues, in particular the increase in type 2 diabetes in children, especially among Aboriginal children. High blood pressure is also a concern, and researchers are looking into the early development of cardiovascular disease. There is also fear that obese children will become obese adults, with all their related health problems. Newspaper headlines have suggested, without any scientific basis, that the current generation of children will be the first to have shorter lifespans than their parents because of childhood obesity. That the headlines are believed and remembered reflects the panic surrounding childhood and youth obesity. In addition to the concerns about physical health, psychological health is deemed at risk, leading to low self-esteem and underachievement.[28] Moss Norman's research on Canadian boys is original; he looks at Canadian boys, not

Infant, Child, and Teen Obesity 185

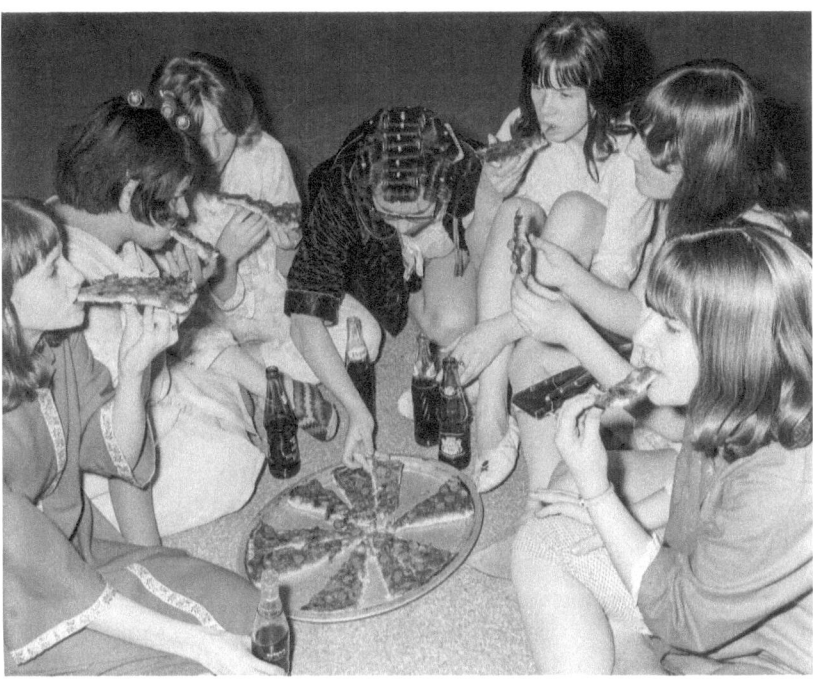

Older children and teens had some agency in determining what food they ate outside of the home, and their scope increased significantly in the 1950s and 1960s. Soda shops and pop stores catered to children and teens. Food provided in school cafeterias or in vending machines would not necessarily meet with parental approval. Eating pizza and drinking soda were part of the food culture for girls (and boys), as shown in this 1960s photograph of a girls' pyjama party. Source: 196-?, 10009433.jpg, Archives of Ontario.

all of them fat, and listens to them talk about their own bodies, other boys' bodies, and men's bodies. Certainly, the research explores fatness, but it also examines obesity.[29] As with adults, there are many challenges to coupling health risk and obesity for youth.[30] Similarly, in challenging overnutrition as the cause of obesity, some studies saw little difference between the eating patterns of overweight and obese children and those of other children. Only very obese children were linked to overeating, especially in the amount of protein consumed.[31]

Recognition of Obesity

Most of those who write about obesity in children and teens see the phenomenon as relatively new. While not a great deal of historiography exists on the subject, references to youth obesity are part of the broader history of obesity.[32] *Childhood Obesity in America* by Laura Dawes is the main history on the topic, covering the late nineteenth century to the present. The themes of her book are the measurement, diagnosis, causes, and treatments of obesity in children; the book also examines how the obesity epidemic came about. She especially looks to the sciences for causes and treatments. As Stearns did, Dawes sees the United States as different from other countries. For example, she sees American discourse on obesity in children as presenting the view that individuals should be "required to treat their own condition," whereas some consider Canada's discourse to focus on the social and economic factors that underpin rising obesity rates."[33]

Unlike obesity in infants, obesity in children and teens was a much more obvious concern in the past. While it is a significant time, infancy is a short period in life compared to childhood and adolescence, and for many parents, infant fat didn't cause unease. After all, as infants became children, the baby fat would disappear. If it didn't, practitioners could look to studies of families and the nutritional needs of each member or to ongoing surveys of children's and teens' growth through school to assess their nutritional health. Although weight chart standards existed for children and teens, how the measurements were taken varied: some children were weighed wearing clothes, others were not; some surveys judged age by the last birthday, others by the nearest birthday; and some studies surveyed groups of children of various nationalities. All were at the mercy of the observers' skills. Even more problematic was the question of what the charts actually measured. In 1929, an article in *The Canadian Nurse* suggested there was a difference between a malnourished preschool child and a healthy child who was underweight because of heredity.[34] Weight, then, was not necessarily a measurement of health. The authors of a 1947 article in the *CJPH* were also not convinced that a normal weight for children was a sign of health. A year later, Pett and his colleague F.W. Hanley noted the uncertainty about the use of charts for children and teens. Children's growth patterns were so quick and individual that it was better to follow their own unique development through time than to compare them with others their own age.³⁵ Stanley M. Garn from the Feis Research Institute, Ohio, advised readers of the 1965 *CMAJ* that the best approach for those interested in children's health was not to compare children's growth patterns to "average values" but to use heredity, that is, "parent-specific or parent-corrected size standards."³⁶ All the debates on standard measurements reflected an interest in what could be considered a healthy weight for the young.

In his first (1893) edition of *The Principles and Practice of Medicine*, William Osler noted that obesity in young girls and boys was not "uncommon" in the United States. By the 1912 edition, he was referring to the "extraordinary number of very stout children." Alan Brown, in his 1923 edition of *The Normal Child* on raising and feeding children, seldom mentioned obesity, although he acknowledged children could be overfed. A Winnipeg study of girls in domestic courses from grades 8 to 10 referred to weights of 10 per cent underweight or 20 per cent overweight as "danger points." The lower margin of underweight reflected the serious concern that being underweight presented to Canadian children compared to being overweight. Alton Goldbloom proposed an actual weight as the measurement of the norm: 26 to 27 pounds at age two; 31 pounds at age three, and 65 to 66 pounds at age ten, with a height of 52 to 53 inches. For older children, Brown differentiated based on height, sex, and age.³⁷

In 1941, Dr Lionel M. Lindsay of Montreal published "The Overweight Child" in the *CMAJ*, which was one of the first overviews of obese children in Canada and used 20 per cent over the normal weight as a standard. He also adopted the classic division of obesity in adults for children, that is, exogenous or endogenous obesity (the latter referred to as "endocrine disturbance"). Rather than giving a sense of which type of obesity predominated, he argued that children generally fell between the two extremes, and in doing so negated the separation of the two categories. Elizabeth Chant Robertson explained to her *Chatelaine* readers that a child was "overly fat" if he or she was over 20 per cent of the average weight or if pinching the waist revealed a "thick pad of fat." Interestingly, she didn't use the word "obesity," even though others did. Lindsay recognized that not all his colleagues measured fat using standards from weight/height/age charts, but preferred a clinical examination that could determine the distribution of fat.³⁸ Nonetheless, the weight/height charts had been and continued to be the rule of thumb for busy physicians to determine whether a weight problem existed in their young patients.

At the beginning of the 1950s, Dr Bernard Laski, a well-known paediatrician in Toronto, wrote an article in *Health* that addressed the issue of the "overnourished" child. In his opinion, such a child was more at risk than one who was underweight, an interesting view given the decades of concern about the latter. By the late 1950s, the issue of obesity came to the fore. The baby boom began in 1946 and continued throughout the 1950s. Families had more children growing up in an economy that allowed families, including the children, to eat more. The expert on children and their weight was Hilde Bruch, and her work was based on child obesity in the United States. Her findings, which addressed children's "nutritional excesses," were reviewed in the 1957 *Ontario Medical Review*, as well as in other medical journal articles. However, it wasn't only the physicians and health experts who were discussing the problem of children and teens being overweight. Articles were appearing in popular magazines. In 1966, *Chatelaine* published "Miss C's Diet Book"; an advertisement for it asked the reader: "Is Your Daughter Overweight?"[39] Basically, mothers were being asked, "How could you let this happen?"

While the standard measurement of obesity in children and teens remained at 20 per cent over the average weight into the 1970s, some experts recognized that this cut-off point was an arbitrary figure. As with adults, others insisted that calipers were a better tool for charting fat, but added the point that weight did not work as a benchmark for children "growing in height and musculature."[40] The panic over adult obesity transferred to children and teens. Some statistics suggested that 80 per cent of children whose parents were obese would become obese adults. In 1974, Toronto professor and physician A. Angel was willing to accept the American statistics showing 2 to 15 per cent of children in Canada were obese. The broadness of the statistical assessment was striking and suggested a weakness in both the definition of obesity and the data collection. By the end of the decade, the obesity estimate for Canadian youth between five and thirteen years of age was 8 per cent.[41] Clearly, there was a consensus that children's and teens' weight should be monitored to make sure it remained within a healthy weight spectrum.[42]

Health

The concern over obesity in children and teens centred on its health consequences. Despite the chubby body image for young children promoted in the 1930s, some health experts were querying the concept and arguing that being fat and flabby was not healthy – it denoted malnourishment, and with malnourishment came lack of intellectual concentration. Other problems included fatigue, increased strain on young bodies, and rising number of accidents. Obesity was a "handicap." In a paper presented to the Canadian Medical Association in Montreal in 1939, E.P. Cathcart of the University of Glasgow admitted that "most clinicians would prefer, from a prognostic point of view, a thin wiry child rather than a heavy obese child as a patient suffering, let us say, from pneumonia." "Wiry" suggested fitness; the image of obesity did not.[43]

Lindsay noted that parents seldom brought children to his office because of their obesity per se, but rather for advice about or treatment of a "handicap, mental or physical" perceived as being a result of their fatness. Given the concern about malnutrition and poor health in children, Lindsay found fat children experienced few health problems, although he admitted that some experienced symptoms ranging from "dyspnoea [laboured breathing] [to] pains in … legs and feet." More serious for him were psychological problems due to the "taunts" of other children; the children's sensitivity to their appearance (for girls, this was especially a problem); and their inability to join in games, which simply made them less active and even heavier. While sometimes stronger than other children because of their size, children who were fat could also be "somewhat cumbersome." More to the point for Lindsay was the possibility that obesity might lead "to definite personality changes or behavior problems," which could determine the child's future, that is, obese children didn't "fit" into society and paid the price for it. Lindsay, however, found that parents saw obesity in their children "as a sign of good health and digestion, and indeed the child may appear so robust and cheerful that any criticism of his weight is resented." Lindsay himself saw overweight children as attractive, with "their round, rosy faces … a pleasure to behold." Unfortunately, not all held that view, and some regarded the obese child as "comical" or "pitiable."[44] In the 1950s, others also saw the psychological effects of obesity on children. Jean Grignon, L'hôpital Notre Dame in Montreal, even warned colleagues that obesity beginning in childhood could retard puberty in both sexes.[45]

In a 1961 article published in the journal of the Canadian Association of Health, Physical Education and Recreation (CAHPER), Sam Landa noted that obesity was a common reason for teens to consult a physician. Concern about childhood obesity was partly motivated by the fear that it was a precursor to adolescent and adult obesity. But obesity in a child could not only lead to future obesity – it could also be a sign of later anorexia nervosa. In 1966, Drs R.F. Farquharson and H.H. Hyland reported on fifteen patients with anorexia nervosa whom they had treated twenty to thirty years previously. Many of the cases they described had one aspect in common: the child or young person had been fat, had been ridiculed, and had consequently refused to eat. Without obesity, anorexia nervosa might not have been so prevalent. In addition, obesity, in and of itself, was worrisome, and its rise in children and adolescents was increasingly considered to be a problem for a developed nation.[46] In the 1970s, the list of obesity-related complications that had long been of concern remained: respiratory infections; slower than the normal motor development; heart problems, such as hypertension; and feelings of inferiority. And the decades-old fear that obesity in children would lead to obesity as adolescents or adults still persisted.[47] Obesity was a vicious circle that caught a child or a teenager in its grip. For practitioners to be able to help, a clear vision of causation followed by treatment was required.

Cause of Obesity

Today, the perceived causes of obesity in children and teens are numerous, encompassing a wide spectrum of physiological and psychological aspects, behaviours, and the environment – social, cultural, and material – in which they live. Causes of obesity in children and teens in the past, however, were thought to be the same as those of adults: food intake, family environment, which more often than not was seen to be the origin of psychological causes; heredity; physiological causes; and lack of exercise. What differed was that obese adults were blamed for their condition, whereas blame was softened when looking at obesity in children and teens. There was a sense that children, and particularly teens, had not been properly disciplined and as a result weren't accountable. It was considered the mother's responsibility to make her children understand what was best for them.

Poor eating was considered the main cause of obesity in children and adolescents. As one commentator noted in the *The Public Health Journal* in 1928: "[O]ften the child's menu will consist of porridge for breakfast, bread and jam for lunch and more jam and bread for tea; fattening, we will admit, if served in sufficient quantity, but not giving the healthy fat that resists disease."[48] There was no doubt in Lindsay's mind about the cause of obesity in children: they ate too much. An article in *The*

Canadian Nurse recognized that children as young as eight, especially boys, began to eat more than they needed, with some becoming obese. Control over the size of food helpings was needed. Brown and Robertson in their 1948 and 1958 editions of *The Normal Child* deemed fat and flabby teenage boys to be the result of too much sweet/starch consumption.[49] In the 1960s, snacks were especially popular among the youth. One advertisement for Preludin let its medical readers know that youth ate too much "CANDY SODAS SUNDAES SNACKS." Certainly, there was a sense that too many teenagers "overload[ed]" on the wrong food. Indeed, it was a sign of youth culture. Doughnut-eating contests didn't help children's weight either.[50]

Eating, however, was more complex than it looked. In 1967, John R. Beaton authored an article entitled "Energy Balance and Obesity" in the *CJPH*, which used a 1956 American study to tell readers that obese high school girls did not eat as much as their peers who were not obese. The situation was different for obese children, whose food intake was more than that of average-weight children. Society also played a part in food intake. In 1967, A.M. Bryans, writing in the *CJPH*, blamed "the advanced technology of food production and distribution" for encouraging young Canadians to eat more than they needed. Discussing the shift from Canada's Food Rules to Canada's Food Guide, J.E. Monagle, chief of the Nutrition Division of the Department of National Health and Welfare, observed that one of the problems with the rules had been "that the quantities recommended resulted in calorie excess for young children."[51] The result could be weight gain to the point of becoming overweight or obese.

Understanding food intake was becoming more sophisticated. As the section on infants indicates, the concept of developing fat cells due to overfeeding became popular in the 1970s. "Juvenile-onset obesity" was an extension of this idea. Such cells never disappeared; only their size lessened if weight loss occurred. While this theory certainly represented a physiological reason for obesity, it could only happen through overeating.[52] The intake of food and fattening food was the most accepted cause of obesity. A Winnipeg school study suggested lunch programs in schools resulted in "excessive" weight gain among some children. Added to that was the poor food selection offered in school vending machines and cafeterias. Neither did nutritional education seem successful. Experts were still complaining that Canadians didn't know what foods to eat. Children were still eating too many candies or sweets.[53] Why? Was it because there was no promotional crusade that could rival what children and teens heard on the radio, or saw on TV, on the billboards, and in the stores? Could the nutritional crusade not compete with childhood lore learned at the family dinner table? Or was it because the advice kept changing? Was eating even the culprit? Certainly, some argued that obese children did not indulge in eating sugar – empty calories – any more than thin children did.[54]

If some obese children (or teens) didn't eat more food than others, something else must be at work. While research was ongoing, physicians could only offer limiting food intake as a solution to offset the body's "problem." Unlike adults, children and teens were not totally in control of what they ate, and their family situation had, of necessity, to be of interest. In the early decades, as noted in chapter one, mothers were blamed for the malnutrition of their children, both the malnutrition associated with being underweight and, at times, with being overweight.[55]

By the 1940s, the work of Hilde Bruch with fat children in the United States and her focus on mothers and the psychological relationship between them and their children was introduced to Canadians. In an article in the February 1948 issue of *Chatelaine*, Chant Robertson described to readers how Bruch determined that many of the fat children she worked with had never learned to eat properly. Mothers were to blame: they tended to keep their children bottle feeding too long and to be overprotective. Immigrant mothers gave their children too much food as a sign of love and a symbol of their determination to make sure their children would not experience the kind of deprivation they had lived through. A news brief on Bruch reported her view that for some fat children their size gave them "a feeling of strength, safety and power,"[56] a reason to eat even more.

Bruch's work became recognized as the most significant contribution in the field of childhood and teen obesity, and her psychological perception of the family and eating was taken up in the Canadian medical literature. An editorial in the September 1955 issue of the *CMAJ* reported on an American study that presented two family scenarios involving obese children. The first featured a family in which everyone was obese and accepted the fact. The second described a fat child with a thin mother who both criticized her child's size and encouraged her child's eating habits. The first scenario was a "harmless situation"; in the second, there was a psychological cause stemming from an unhealthy dynamic between mother and child revolving around food. The second scenario was one that Bruch had popularized.[57] Whether Canadian practitioners accepted the full depth of Bruch's psychological approach was doubtful. Their hesitancy didn't mean that they rejected her work, just that they accepted more traditional mother-blaming, based on the dominant role the mother played in children's lives – fat or not. And in the 1950s, more mothers were working outside the house. Certainly, doctors recognized the cultural factors affecting families. For example, one Toronto study mentioned Jewish children, who constituted 38 per cent of the students in the study. The study's summary of these children concluded: "Eating habits and social attitudes tend to make many in this group overweight."[58]

Daniel Cappon, an associate professor in the Department of Psychiatry, University of Toronto, was very familiar with Bruch's theories. In 1958, he reported to his colleagues her argument that the dominant figure in the lives of obese children was the mother who was "incapable of giving her child love" and consequently "substitute[d] food" for love. While finding Bruch's work "brilliant," he did question her research methodology. Where were the controls in her study? Where was the "proof that any one family constellation of interpersonal dynamics and values [would] result in obesity"? Instead, Cappon accepted Freud's theories as proof of a situation more or less standard across families. For example, in explaining obesity in girls, he argued: "A girl's overeating may result from penis envy expressed ... with the phantasy of incorporating the male phallus ... To the child's mind, rather logically if the baby is in the tummy, it gets there through the mother's eating too much."[59] In his view, overeating in girls could be the expression of a desire to have a child and be like their mothers. The psychological cause could be complex and multifaceted. Whether the psychological was the cause or the consequence of obesity was never clear.

The psychology of the family had become an interesting aspect of obesity literature and continued to be into the 1960s and 1970s. Picking up on Bruch, Sheila Kieran in *Chatelaine* referred to food being a mother's substitute for love of her children; children also learned that food was a reward for certain behaviour.[60] The medical and health literature accepted psychological factors as a source of obesity, but made the point only in passing, perhaps because most practitioners were not adept at working with or understanding the psyche of their young patients. In the later years of the 1960s and the 1970s, many teens seemed to embrace a culture that was contrary to family and society – in fashion, music, and even politics. An article written by Maurice Jetté, William Barry, and Dr Lyon Pearlman, Department of Paediatrics, Children's

Hospital of Eastern Ontario, focused on psychology. Obese teenage girls had problems with the "adolescent female role," while obese teenage boys "show[ed] few masculine interests." Both sexes tended "to have fewer successes, function poorly in the academic setting, and have a high failure rate along with acute attendance problems."[61] As in earlier years with malnutrition, obesity became a signifier for youth's other problems. Such a listing of difficulties could only produce anxiety for Canadians about child and teen obesity.

More common than psychological assessment was the perspective articulated by Mrs Ruth Mowat, from Burlington, Ontario, a member of Calorie Counters: "[N]othing ... breaks my heart more than to see an overweight child. There is no excuse for it, and it definitely reflects on the parents." But just as children didn't have control over their food, neither did the individual family. Parents were bombarded with advice about proper and sufficient nutrition. In their efforts to ensure the latter, some families were encouraging their children to eat more, believing that there was no optimum situation – a "more is better" syndrome. Adelaide Daniels, the founder of many Canadian Weight Watchers groups, heard the same story from obese adults: "'My mother forced me to clean my plate as a child.' 'My mother gave me chocolate cookies when the boys bullied me.' My mother this, my mother that. They don't understand that although mother meant well, she was misguided by today's standards."[62] Yet standards for eating kept changing, so what had been learned at one point in life didn't remain the "best practice."

When mothers were blamed, it was usually with little analysis of the reasons. Most mothers certainly did not overfeed their children through malice, so pundits looked to their ignorance of nutrition, ignorance that some physicians shared. And if mothers were not ignorant, they were seen as "frustrated," "demanding," and fussing over their obese children.[63] But even when mothers knew what to feed their children, it wasn't always easy to get the child or teen to eat it. Their agency may not have been an adult's, but they did have ways to get what they liked to eat. Indeed, families had their traditional foods. Different families ate different foods, ate the same food differently, and saw food in different ways. Food was enmeshed in a heritage that was central to how a family saw itself. Eating habits were not going to be easy to change.

Given the psychology surrounding youth and eating and mother-blaming in the literature, it's not surprising that practitioners and families looked to something beyond blaming individuals. Certainly, Canadians were aware that weight seemed to be characteristic in some families. Yet, seldom in the early decades was heredity discussed beyond listing it as a cause of obesity. In the mid-century, many physicians, such as Laski, realized that genetics was a possible factor in accounting for childhood obesity, but they also recognized that children learned eating behaviour from their parents. The nature/nurture debate was difficult to disentangle. Nevertheless, as described in chapter three, heredity was given some importance when statistics were attached to it. In 1963, W.W. Hawkins, National Research Council, Atlantic Region Laboratory, Halifax, described the common conclusion reached by surveys of obesity: studies saw a positive correlation between obesity in children and in their parents. However, he and others warned that environmental aspects of obesity causation were so numerous and complex that separating heredity from them was "nearly impossible."[64] Despite naysayers, heredity continued to be listed as a factor in obesity through the 1970s.[65] What it didn't explain was the growing rate of obesity in children and teens.

Faced with an obese child or teen, practitioners' first question to answer was whether there was a physical disorder causing the obesity. In the 1920s, physicians were quite taken by a number of cases of obesity in children that seemed linked to the failure of their endocrine system. An example was Alfred Froelich's (Fröhlich) syndrome, which was caused by a pituitary disorder and resulted in obesity more often in boys, with genital smallness, and a more feminine demeanour. While it was a popular explanation, even Froelich believed the syndrome was relatively rare.[66] Bruch recalled that when she came to the United States in the 1930s, the endocrine theory dominated, with its focus on the pituitary gland. That being the case, she was struck by not finding endocrine problems in the fat children she saw: most of them were quite tall, physically mature, and well nourished, unlike what the conventional endocrine theory suggested. While Bruch's work wasn't well known in Canada until the 1940s, there were physicians who had already rejected the endocrine cause of obesity.[67]

By the 1940s, the endocrine cause of obesity in children was coming under major criticism, as it had for adults. Yet, many physicians were not willing to renounce a physical cause. More often than not, they focused on some kind of disturbance of the thyroid or another part of the endocrine system. While Lindsay in 1941 believed that most overweight children fell between exogenous and endogenous weight gain, he did write that all obese children "are the result of a peculiar metabolism, which in the last analysis is probably governed by glandular action." How this conclusion was going to help in treatment was unclear, but the evidence he cited for his conjecture was the weight that young people gained at puberty. Lindsay's willingness to even consider endocrine obesity seemed unusual for a time when many physicians were rejecting it as a significant cause in adults. Perhaps his was an optimistic perspective that such a cause in youth would be outgrown or that medical science could manage it.[68]

Nine years later, Laski noted that in the literature on childhood obesity there was still a tendency to emphasize endocrine obesity in adolescent boys whose genitalia seemed small due to endocrine (pituitary) "underfunction," seemingly a reference to Froelich's syndrome. Laski, however, dismissed such a view. He pointed out that obesity rates in the sexes were similar and that many cases of small male genitalia were the result of a growth pattern factor that would soon right itself. Nonetheless, the belief in some kind of glandular cause remained, and drug companies advertised products containing thyroid extract to suppress overeating in children.[69] The use of such products either confirmed a belief in a glandular cause or manipulated the metabolism of an individual's healthy thyroid.

After the 1950s, little was written on endocrine causation. The interest in metabolism, however, seemed to increase in the 1970s, keeping in mind that the endocrine system was linked to metabolism among other aspects in the body. Dr S.S.B. Gilder, in an attempt to be sympathetic, described the overweight child as handicapped, metabolically speaking. A reviewer commenting on a book of essays on adolescent nutrition noted that some of the papers on obesity in the collection raised the issue of metabolic abnormality, although not all authors in the book agreed. Also introduced in the 1970s was the issue of hyperinsulinema (too much insulin in the blood that could be linked to a metabolic disease) in children.[70] But whether it was a cause of obesity or the result was not clear.

If the issue of children and teen eating appeared complex and enmeshed in family dynamics, heredity, and disorders of body, exercise seemed to be much more straightforward. Children and physical play naturally went together. But even exercise had different goals. In the 1920s, Brown encouraged mothers to let their children play outdoors rather than indoors, which he connected to modern living conditions. But his was not a reaction to weight, but more a concern for children's general health. Similarly, a feature article in the 1937 *Canadian Home Journal*, "As the Twig Is Bent," displayed exercises for children. Some were for posture, others for flexibility, and one of them was to create flat tummies. In the examples, three of the four children doing the exercises were girls, suggesting that such exercises were designed for girls to make their bodies attractive. Regarding teens, there was a sense that youth were living dissolute lives, driving around in cars and too often not getting enough exercise,[71] which was perhaps a concern more about morality than weight.

Nevertheless, some Canadians were so worried about the lack of conditioning in young people that Lloyd Percival established a Sports College in 1944 to train youth and those who worked with them. While those involved in physical education were concerned about lack of exercise, physicians such as Brown and Chant Robertson still saw exercise as a health issue, not linked to weight. In 1958, however, Chant Robertson informed her readers in *Chatelaine* that exercise could prevent becoming overweight. Indeed, the activity difference between average-weight and overweight teenage girls was significant – the average-weight girls engaged in strenuous physical activity over three times more often than did the overweight girls.[72]

Concern about lack of exercise in the young increased. In the 1960s, studies conducted by the Canadian Association of Health, Physical Education and Recreation using the Physical Work Capacity test found fitness in children "inferior to that of other groups studied." Commentators on exercise in the young, however, queried how feasible it was to encourage activity in children if society as a whole was not supportive. For example, when interviewed about their fat adolescence, women adults remembered being "dissuaded" from exercise by the stress of the changing rooms at school where other teens could look at them – teens didn't have privacy.[73] Concern about exercise in children and teenagers peaked in the 1970s. Advertisements for ParticipACTION and the supposedly poor health of Canadian children, as compared to Swedish children, dominated the media's perception of the young. A popular insert in many Canadian newspapers showed a "photo of a young, double-chinned boy wearing a t-shirt with the Canadian flag emblazoned on it, slouching in a chair with outstretched legs, holding a pop bottle and eating a hot dog." The caption reinforced the message: "Middle-Aged at 12." Lack of activity would make children "prone" to obesity and all the health problems that came with it. Obesity in children would also weaken their future citizenship and thus the nation[74] at a time when the Cold War was still a danger.

Society had changed, and the activity of children had changed as well. Too often children no longer walked to school, but received rides from their parents or took buses. They also spent more time watching TV, modelling themselves on the behaviour of adults. Instead of playing in a "self-generated" way, children were often engaged in organized activies, especially when they participated in physical exercise, which didn't give each child much free activity time. While it was impossible to say that the decline in activity was a cause of obesity, it was an associated factor.[75] Such linkages, however, led Canadians to draw cause and effect conclusions. Of course, the opposite could also be possible, that is, lack of exercise was not a cause of obesity, but rather obesity resulted in a decline in activity.

In 1975, A.W. Myres explained the complexity of weight in children. What needed to be considered was the "total environment ... social, cultural, medical, economic and psychological." He was not the first to say it. In 1967, A.M. Bryans concluded: "Juvenile obesity is probably a reflection of undefined, complex, and inherited and metabolic factors, aggravated by diet, lack of exercise and other environmental influences. There seem to be both psychological and physiological reasons which make obesity, once established, a self-perpetuating entity."[76] Where that left the obese child, his or her parents, nutritionists, and physicians is unclear. But at least every possible explanation had been covered.

Treatment of Obesity in Children and Teens

Today, the concern about child and teen obesity leads to grasping at any possibility to offset it. But what works? Too often dieting is advised. Yet, what kind of impact does dieting have on a young body? Others concentrate on making sure children develop positive body images, no matter what their weight, because those who have confident, strong body images tend to eat better than those who don't. Counselling young people is popular. Surgery has become a treatment for some teens, and the age at which surgery is allowed is likely to go lower.[77] In the past, treatment of overweight or obese children and adolescents was based on methods used for adults, but adjustments were made due to the youth of the individual being treated. For example, at times no treatment was given for overweight or obese children. Lindsay believed that when children seemed healthy and strong and not worried about how they looked, keeping them under observation was enough. After all, children's growth patterns were individual, and with growth the problem of obesity might disappear. But if the child did complain, either

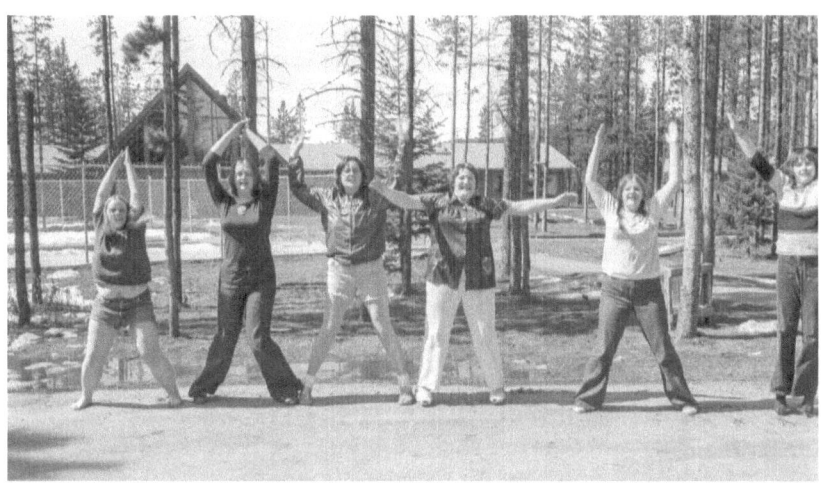

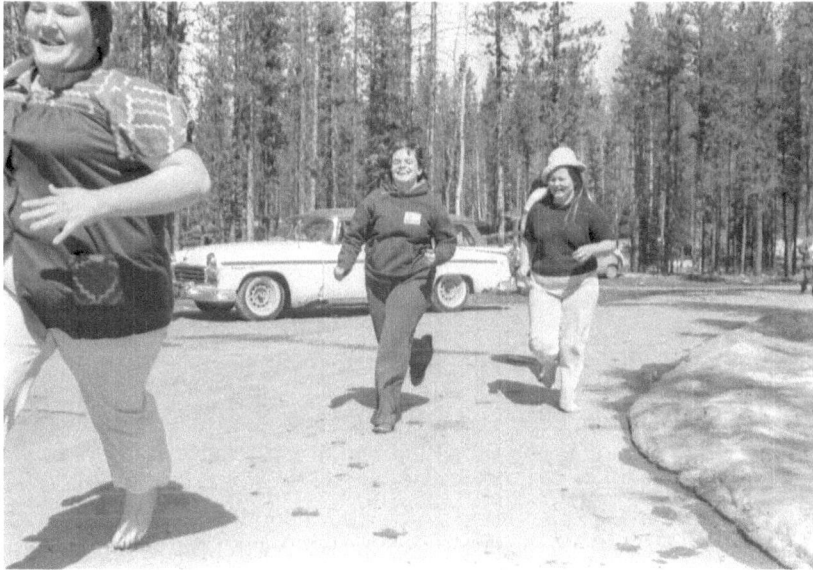

Most teens were sensitive about the appearance of their bodies and particularly their weight. These two photographs of girls exercising accompanied an article in the *Calgary Herald* on 10 April 1974. The top one showed girls "exercising on the spot to slim themselves" at Camp Slim-Teen, and the bottom one pictured girls running "like a page torn out of an army fitness program." Source: Photographer, Ken Sakamoto, *Calgary Herald*; NA-2864–25088a&b (two photos were put together), Glenbow Museum.

about physical problems or psychological issues, treatment should be considered.[78]

Even though dieting was considered the main treatment for adult obesity during the 1920s and 1930s, children and adolescents were not to be put on diets. However, Toronto's Walter R. Campbell made an exception to this rule if the child or teen was "grossly obese," that is, 25 per cent above the normal weight. Dr Dafoe didn't wait for the Dionne quintuplets to become obese before he shifted the food they were eating – specifically limiting starches and sugars. Little changed in the medical view of dieting during the 1940s and the 1950s. The young were not to be placed on reducing diets, especially when they were growing quickly. Altering what children and teens ate, as Dafoe did, was considered a better strategy. For Lindsay, cutting back on fats and carbohydrates and ensuring that protein and green vegetables were consumed was the only recommended "diet" for the young. Chant Robertson noted that changing food habits was easier with younger children; once eating habits had been formed, change was more difficult, perhaps due to "some derangement [in] ... the satiety centre in the brain." In an optimistic tone, however, she suggested "appropriate diets" might offset that issue.[79] But would teenage girls and boys follow an "appropriate" diet?

In 1946, Adele White told her *Chatelaine* readers that teenage girls who had a weight problem needed to "slim down," not through dieting per se, but by eating differently. She advised that ignoring breakfast was not wise, but whether White's idea of breakfast would appeal to teenagers was another issue. She recommended the following: lemon juice slightly sweetened with sugar, accompanied by a spoonful of wheat germ, as a start to the day; followed by an egg (boiled or poached), Melba toast, and skim milk or half coffee and hot milk. In the 1950s, medical journals suggested the Oslo breakfast, a cold breakfast of milk, cheese, salad or fruit, wholemeal bread, and butter or margarine. The goal was to replace "bad" food with "good" food, which meant teens were not to eat their favourite foods. Low-calorie food was also on the market, and L.S. White advised it as a help for those who had to watch their weight, including children. But others considered the real solution to be educating mothers to understand what foods children needed to eat to be healthy.[80]

Changing eating habits was not going to be easy; certainly, once obese, children and adolescents were difficult to treat through diet.[81] In 1962, Mrs S., from Côte Saint-Luc, Montreal, wrote a letter to the

Nutrition Division in Ottawa asking for a calorie chart so that she could keep track of her eleven-year-old daughter's eating. The girl was fat, but didn't seem to eat much, although Mrs S. did admit that her daughter ate six or seven candies at home each day. Mrs S. also noted that her husband's family put on weight easily. Yet, her older daughter wasn't fat, and the mother wanted her younger daughter to "have a nice figure when she grows up to be a young lady." J.E. Monagle answered the letter and basically advised the mother to take her daughter to a physician for advice and to follow the Canada's Food Guide. He did mention the number of candies the girl was eating, and warned that, unless "these are extraordinarily small candies," they would weaken the girl's nutrition and/or her "dental health." The mother was considered to be the key to changing the child's eating habits. Teenagers, however, were notorious for their bad eating habits, and *Chatelaine* responded with an article entitled "Your Diet That Lets You Eat Your Cake and Look Slim, Too." The article proposed a balanced diet designed to allow for "delicious snacking." From a list of bonus foods, the teen could choose one snack a day: 1 Coke, 8 ounces of ginger ale, 12 potato chips, 16 peanuts, 10 cashew nuts, or 3 marshmallows. Prohibited were milkshakes, malted milk, chocolate bars, doughnuts, and chocolate cake.[82] Whether a teenager could keep to twelve potato chips was anyone's guess.

Severe dieting for the young seldom met with approval. One unattributed article in the 1975 *CMAJ* referred to the use of Simeons' 500-calorie diet along with injections of human chorionic gonadotropin (HCG). As the physician reporting on this treatment stated, the whole method was questionable. The diet did not "support the child's growth needs," and neither was it clear what effect it would have on puberty. An editorial in the *CMAJ* also warned against young children's use of saccharin because of its potential carcinogenic nature.[83] Some diets, however, were deemed necessary, especially when children had other health issues. Obesity was a factor for children with mild hypertension, so placing them on a diet, especially one that lowered salt intake, was deemed important. Of course, such a diet was easier to manage for children than for teenagers.[84] Looking at the family, Gilder suggested that it was not fair or even feasible to put a child on a diet and have everyone else in the family eat in a normal, or even an abnormal, way. The "family must help and regard the child as handicapped." The family's responsibility was to adopt the eating lifestyle that the child needed in order to lose weight and maintain that loss.[85] Missing in the advice was how other children in the family might react to having their food habits changed, or how a mother would be able to make this change if one of her other children needed to eat more. The complicated balancing act of feeding the needs of each child was overlooked.

Two adjuncts to dieting for adults, psychological therapy and drugs, were also tried with children and teens, although there wasn't a lot of literature on treating children with therapy. Certainly, physicians counselled their child patients. They tried to determine from these children and their parents (mostly the mothers) what their home life was like and what factors might be at work to make them overeat. Little psychological/psychotherapy treatment itself appeared before the mid-century, and even when it was available, two problems existed. First, by the time an obese child was brought to a therapist, the child's experiences in the world would have undermined his or her confidence. Second, the child needed the support of one of the parents to commit to the therapy, or the child was not going to be able to face whatever the underlying factors were that led to overeating. Early in the 1960s, Dr Martin Wolfish, associate professor of paediatrics at the University of Toronto, rejected psychiatry, noting that teenagers sent to a psychiatrist were singled out, making them feel strange. What they needed was understanding and common sense, both of which a general practitioner could provide. Neither was behaviour modification as effective as it was for adults. However, doctors agreed that "self-acceptance" was important for youth and that psychological support, whether through counselling or other means, was beneficial.[86] At the very least, as with adults, it would make patients feel that they were not alone.

Appetite suppressants were used on children and teens seemingly more than any kind of formal psychological counselling. As previous noted, the acceptance of the metabolic/endocrine cause of obesity in some children was widespread during the interwar period, with the result that thyroid extract was used to raise the basic metabolic rate, thus increasing energy expenditure. One of the treatments tried for Froelich's syndrome was injections of testicular extract along with pituitary injections, but many were wary of this option. The treatment certainly didn't seem to be used much in Canada.[87] In his 1941 article, Lionel Lindsay was willing to consider thyroid extracts for children at puberty only as long as the doses were small and the child was being carefully monitored by medical personnel. For Lindsay, the use of thyroid extract was "palliative" in effect. It managed to stabilize the metabolic system until "nature ... establish[ed] a more normal balance for the fat regulating mechanism." If that happened, then any psychological problems and physical challenges due to being overweight would be offset during adolescence, leading to a well-adjusted and healthy adult. Lindsay also suggested to his colleagues that benzedrine sulphate in small doses was helpful to encourage overweight children to be more active. The drug stimulated physical activity, and Lindsay had heard that it also depressed the appetite. But not all were happy with the use of benzedrine. In 1946, Leonora Hawirko and P.H. Sprague reported in the *CMAJ* that physicians elsewhere did not believe young people tolerated it well. What they recommended was d-amphetamine.[88]

While Bruch, in her book *The Importance of Overweight* (1957), rejected drugs as "useless" for children and adolescents, Dr Antonio Martel from Quebec City approved of Preludin (phenmetrazine) as safe for treating children. Other drugs, too, were available for children. Obedrin (methamphetamine, mood-lifting; pentobarbital, calming; plus vitamins) advertised that it could be prescribed for children, as did Probese TD & VM, which promoted a new and milder form "for the pediatric case." Dexedrine came out with a lower-dose version for use in treating children and geriatric patients.[89]

In the 1960s, drug advertisements increasingly appealed to the concern about adolescent vulnerability in their formative years. One advertisement for Ambar #2 Extentabs (metamphetamine hydrochloride and phenobarbital) had as its visual an older girl sitting on the sidelines at a dance. The text addressed doctors: "She tries to lose weight – but her emotions won't let her. She becomes irritable and depressed when she doesn't eat, and anxious when she considers her future … 'What can I do?' she asks when she visits your office." The answer for the physician, of course, was easy – prescribe Ambar #2 Extentabs. The drug would stabilize her emotions so she could stay on a diet and suppress her appetite so she would not want to eat as much. The advertisement for such products made losing weight seem easy and the physician's task manageable, promising a successful treatment. Not all drugs, however, were safe for children or adolescents. Advertisements for Durabolin warned that its composition (nandrolone phenpropionate) warranted caution if given to women and children, since they were "more sensitive to any degree of androgenic stimulation and should be watched for signs of virilization." Too large a dose could also "inhibit" menstruation.[90] Older girls often purchased over-the-counter diet Ayds. In the October issue of *Chatelaine*, an advertisement featured the testimony of a teenage girl, who described her fight with weight and stressed that nothing worked until she followed her mother's example and used the "Ayds Vitamin and Mineral Reducing Plan." She continued to lose weight, but was persuaded to stop taking Ayds by her parents. At that point, she put the weight back on. But, by using Ayds again, she lost weight and was "nominated for the Centennial Queen of Leamington [Ontario] Pageant." She didn't win, but in her words "it sure felt good competing with all those other, lovely slim contestants."[91]

Despite the concern of the wider society about non-medical drug abuse by young people in the 1970s, prescribing drugs for children and teens remained popular if the advertisements in the medical journals reflected reality. The marketers of Pondimin (fenfluramine) advertised in medical journals that their product would help teenagers "resist temptation without emotional aggravation." One of its advertisements showed a visual of a teenage girl. In bold type, the ad assured its readers: "NON-STIMULATING ANOREXIANT HELPS TEENAGERS LOSE WEIGHT WITHOUT LOSING THEIR COOL." The focus here was not on obesity per se, but on simply losing weight, keeping a certain figure.[92] As noted earlier, some health experts even supported the use of HCG for "obese, sexually immature young males." It was a tool and not a cure, but for some it did result in "a remarkable reduction in the waist and hips." Canadian youth were fortunate that HCG wasn't one of the favoured appetite suppressants.[93]

The concern about lack of fitness in children and teens, coupled with the "energy in" versus "energy out" equation, meant exercise became a partner to dieting. Mason, in his 1924 article, did not approve dieting for children and only accepted minor exercise. Lindsay's article in 1941 suggested physical activity in the form of swimming or cycling for obese children whose movements were limited and who were indolent because of their weight. But not everyone saw exercise as a solution – imposing exercise on young people was not going to be easy. The concern of teenage girls about their bodies, however, was such that they were often willing to do what was needed, even exercise. For them, it was about becoming attractive, and being fat in their eyes was not attractive.[94] After World War II ended, Canadians were worried about a decline in youth activity. While exercise was something that was good for health, in and of itself, some saw exercise as an aid to losing weight. Dr Richard Goldbloom did. He especially approved of walking, and felt that it was easy for an overweight child to do. He also criticized high school exercise periods – there were not enough of them, and the exercise followed wasn't strenuous enough to help weight loss.[95]

Consensus about the value of exercise for health existed, but as a weight-loss treatment it was contentious. But if exercise wasn't key to weight reduction, it couldn't hurt. With that thought in mind, some healthcare workers developed programs to get obese adolescents involved in team sports to see if group physical activity would improve their self-image and their health. If both changed, perhaps their eating habits would change as well. The whole push for Canadians to be more active throughout the 1970s included youth. That obesity was a problem among the young emerged in separate programs for them such as "Fun and Fitness" at the obesity clinic in Cochrane, Alberta. In this program, children (ages six to fourteen) and their parents received training (separately) about nutrition and eating habits, followed by discussion of the problems the youngsters were facing and then exercise, be it dancing or sports.[96] But there weren't many such programs.

Conclusion

Obesity in Canada's infants, children, and teens in the past prompted an emotional reaction that adult obesity didn't. Adults were expected to control their bodies, but that couldn't be asked of infants and young children or even teenagers. The concern about obesity existed in the 1920s, albeit not significantly, but with each decade that concern increased; by the 1950s, it became a medical issue. The perceived causes of obesity in infants were very contentious, revolving around breastfeeding versus formula bottle feeding. The age for weaning was also debated. For children and teens, the causes of obesity were similar to those in adults, but in a different context. Eating too much was seen as the major cause, but the family environment was more of a consideration for youth. What teens ate was effected by the youth culture – milkshakes, snack food, and soda pop. Physiological causes seemed more significant in the young than in adults, but the reason was most likely variation in the age of development. It was difficult to blame children or even teens for their weight. As a result, a body-based cause – heredity or metabolic/endocrine disorder – helped practitioners to understand how a small child could become a fat child. With the discovery of the fat cells, first in infants and then in the young, a cause that appealed to practitioners emerged, even if the reason for the cells was overeating. Whatever the cause, the mother was seen as the responsible individual to blame.

Treatment for infants was limited to mothers understanding that a fat infant was not a healthy one and that overfeeding infants was harmful. By the end of the 1920s, treatment of obesity in children and teens was largely fixed – limited dieting, drug treatment (usually with thyroid extracts), and some exercise – and remained so throughout the period under review. Drug treatments other than thyroid extracts and very limited attempts at psychological counselling were added, but other than that, treatment seldom varied. How successful treatment was depended on those assessing the treatment. For example, Lindsay didn't think any of the treatments that he suggested – dieting, exercise, or use of drugs – would change the constitution of the child or alter the endocrine system. And, certainly, teens' growth at puberty complicated treatment. The best that could be hoped was that such efforts were palliative until the child grew and the teen matured. By 1975, little had changed vis-à-vis prognosis. Any "long-term" success in treating obesity in children was estimated at less than 20 per cent. Wolfish concluded (or hoped) efforts to "improve appearance, physical fitness and self-acceptance" were much more successful.[97] Certainly, appearance or body image has been central. Older children and teens learned how their bodies compared to others and to ideal body types that formed the "normal" adult image.

7 Body Image

"Whether we like it or not, middle-age starts at about age 26. After that there is often deterioration."[1]

Historians have offered rich and prolific histories of how the body has been perceived, idealized, and treated. Although they have not looked at the fat body very much, central to any study of obesity or fatness is the concept of body image. Over time and cultures, body image has denoted health, age, attractiveness, and acceptance. In the twentieth century, weight has been part of how we evaluate those traits.[2] Health experts, too, have used a patient's body image to assess fatness and wellness along with body measurements. Canadians have done the same, using their own bodies. They ask themselves: "Is my body attractive or handsome?" "Am I fat?" "Am I too fat?" "Does my weight stop me doing things?" "Am I healthy?" Body image is significant in how we see ourselves. This chapter examines how the popular media put forward an idealized body in the past. Indeed, throughout their lives, the media tells Canadians what their body should be. *Maclean's*, *Chatelaine*, *Canadian Home Journal*, and Eaton's fashion catalogues, among others, constructed ways to show people what the ideal body should be through advertisements, articles, fiction, and clothes (including the models wearing them). Most media used the slender, white, middle-class body to attract consumers. Those who were overweight could only see themselves in a few advertisements for specific products and in certain clothes. Obese citizens almost never saw themselves – they were outliers who didn't fit into society. Older Canadians, too, were outside the idealized body. Indeed, media often placed aging and fatness together. Canadians learned from the media that bodies should not be fat. Even doctors, before they were physicians, learned from the media.

The chapter is divided into two sections. The first looks at articles, fiction, and advertisements in popular magazines to show how gender and stage of life shaped the ideal body image. The three narrative forms used bodies to sell products, including the magazines themselves. Through the magazines, Canadians could see what the ideal body was and what it was not. The second section is an analysis of Eaton's catalogues from 1920 to 1976, using clothing sizes, fashion silhouettes, and both men's and women's clothes.[3] Clothes are significant. As Joanne Entwistle reminds us, the familiar body image we see is a "dressed" one. A dressed body is reflective of an attempt at order, and Entwistle maintains that an inability to dress "appropriately" creates an outsider status.[4] By the 1920s, ready-made clothes were available; as a result, the pressure to fit into a specific body size was significant, which meant more attention was given to weight. As discussed in the following two sections, gender, age, and weight/heaviness were symbols of body, and together they created visual personas.

Gender, Age, and Fat in the Media

The aftermath of World War I resulted in a new style, a veneer of a different society in which youth appeared more carefree, self-centred, and engaged with living life to the full. The visual representation of an ideal body shifted. The slender body dominated articles, advertisements, and stories. The fat body could be found but was usually portrayed in a negative way. The slender body silhouette of women was pervasive, accentuated by the fashions of the time, especially for young women. The popular media used women's bodies more than men's to sell products, especially body products. Women seemed the primary consumers of body image. An article in the *Canadian Home Journal*, entitled "Minimizing One's Size: By Wearing Just the Right Clothes," was directed at "mature" women with "well-developed figures." The author argued that "there is no great crime in being large," yet the whole article focused on teaching women how to dress to look thinner. Aging and fat were enemies of women, diminishing their attractiveness. Women were inundated with the tribulations of an aging body. They had to beware the age of forty, when hair started to become grey, chins sagged, and bodies were no longer slim.[5] A Bissell rug cleaner advertisement depicted, in cartoon form, a woman and her mother-in-law, the younger woman shown slender (if rounded) and the mother-in-law drawn with a large bosom, abdomen, and buttocks.[6] The mother-in-law's heavier body signified age. Age was seen as the dominant factor for being overweight. But is it? Could it be that a woman who is fat looks older than one who is not overweight? An article in *Chatelaine* described what was wanted from a woman's body: "curves without fat." In the depths of the Depression, women sitting at a desk all day were warned about developing concave chests and rather large bottoms.[7] Women needed to work on their bodies, and they couldn't begin too young. Walking for girls was a body-shaping exercise of sorts, but they were encouraged to walk as though their head was a flower on a stalk. By doing so, they were told, they would be less likely to develop a dowager's hump when they reached middle age.

The fiction of the time often reflected and reinforced the gendered aspects of society along with the ideal weight and age. Certain themes emerged over time: the association of overweight characters with negative attributes; the beauty of the slim young woman; the inability of the overweight woman to be her own woman; and the absence of overweight people as the main characters in a romance. In fiction, the older fat woman was often a negative character. In the 1929 story "Platitoodinous Hooey," such a character was "the ruddiest, homeliest matron ... fat and ... forty; in fact forty-three or forty-four ... and she was angry ... [a] virago." Her age and her fat meant that she was no longer seen as a woman. The only positive characteristics for an aging woman were being "kind, motherly, and self-effacing," but certainly not attractive or sexual.[8]

The consort of the 1920s flapper was slight compared to young men today. A photograph of weightlifters from the Vancouver Police Mutual Benevolent Association showed young, active, lean, almost thin men.[9] Marketers, however, used muscle on young men to designate both attractiveness and health. Such men were depicted, for example, as water skiers in Canada Dry advertisements. These types of advertisements suggested the hardness, energy, and stamina of the male body,[10] and those men got the girl. The fiction story "Ginger Ale and Pop" was about two young people. Ginger was a debutante who was in the limelight due to her willingness to take risks. Her friend Augustus, also known as "Pop," was a friend who kept an eye on her, protected her, and eventually foiled thieves who were after her diamond ring. Pop was the hero of the story, but he didn't get the girl because he was "a stocky, slow moving youth" – Ginger's mother saw him as a "perfectly

210 Fighting Fat

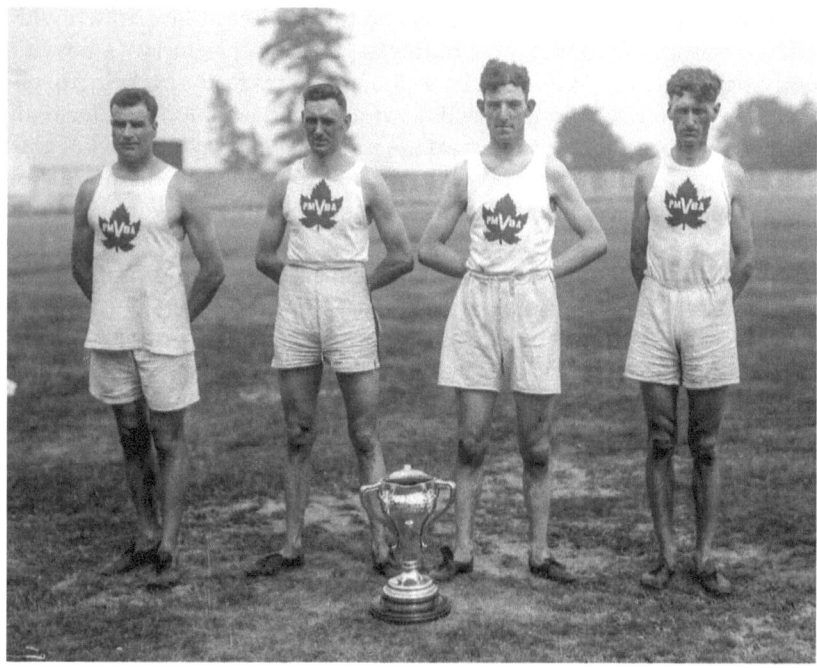

These men's bodies are slender or even thin, although they were champion weightlifters from the Vancouver Police Mutual Benevolent Association in 1923. Their bodies would have been considered exemplary for the time. The contrast with bodybuilders today, who manifest greater bulk and extreme definition of musculature, is striking. Source: Photographer, Stuart Thomson, 1923; AM1535-: CVA 99–1022, City of Vancouver Archives.

nice, perfectly pure-minded bovine." He just didn't have the quality to marry a slim and beautiful girl.[11] Like women, men also aged and put on pounds. In his article "Me-Athlete" in *Maclean's*, Hugh Grant Rowell warned that too many men worked at a desk and lived a sedentary life. Even men who still laboured with their body were using more machines.[12] Rowell's article was published during the Depression when too many men were losing their employment. Those men who had jobs were lucky, but their manhood still needed a strong body. Unlike fat

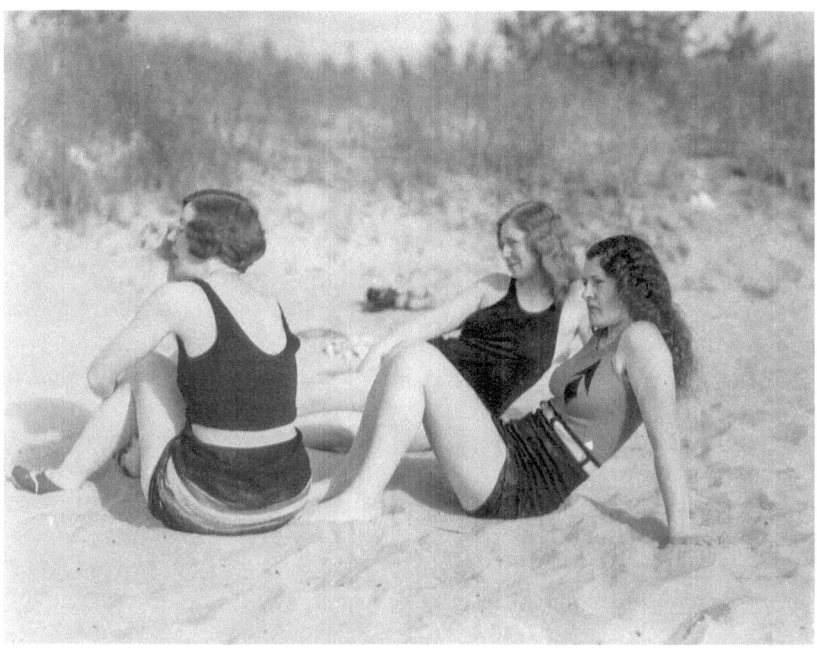

These young women's bodies conform to the slender image of the flapper era of the 1920s, and their swimming suits highlight this slender image. Source: 1925, 10012507.jpg, Archives of Ontario.

women in stories, fat men were given all sorts of character traits. Overweight men and men who were no longer young and slim could still have a positive image. A story told of Mrs Grange, who was contemplating leaving her husband because he was "growing a little stout." But at the end of the story, Mrs Grange learned that she still loved him. The story might have had a happy ending, but readers could draw the lesson that husbands should not get fat in the first place. Other fat male characters could be found: benign fellows, villains, men with a happy disposition and willing to use their experience to help others, and successful older, portly men.[13] Fat men could see themselves in many fictional personae.

World War II added certain perspectives to body image. For men, the ideal was the soldier – a young man who was healthy enough to be accepted to fight for his country. But even older men could become heroes. A story described the actions of retired Captain Mannering, who with his young grandson went to Dunkirk to help the British soldiers stranded there. He subsequently went on a military mission where he was killed rescuing a wounded soldier. During the mission, Mannering lost the extra weight he had gained over time – "the paunch that gave majesty to his figure," but a "majesty" that was no longer positive in war.[14] During the war, young women were taken to task for their fixation on being underweight – their country needed strong women to take men's places in the workforce. But a strong body didn't mean being overweight. Women working in sedentary war work had to keep track of their weight.[15] Women still needed to be attractive. Middle-aged women who were not sedentary in their work could comfort themselves that standing most of the day would prevent "middle-aged spread."[16] Being attractive was even measured. For example, *Chatelaine* had a list of measurements for the ideal body against which young women could compare their own bodies.[17]

How could men show their manhood once the war was over? Some advertisements surrounded men's bodies with the accoutrements of success, such as cars and young slender women. Other advertisements encouraged men to purchase chest expanders, among other body developing aids, the fear being that the increasing number of sedentary jobs available to middle-class men would weaken them.[18] Middle-aged men, too, had problems because of their aging bodies. In one story, Ellen Tate found out her husband Leonard was having an affair with a much younger woman. When the young woman came to see Ellen to work out their situation, Ellen scared her off by letting her know that Leonard kept putting on weight and was losing his hair as well as using hair colour. The message was clear – having an affair with an older man was understandable, but not with a man who was starting to look older *and* overweight.[19] Men like Leonard had to deal with their bones becoming "more brittle, muscles los[ing] resilience, and the fibres of the arteries [growing] less springy." Not a happy image. No wonder some men looked to a "magic potion" – testosterone – to renew their youth. But, as Sidney Katz explained to his *Maclean's* readers, it wasn't the hormone level that was the problem, but too much eating, overuse of alcohol, overwork, and emotional problems.[20] The various factors meshed with one another. The concept of men's body image permeated society no matter the decade, and while the ideal of that image might alter somewhat, its significance didn't. Men were still being told to remain the same weight as when they were twenty-five years old. At the same time, they had to try to offset the problems that came with being forty.[21]

After the war, women had lost their war jobs, and many had to find other employment. But some jobs looked only to slender, young women. For example, airlines hired female attendants to present a certain impression and gave their attendants lessons in charm and how to keep their weight under control.[22] *Chatelaine* told women to look at their bodies and be honest about "its bulges and sags." Stenographers learned that hips should never be more than four inches larger than their bust. The message went out – fat was ugly, dangerous, and associated with age.[23] No wonder some women saw fatness as negative to the point they felt the help of a doctor was needed. No matter the age, women were warned about problems that undermined their bodies. Articles on weight informed readers that fat was a "beauty defect" and that winter was a particularly dangerous time for weight gain. By April, they needed to "take stock" of their figures and begin to lose weight, work at slimming the waist and derrière, and not forget the upper arms and elbows. Women's lives were brought into line with the cycle of nature, a metaphor that was commonly used for women. No matter what the problem – "Top Heavy ... Thick Waists ... Hips Away ... Problem Legs" – women received endless advice about their bodies.[24] The central character in "The Bequest," a 1958 short story by Yves Theriault, is Edwina, an older, fat, wealthy woman married to Clarence, a much younger man who married her for her money. He begins an affair with Doris, who is much younger than he is. When Edwina dies of cancer, he rushes to Doris to let her know, but she has gone, leaving behind two notes for Clarence. The first is from Doris herself, making it clear she is not interested in being "with a man your age." The second is from Edwina, telling Clarence that she had known about the affair and consequently has left her money to Doris, knowing that Doris would reject him.[25] Edwina was smart and had a strong character, but it was only in death that she was able to get her revenge on Clarence. The story saw Edwina's age and weight as stigma.

Many of the themes continued into the 1960s and 1970s. Both men and women were told that a trim waistline was necessary. Beauty contests depicted ever-slimmer women as a women's ideal body began to weigh even less, although women under the age of thirty had actually become heavier. And, as it had been in the 1950s, the right kind of shape or the right look had implications for women's jobs. A study of full-time workers at York University revealed that in 1977 those who were "good looking" made substantially more money than those who were not, when other variables were held constant. Suzanne Thyer, an artist and illustrator at age twenty-five, was constantly at war with herself. She considered herself a thin fat person, that is, someone who had made herself thin, but was "naturally" overweight. Her battle to keep slim was ongoing, and it didn't seem to make her happy, but then being overweight didn't either.[26] She was in a no-win situation, since an overweight woman is pressured in a negative way by the ideal body image.

Stress was even greater if the woman was middle-aged. June Callwood told *Chatelaine* readers that she was 3 pounds overweight and, as a result, was watching what she ate, eating only an apple for lunch. She felt uncomfortable when overweight, and her clothes felt tight. Her punch line made the point that "the fat that you put on when you're over forty, as I am, is soft ugly fat."[27] Callwood was telling readers that 3 pounds over their "best" weight was a sign of fatness. No wonder more women than men looked to doctors to help them lose their pounds. In stories, older women seldom played a central role. But in one story, an older woman did. In the 1962 December issue of *Chatelaine*, "The Cleverest Christmas" had as the heroine Mrs Stirling, a widow from Saskatchewan visiting her daughter and son-in-law in California for Christmas. Mrs Stirling was "small and plump, wore flowered print dresses and her soft curly hair was plain untinted grey." She was not the kind of woman her son-in-law thought would impress his friends, but it turned out the California set loved her down-to-earth attitude and her belief in what Christmas was about.[28] But then she was "plump," not fat. Words chosen about fat mattered.

Variation in men's bodies still seemed to be more accepted compared to women's. Even when a man was overweight, wearing a business suit could offset (or hide) any weight issues he might have. But there were limits. Indeed, for their health as well as their looks, men were still expected to stay at the weight they were when twenty-five. Even the popular actor Al Waxman had to obey a network directive to lose weight in order to keep his television show *King of Kensington*.[29] *Maclean's* Dorothy Sangster warned that the middle-aged man was at risk for cancer, diabetes, heart problems, and arthritis. Even without any of those health problems, a middle-aged man peering at himself in a mirror with his diminishing sight would see an "expanded" waist and thinning or greying hair. Canadians may have been trying to keep their weight down, but, by the 1970s, some boomers were reaching thirty, and their bodies were changing. John Hofsess in *Maclean's* told readers that the years between twenty-five and thirty-five were years of deterioration, especially for men. By letting their body decline, men lost "self-respect."[30] In chapter four, we saw advertisements promising men a hard, firm body with only seventy seconds of exercise a day. A similar advertisement in the 1970s promised a "rock-hard lean stomach" that could be achieved in seven minutes a day through synometrics (muscle contractions). For men, body building aids and equipment were popular: chest expanders, protein powders, and the traditional barbells and benches. Ben Weider's protein tablets, associated with male bodybuilding, were widely advertised. A simpler solution was to develop a good posture that would make a man "more vigorous, youthful and lively."[31] The body had become a battle ground.

You wouldn't think that an automobile advertisement would be germane to a study on obesity, but the 1979 Honda Accord sales pitch was. In big, bold letters it exclaimed: "**TWO LUXURY CARS THAT AREN'T OVERWEIGHT, SHORT OF BREATH AND OUT OF SHAPE**." The advertisement referred to other luxury cars as being "marshmallows on wheels," but assured readers that performance cars – the Honda Accord Hatchback and Sedan – were what they wanted. Making reference to the size of luxury cars and their performance (or lack of) played into the image of fat people at the time.[32] Too often, being fat was an isolating and stigmatizing condition. Those who were overweight were referred to as the "overweights," as if being fat was their identity and designation.[33] In looking at the media's ideal body, most readers didn't see themselves. Who could ever have an ideal body? But outliers from the norm would see much to remind them what they and others saw as negative – being fat or being older, or both.

The advertisements, fiction, and articles of the media used the idealized body image to get Canadians' attention. The image, however, was not possible for most people. Indeed, the media employed the negative aspect of the body – aging and fat – to give a sense that Canadians should do something to get over the negativity. But it was also through the media that readers "learned" what the problems of their bodies were and how they might overcome them. For sixty years the problems did not go away – only different people aged and felt they were fat. Many Canadians got an education of a kind through the media, and doctors received some of the same education.

Body Image and Clothing in Eaton's

All the effort to create an attractive body was for nought if clothes did not show it off.[34] The Eaton's catalogue was a touchstone for Canadians. Its pages depicted an idealized body for both men and women. To sell clothing, Eaton's used illusion, offering their customers a dream of how they would look when they wore Eaton's clothes, even though the clothes were largely for everyday use. Clothing is a consumer product that allows the individual to choose a particular image she or he wishes to project. But the choices were constrained by what was available, especially for fat people. Everyone needs clothes, and not being able to find clothes that fit could emphasize that your body was not right.

In understanding body image, sizes of clothes are important. Eaton's catalogues had sized clothes for bodies – short, medium, or tall; and small, regular, or large – based on measurements of chest, waist, and hip. The result was a myriad of clothing categories: half-sizes, misses, junior, women's, young men's, regular men's, king, and stout, among others. Sizes for children and teens were also available. The measurements used for a size kept changing, especially for women, and various sizes could overlap in different categories. Eaton's clothing sizes had standardized measurements, but if you did not fit the standard measurements for your size, you would have problems finding clothes that fit well and the clothes would instead call unwanted attention to your body and body weight.

While standard sizes of clothes had to acknowledge the reality of bodies, the message surrounding clothes was one of fashion and transformation. The visuals of models were drawn before the use of photographs became more common. Drawings of women were especially elongated – overly thin ankles, long slender fingers, long torso and legs, and ethereal-looking arms. These visuals were an illusion. While the 1920s was a golden age of sport for women, the drawings didn't show strong women. Men did not escape the emphasis on being slender, but the visuals were quite different in nature. For one, the drawings of men gave them much more substance than women. In the 1920s and 1930s, photographs of men in the catalogues outnumbered those of women, and the photographs reflected reality to a much greater extent than the drawings. When photographs of models became the norm, from the 1940s on, both men and women looked larger than what the drawings had depicted. Basically, the photographs reflected reality more than the drawings had. The more frequent depiction of older men also stood out compared to older women. Indeed, the age spectrum for men in the catalogues was more varied than for women. While in the 1930s and subsequent decades the age spread of women portrayed increased, older women remained a small minority; elderly women were non-existent. For women, youth was fashion's norm. Men's faces also showed more variety in the drawings and in the photographs: they had hard-looking faces, sometimes craggy, sometimes with a hooked nose or a moustache. Their faces had character and strength. Even their hair seemed more individual and not just a fashion statement. Hair on men could be full, thinning, or even bald. The drawn visuals of women usually had the same evenly shaped faces. The variation and individuality of men's visuals reflected an ironic dichotomy. The fashions for men were more limited compared to those of women, but the visuals depicting them were more varied.

Gender emerged beyond the fashions and their visuals in the catalogues. In the late 1930s, a made-to-measure system for men's suits and overcoats was available for the average figure and for the "hard to fit" ones, including stout figures.[35] For women, this option was not offered until 1944, and didn't last long or apply to large sizes. Men also seemed to have had access to more personalized sizing. Through to 1976, Eaton's always asked male customers to provide height and weight measurements when ordering certain clothing.[36] While gender dominated in the catalogues, it differentiated between young and older men and young and older women. Weight, too, was a strong issue in that older men and older women were overweight more often than younger adults. Age and weight were also connected to visuals of working-class men and women.

Men's Sizing and Clothes

Men's sizing was generally consistent and logical over time, although measurements of the sizes could differ. From 1920 to 1976, regular men's sizing (36–46) was based on chest measurements: a size 38 meant a 38 inch chest. No hip measurements were given until 1965. Between 1965 and 1976, waist measurement gave a 3-inch range for each size. Stout sizing gradually shifted as well. In the 1920s, the size range was 38–46 and remained a consistent 40–52 from the late 1930s to 1971, when it contracted to 40–46. However, in 1974, king sizes replaced stout sizing and offered sizes 48–54.[37] The body profile was largely consistent as well: rectangular with chest and waist seemingly the same measurement until 1965, when the waist could be smaller than the chest or a bit larger, creating a slight inverted triangle body or a pear-shaped body, respectively.

Boys' sizing ranged from 6 to 20 before 1956; after 1962, there was no size 20. With time, there were changes in waist and chest measurements. Some of the shifts reflected the maturity of the body. For example, the age of puberty became younger between 1920 and 1976. With sizing ranging from a chest size of 24 inches (size 6) to 36 inches (size 18) in 1920 and from 26 inches (size 7) to 34¼ inches (size 18) in 1976, there was a rather broad age group that would go from young boys to youth on the verge of puberty. A significant change in boys' sizing was the husky size, introduced in 1956. Husky was different from regular boys' size in that the waist size was 3 to 4 inches larger. By 1976, the chest measurement for husky size 7 was 3 inches larger than the regular boys' clothing, the waist 2½ inches larger, and the hips 3½ inches larger – all in line with the measurements of a regular size 12. That a husky size 7 boy wasn't simply wearing a regular size 12 suggests a different conformation due to height and perhaps style due to age.

The silhouette of clothing in regular sizes represented the standard of how a man was supposed to look. In the 1920s, clothes suggested a body that was straight from the shoulders to the hip. And the clothing style that best represented this image was the suit. Generally, the suit in Eaton's was a sign of a middle-class professional or a white-collar worker. Regular men's size suits were close fitting, with a single-breasted coat for young men and a more conservative cut for older men. For example, in the 1920 Spring/Summer catalogue, the suits for young men emphasized the appearance of the suit, while for older men the character of the suit was emphasized. The silhouette of the thirties moved away from the more linear look of the 1920s to one that emphasized the breadth at the padded shoulder, which, as a result, accentuated a rather narrow waist. As the representation of the masculine man, the inverted triangle silhouette was the fashion until the 1960s, providing men with a consistent image.

In the 1940s, men in the drawings often had granite-type chins, and some looked like caricatures of comic book heroes; this style was echoed in the language of the text. An advertisement for a two-button single-breasted style of suit described the "square cut shoulders and a collar that hugs the neck … giv[ing] you that masculine look," leaving the potential consumer with the notion that the suit was made for a "real" man. While ages were diverse in the 1940s, young slender men dominated. In the Fall/Winter 1947–48 catalogue, the heading on one page of suits read: "Styled for Young Men and Men Who Stay Young," the latter assuming older men's desire to maintain the allure of youth. By the end of the 1950s, shoulders of suits were not as square as they had been, but trousers were becoming slimmer, closer to the body, thus still maintaining the inverted triangle silhouette.[38]

The silhouettes in the 1960s and 1970s changed more than they had in previous decades. In the early 1960s, there was a narrowing of the body, in particular from the waist downward. While trousers for men were still pleated in the early 1960s, plain fronts were also popular. And suits shoulders seemed slimmer. Slacks for boys and youth emphasized the slimness of body, letting the "true" body show itself. By the late 1960s and in the 1970s, the presence of young men increased in advertisements, but was always offset by the ubiquitous suit that limited how youthful men wearing it could be. The suit was the male uniform and represented the gravitas of citizenship attributed to men; they had been and could still be asked to make the ultimate sacrifice in war, and they were to be the support for their families. Young men might have been the ideal, but they weren't fully adult until they took on responsibilities. Nevertheless, by the mid-1970s, "leisure suits" were available, casual in style and hardly suits, except that they had a jacket and pants that went together. There was also the introduction of flared pants and those with a "close-fitting thigh and hip." Advertised for the "mature man," however, was a "full-cut model ... a roomier cut with standard leg styling."[39] Regular size clothes helped men to maintain a manly body image. But while young men dominated in the catalogues, all ages of men were pictured; indeed middle-aged and older men were often projected to be a success in their suits.

Fat men in the catalogues were often described by the word "stout," as late as the 1970s. Unlike the sizing for regular or young men's fashions, the sizing for stout men depicted a two-dimensional rectangle, equal measurements for chest and waist, indicating that weight was centred on the abdomen. Rarely did stout men get a page of fashions devoted to them, which suggested that their choice of clothes was limited. One page in the Fall/Winter 1920–21 catalogue showed night shirts and work shirts. One of the shirts was described as a "very satisfactory Shirt for stout men ... Cut from a large roomy pattern, allowing full freedom of movement and comfort to the wearer." If the goal for young men in regular suits was appearance and for older men character, the goal for the clothing of stout men was both comfort and fit, with emphasis on comfort.[40] The message embedded was that the problem for the stout man was finding clothing roomy enough to let him move with ease. Big men simply put more strain on their clothes, and too often the clothes, if not fitted properly, put too much strain on the men. Stout clothes allowed overweight men to get on with their life and focus on their job. Jobs were what made them men.

In the same 1920–21 catalogue, the "Blue Serge Suit for Stout Men" advertised its slimming properties: "This suit is designed especially for the man inclined to stoutness … to relieve his figure of any appearance of corpulence." The careful way of noting that a customer might be "inclined" to be overweight allowed the customer to feel that he wasn't stout yet, only inclining that way. Wearing clothes was a magic act that would make the wearer appear to weigh less. While measurements for the stout body looked straight – the chest and waist were similar – the body in three dimensions didn't. It was this reality that posed a difficulty – a protruding abdomen breaking a flat look. In spite of that, it was claimed the suit would take "away much of the stout appearance at the same time providing plenty of room where needed."[41] The suit dealt with both the problem of the appearance of stoutness and the special needs of the body for room due to the reality of stoutness.

The visuals of stout men were somewhat heavier than average men, with emphasis on the roundedness of face and the stockiness of body. What is interesting, however, is how such visuals connected with various classes of customers. For example, in the 1923 Spring/Summer catalogue, workwear was advertised with some men drawn with jowls, whereas those wearing leisure clothes for golf or riding were depicted as quite slender. Work garments for men didn't have sizing for stout men in the 1930s, but the drawings of work fashions indicated heavy-set men, with large sizing of some trousers and tops. The faces of the working men were drawn larger, and they appeared somewhat older than those wearing suits,[42] suggesting a connection between older men and weight. Part of this was class based, but also age based. Overweight males were seldom portrayed as young.

Stout styles were similar or identical to those offered to other men. Trouser styles were loosely pleated in the 1940s, and they added to the visual size of all men. Shirts, too, were advertised "for the man who values his appearance" and included both regular and stout sizes under that description.[43] When a photograph of regular size man was placed next to a stout man, the latter was clearly heavier and bigger in the midsection and the hips. A drawn man of "generous proportions" in the

1950 Spring/Summer catalogue had the same masculine face features of other models, but he seemed older, with facial lines and a sense of a neck that was somewhat jowly. Otherwise his body didn't seem to differ from the regular size men portrayed. If the profile was provided, the size of the abdomen was slightly curved, but not overly so.[44] With work clothes, there was a move to terms like "oversize" and "big," but unlike in the medical literature, which saw fat men as sedentary, the "big" men in work shirts were seen as active. Indeed, the language describing one set of trousers was "robust" and another as offering "generous dimensions that shouldn't restrict the movements of men with larger proportions."[45] Again the message was that fat men were still active men.

The 1960s saw more appeal to stout men as revealed by the Eaton's creation of a "Stout Man's Shop" for the "big man in 'hard to get' sizes … chests to 54 ins … waists to 52 ins."[46] The emphasis of the fashion text remained, as it long had, on the quality of the clothing and its value. Slimming was not a focus except in noting the plain trouser fronts, and it was left to the consumer to connect slimming with plain fronts. Despite having their own shop at Eaton's, fashions for large stout men were rather limited. Suits for stout men were still available in 1971, but were found on the page with regular suits, and the sizing for stout men seems to have taken a downward turn. By the mid-1970s, use of the word "stout" had ended, and references to "king size" replaced it. "Stout" was a word that had perhaps become outdated as it suggested an older man who was overweight. Men had become larger, and it was not always due to fat; sometimes it was simply muscle from working out. "King size" was a term that could be seen to include fat men, but not only fat men, which made a better marketing phrase. In suits, there was a king regular and a king tall size. It is interesting that the sizing was the same, 48–54, with the size 54 having a chest of 52 inches and a waist at 50–52. King tall (5'11" to 6'2"), however, might not really be the stout size that the king regular (5'7" to 5'11") was. King sizes had their own page in the 1975 catalogue (something that large women's fashions didn't have). Quality and comfort continued to be the significant themes. Of the two models shown, the shorter and older man was perhaps overweight, but certainly not fat. The larger man was simply that, larger.[47] Compared to women's fashions, those for men showed off their bigness.

"Husky" boys' clothing was offered in 1956, the first time the heavier boy was singled out. In the past, the word "husky" had been used to describe a regular active boy. It was a positive description, so when used to describe the overweight boy, it didn't have the same negative connotation that "chubbies" would have for overweight girls' sizes. As noted, the most significant difference between the husky boys' clothing and the regular boys' clothing was that the husky sizing had a larger waist. The depiction of the difference between the two was muted, however. In a drawing showing two boys playing baseball, one slender and the other heavier, the visual message was that a boy was a boy, and an active boy at that, no matter what the weight. In the 1959 catalogue, the husky size was advertised with the regular sizes, and was described as a "build" size rather than a weight size.[48] The word "build" had the connotation of permanence, that is, this was a body determined by heredity. The language was more matter of fact than critical, which, as we will see, was quite different from the descriptions of girls wearing the chubbies line. Those boys who were depicted as "husky" in the 1960s were slimmer in the drawing than they had been, but that changed in the 1970s, with drawings seemingly more realistic than in the late 1960s.[49] And when these boys became men, they would have the stout man's clothes – comfortable and well fit.

When the body was exposed as it was in advertisements for underwear or athletic wear, it would appear that regular size young men had muscular upper bodies with broad necks, which were somewhat accentuated.[50] Advertised in Eaton's Fall/Winter catalogue for 1938–39 on a page for athletic clothing was the "Bracer" underwear for "sport and daily wear." Available in sizes 34–44, the Bracer was not designed for stout men. What it did offer was "correct fit without the slightest discomfort." When advertised in *Maclean's*, however, the Bracer was promoted as a way to lessen the appearance of the abdomen, a hint that men were concerned about their figures. For example, in one *Maclean's* advertisement the text read: "Men! Here's a supporter belt that gives firm, adequate support without discomfort. One that keeps you slim, youthful, athletic. It's the Bracer!" Clearly being trim was important, but not at the loss of comfort. Another advertisement emphasized that for a man nearing forty the Bracer would help with the "mid-section sag" that made him look older.[51]

If the 1930s advertised the "Bracer" for men, the "Holdrite" support garment took its place in the 1940s. The Holdrite was designed for a young man who undertook "strenuous forms of sports"; it was also a "boon to men of mature years who are putting on weight" and would help "control the figure." The before profile was of an older man with thinning hair whose abdomen looked large enough for him not to be able to see his toes. The after profile, when he was wearing a Holdrite, showed how his abdomen had miraculously disappeared.[52] Looking slim had become easy, although comfort was not mentioned with the Holdrite, unlike the Bracer.

Men's briefs in the 1960s included the Harvey Woods "5BX" Reducers with a "5-inch elasticized waist-band plus 1¾ inch band of rubber [that] pulls in abdomen." Certainly such apparel would give the wearer the appearance of a smaller abdomen and having control over it, appealing to men's body image. The briefs came in small, medium, large, and oversize sizing with large being 40–42 and oversize being 44–46, big perhaps, but certainly not to the degree of stout fashion waists that went up to size 52 at times. Indeed, they seemed more for average men's sizes with a specific emphasis on the higher range. In 1974, one of the men's briefs was advertised on a page with athletic/reducing equipment. The brief had a high waist that promised to give "firm support to your back ... [and] holds stomach bulge in place."[53] Bulge certainly was not something that any man would want. These were not athletic supports at all, simply body supports. They were foundation garments, akin to the Bracer.

What strikes a historian looking at the depictions of men's fashions in Eaton's catalogues is that they did not change that much. Suits dominated the men's pages, and there wasn't all that much that could change with them – padded shoulders, a more tapered line to the waist, double- or single-breasted, pleated or flat front trousers. If clothing was a reflection of identity, men's identity was largely stable, and the choice of the suit suggested a successful person, open to more men than "in vogue" fashions would be for women. Despite the limits on men's clothes, the visuals depicting men were individualized through a broad spectrum of ages, facial types, and hair. Stout men who were depicted rarely looked fat, simply curved. Throughout the decades, aging and more weight went together. While the message of slimming in the clothes' text existed, it did not dominate when compared to the emphasis on value and comfort. Indeed, there wasn't an undertone of the stout figure being one that needed to be altered. It just was, and so needed to be accommodated. Some underwear garments were the exception, as they claimed to have the ability to reshape the body.

Women's Sizes and Clothing

Women's fashions pose more challenges than men's. Unlike the silhouettes for men's fashions that didn't shift significantly over time, the silhouettes for women's fashions did. The variety of fashions was much greater for women than for men, as were the various categories and sizes, which changed over time. For example, among the categories were women's regular, misses, junior, extra (or large), half-sizes, girls', and more. But there was no consistency to what each one meant over the time period. Nevertheless, size was important to a woman; it said something about her, and going up in size or having her normal size be tight could easily alter the way in which she looked at her body. Fashions themselves signified much about society and a woman's place in it, and were an emotional investment for the individual who was wearing them. Youth dominated the fashion pages for women. This domination, along with the slenderness of body portrayed, denied the future facing the majority of young women – marriage, childbearing, motherhood, aging, and for most, putting on weight.

From 1920 to 1976, women's regular sizing varied within sizes 32–54, depending on the time period. The larger sizes, 46–52, began in 1956; by 1976, Eaton's introduced an additional category, "larger women's," which encompassed sizes 48–54 and overlapped with the larger range (extra large) of 46 to 52 in the women's regular category. From 1920 to 1962, sizes 32–52 were determined by chest measurement, that is, a size 34 had a 34-inch chest. In 1965, however, sizes 34–52 (no more size 32) increased the chest measurement by 3 inches, so that a size 34 had a 37-inch chest. Waists measurements for size increased in 1950, 1965, and 1971. Thus, a woman could comfort herself with the delusion that her size remained the same, even though she had increased in girth. Misses sizing (6–22) and junior sizing (women, 5–19) had different measurements over the years, just as regular sizing changed. Misses and junior sizing dominated the fashion pages and appealed to a younger demographic willing to spend more on clothing. Since the 1920s, half-sizes appeared under names such as "short-stout women" or "short-stout misses." In 1956, half-sizes became a section on its own, beginning at size 12½; these clothes became the most frequent recipients of slimming messages. Half-sizes didn't have the largest sizes, but it was the category for "overweight" customers. The categorization and the sizes of women's clothing is a quagmire.

Teen sizing began in 1950, and, depending on the time period, went from size 8 to 16. As with other categories, some change in measurements occurred. Girls' sizing (7–16) was linked to age (6–14) from 1920 to 1932. In 1941, the sizing was determined by chest measurement, and sizes remained linked to age as indicated by the chest/waist measurements. In 1959, for example, sizes 7, 8, and 9 had differences between

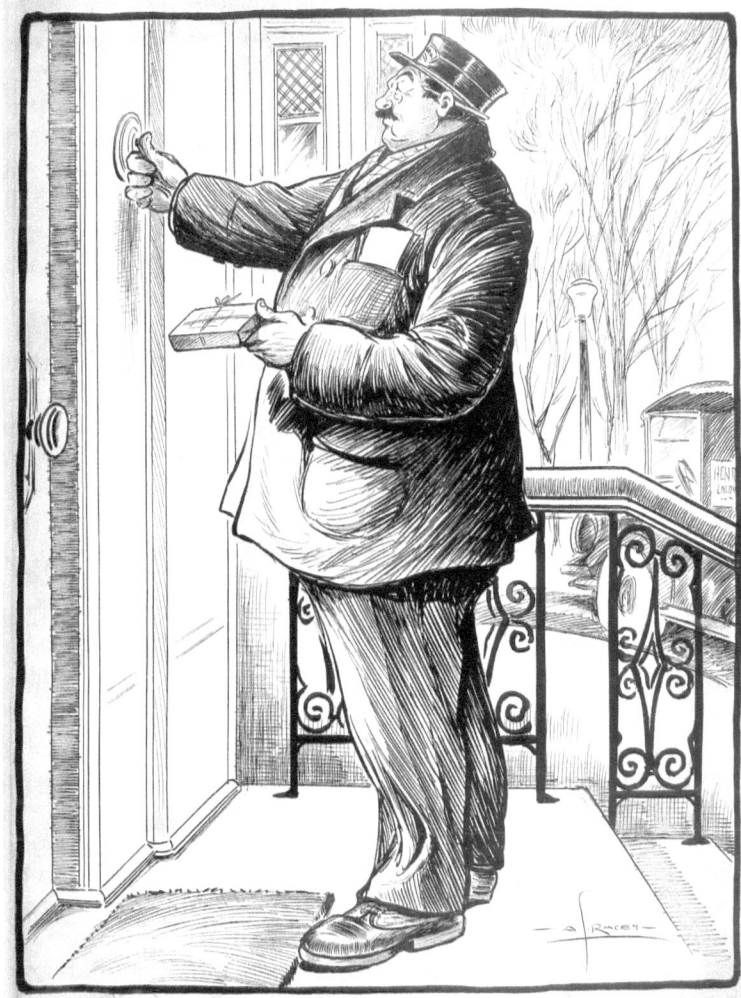

Fashions were created for slender women or women who wanted dresses to make them look slender. In the 1920s, many Canadians did not like the new fashions, which revealed more of a woman's body than had been conventional earlier in the twentieth century. This 1927 cartoon shows a very fat, older mailman delivering a very small package – "Her New Easter Dress Arrives" – indicating that the dress in this package would show more of the body. Source: 1927, Gift of Mrs Susan Racey Godber and Mrs Margaret Racey Stavert; M2005.23.73, McCord Museum.

chest and waist of 2, 2½, and 3 inches, respectively. By size 14, however, the difference was 6 inches, and for size 16, it was 7 inches. Sizes 14 and 16 were cut to fit adolescents with a significant inverted triangle rather than reflecting a child's silhouette. Chubbies, another category for girls, was introduced in 1959. Chubbies sizing was designated in half-sizes (8½ to 14½), but there was no connection between chubbies sizes and equivalent regular sizes for girls. For example, a regular girls' size 10 measured 28 inches for chest, 24½ inches for waist, and 29 inches for hips. A chubbies size 10½ measured 31 inches, 28½ inches, and 34 inches, respectively.

For women, the 1920s began with a silhouette of "long straight lines" and hems at the calf level, emphasizing the youthfulness and slimness of the cut in many of the fashions. By the end of the 1920s, the silhouette was more tapered towards the hip, but still in a line. At the end of the 1930s, waists were being emphasized; dress skirts were fuller and not as close to the hip. But the slenderizing message remained. The focus on youthfulness was also strong, especially in the misses sizes, but it was clear that the advertisements were pushing these fashions towards any woman who could wear the misses sizes.[54] The pitch was that youthful styles were becoming to a woman of any age if she could wear them, which meant that youthfulness dominated women's style irrespective of age. This orientation was quite different from men's clothes.

The trim body image in women was one that society seemed content to follow throughout the decades. What changed over time was only the shape of the slender silhouette. In the 1940s, the very fitted waist accentuated the hourglass figure. In part, this was a consequence of the use of padded shoulders that made the waist look smaller. In turn, the "smaller" waist made the hips seem larger (and more curvaceous) than in previous years. At times, the models wearing regular size clothing looked quite thin, perhaps due to some doctoring of photographs or perhaps because of the influence of the Christian Dior couture style after the war. At mid-century, the fashions catered even more to the curvaceous silhouette for women, reflecting the domestic life after years of depression and war, and the increasing birth rate. It could also be that it was now permitted to depict women's sexuality. Waists continued to be the focus as skirts became larger and fuller. By the late 1950s, however, the sack dress emphasized a slim profile. Slacks, too, were more visible in the catalogue, but not for the extra size woman. In the 1950s, the models in regular sizes seemed older – in their thirties and forties – than they had been, with the text admitting that they had "more mature" figures, although seemingly looking slender.[55]

The 1960s in Eaton's began with the junior sizes showing a sheath dress, a "slim look," and slacks made of stretchy material and close to the body in style. Photographs of women in the fashion pages became more extreme in their thinness, with some looking almost anorexic around the neck and arms.[56] The fashion model had become an ideal to emulate. By the end of the sixties, the best-known fashion model was Twiggy, an icon of slenderness and the model who, in the flesh, reflected the ethereal drawings of "women" common in the fashion papers. The late 1960s was an era when the first of the boomer generation arrived at young adulthood, and the public image of many young women was challenging the established norms in the society. Making women ethereal in fashion with the mini skirt could offset young women's increasing power. In 1968, Eaton's marketed Twiggy's brand name hosiery. It certainly provided a youthful look, coming in colours such as pink and apple green; it would have been difficult, however, to regard women wearing such fashions as "adults." The whole phenomenon of Twiggy was noteworthy. She was 5 feet 6 inches tall and weighed 91 pounds; if she was the ideal, even approaching the ideal was obviously quite impossible for most adult women.[57] But then Twiggy was not an adult; she was an adolescent whose body had become the icon of femaleness, even adult femaleness. The late 1960s and early 1970s continued with mini skirts, but added the midi and maxi as well. Choice was the name of the game. Given that the mini was still popular, a thin body was needed to make the fashion clothes look as designed.[58]

The regular body fashions from 1920 to the 1970s had two aspects: the clothes needed to make women slender and look youthful. Stout women and fat teens were going to have a hard time finding clothes that fit or being seen as slender or youthful. Early in the 1920s, an article in *Maclean's* reminded readers that "the stout woman has probably the most difficulty in her choice of clothes." Especially problematic was the short and stout woman with "an appearance of dumpiness, looking almost as broad as she is tall," and her colour palette limited to dark colours, navy blue and black.[59] Any fat woman reading that description would wonder what clothes would be best. Nevertheless, when you look at the extra size women's clothing in the 1920s, the stress was on style, unlike the comfort and fit value that were the advertised attributes of stout men's clothing. The emphasis was on hiding the fat woman's body rather than accepting it, which was the orientation of

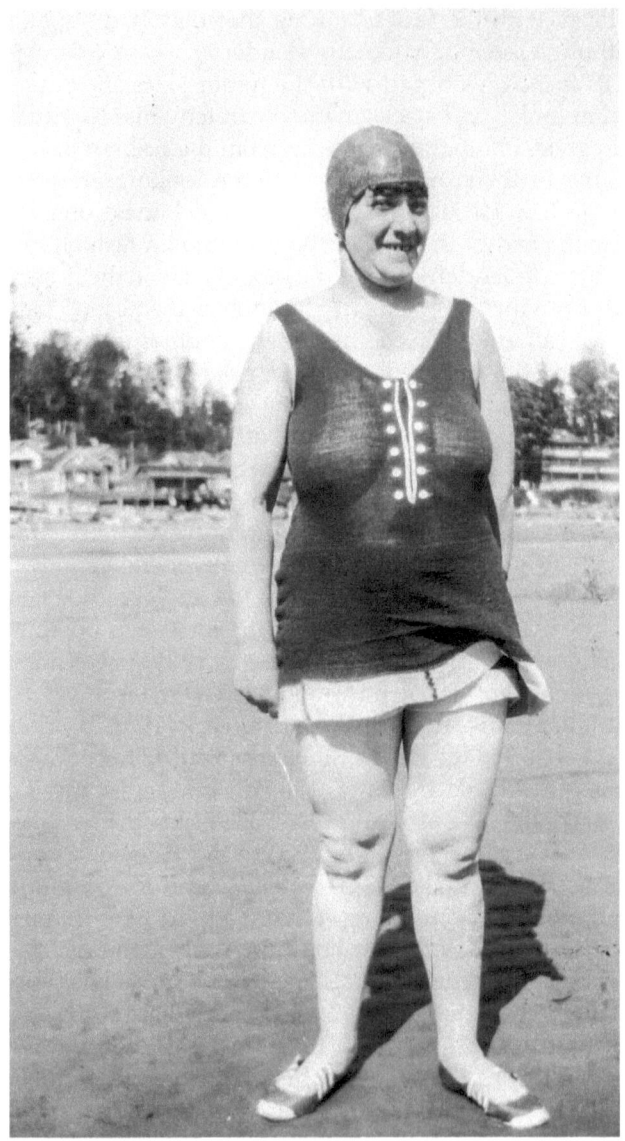

Not every woman's body was slender or young, as seen in this photograph of a mature woman at a Vancouver beach, c. 1925. Older women and overweight women often had difficulty finding flattering clothes. Source: 2748a; © North Vancouver Museum and Archives.

the large man's fashions. The fat woman needed to look smaller, and the fashions would correct the appearance of her body and let her look slimmer and taller. In the 1923–24 Fall/Winter catalogue, there was a suit for the "large" woman on a page of suits for regular sizes. The text of the large woman's suit was clear: "It is a well-known fact that the large woman looks her best in a suit, and this smart one … is cleverly tailored to give the effect of slimness."[60]

The drawn visuals of extra large women showed them heavier than the regular and misses size women, especially in the bust, more rounded faces, and double chins. Nonetheless, their ankles and lower calves were depicted as disproportionately thin, just as those of the regular size women were. And while the visuals might suggest slightly overweight women, nowhere was there a drawing of a woman who looked fat. In the Spring/Summer 1932 catalogue, large size coats and misses coats and suits were shown on the same page. It was next to impossible to discern the differences between the drawings of the models on the basis of size. This lack of "reality" was quite common. However, the descriptions of the clothing were noticeably different. The text for large sizes mentioned the fashions' slimming quality, whereas the text for misses sizes didn't need to use the "slim" word.[61] Captions in the 1938 Spring/Summer catalogue caught the magic of both the images and the fashions in larger sizes: "Frocks help you to look slimmer than you are. Clever Styles Stress Slenderizing."[62] The push for illusion became more blatant and, at times, surreal. However, a look at the text of fashions revealed the hint that youth and large sizes did not go together – rather, the goal for the larger women was to wear a "dignified frock." The words "grace" and "graceful" were used in descriptions of clothes for larger women and continued to be into the end of the catalogues. Not surprisingly, the word "matronly" was associated with the large size, denoting both age and heaviness. Other terms used to describe such women were "of ample proportions," "stylish stout," "above average size," and "of large dimensions."[63] Unlike for men, however, the use of the word "stout" for larger women lessened by the late 1930s.

Made-to-measure suits were offered to women in 1944, but the larger woman wasn't considered, even though this service was offered to stout men.[64] While in the popular mind the image of slimness and youth went together, fashions in the 1940s for larger women often promised the former, with the clothing itself described as youthful. For example, a dress might be called a "youthful printed frock," designed for the woman who was "youthful-minded" even though a matron.[65] The larger body was not a young body. In 1956, Eaton's regular sizes absorbed sizes up to 52. Even with regular sizes taking over the large woman sizing, clothing choices for large women did not increase, since the regular size didn't always include the full range of sizes to 52. Given that the large sizes were now combined with the regular sizes, a connection between the overweight and "regular" woman occurred. This combination made being a regular size negative. Certainly, the descriptions of the fashions had been doing this for some time with the slenderizing theme, and this pattern continued.[66] For older and heavier women, the text for the fashions offered "maturity" and a dignified "stately figure."[67] Nevertheless, the models wearing the fashions seldom looked older or heavy. While women wearing half-sizes would be heavier, not surprisingly there was little sign of this in the models wearing the clothing. The models, however, tended to look more mature in their late twenties or thirties. When the half-size and women's/larger women's dresses appeared together, the problem areas of each were made specific. For the woman needing a half-size, the problem was that she was "not so tall." For the other two, it was that they had an "average" figure but were "not so-slim."[68] The descriptors were focused on what a woman was not rather than what she was.

In 1959, chubbies sizing for girls was introduced. Despite the chubbies sizes being outside the comparable girls' size measurements, drawings and photographs of the girls in the two categories didn't differ much.[69] The photographs of girls depicted in the 1962 Spring/Summer catalogue wearing chubbies clothes did not look chubby. Indeed, the body difference among girls can basically be put down to age and development. The ones who looked a little heavier in the waist also looked younger and underdeveloped compared to those who were thinner. It would seem that being chubby was about more than weight. Indeed, none of the models appeared overweight. By 1965, chubbies fashions became integrated with girls', with no special headings and fewer choices,[70] after which chubbies fashions declined. This change meant that clothes for young overweight teens had to be found in women's fashions. Indeed, any teen sizing would not fit fat teens. One woman remembered what it was like to be an overweight teen at the time: "As an Eaton's customer from a rural community in 1971, I can verify how small the fit was. An overweight teen had little hope of finding apparel in teens' or even the juniors' section. I occasionally ordered items from the half-size section, but they were generally too mature-looking for a 15-year-old, being more suited to someone at least 35 and up."[71]

In 1965, a "slimline dress," one that had a "flattering bodice," was introduced for in half-sizes for women.[72] The photographs were of older women, but other than not having the body of a teenager or a very young woman, the models didn't fit the image associated with a heavier body. Similarly, the description of women's sizes (34–52) highlighted the slenderizing properties of fashions in captions – "fashion decrees a slimmer, slightly flared silhouette." "Marie Dressler Slender Stouts" offered larger sizing (38–52), and the contradictory message of slenderness being a characteristic of "stouts" clothing was only surpassed by Dressler's name on the brand as a guarantee of looking slim. Dressler was an actress who was not slim in life, nor were the characters she played. Nevertheless, fantasy was what was in the catalogue, with two very slender models wearing Dressler dresses.[73]

Clothes for large women were actually becoming more difficult to find. By the end of the 1960s, the only new fashion for heavier women was pants offered for extra size women (46–52).[74] Little attention seemed to be paid to style with the larger sizes, and the emphasis on slimming was somewhat indirect. Age and weight still went together throughout the 1970s. The day dresses in the catalogues were cheaper and less stylish, and the fashions advertised in the larger sizes featured older models and the occasional model who actually looked heavy.[75] Their hips were larger, and it seemed as though their stomachs were more rounded, although not as realistic as the plus size models of today.[76] It all seemed to send the message that large size women's clothing was not important to Eaton's.

Foundation garments played a much larger role in women's fashions in any size than they did in men's. The only fashion section where older and larger women were significantly visible was in corsetry. Indeed, the overweight woman in a corset was the predominant image of aging women in Eaton's catalogues. Looking at the foundation garments and reading their texts introduces a range of unpleasant feelings: the discomfort of most garments; pain from wearing some of them; the sense of a body under restraint; the awareness of control with every breath; the overriding perception that no matter what you looked like, you would not measure up; and the fear of having to try girdles or corsets on and look at your reflection in the mirror. The language, as always, was key. Item 98–3827 in 1920 was "for stout figures ... specially adapted for full-bust figures who desire a firm support and a neat appearance." A woman without such a brassiere would have a sloppy appearance and a body out of control. The drawings of brassieres for the "stout figures" were of women who were full-busted, but otherwise they were not particularly fat – indeed, quite the contrary if their arms were examined. The message to the reader was that by wearing such garments, she too could look like the drawings, that is, she would not look how she really appeared. In the 1923 Spring/Summer catalogue, women, including stout women, were offered a "Boysform Brassiere" to give them "that trim boy-like appearance." Remarkable contortions and plasticity are asked of the female body – the sloppiness could be contained and the body reshaped.[77]

The advertisements for corsets made it clear that all women needed to "mould their figure," even girls and youth.[78] In 1922, the *Canadian Home Journal* printed an advertisement for Gossard Corsetry noting that the ideal body was not attainable for most women: few were beautifully proportioned, and even if they were, it would not last since the ideal was focused on a "slimmer type for the young girl who goes in for athletics." Once past age nineteen, the young girl, too, would have to work at keeping slim. To make the impossibility of beauty concrete, the advertisement listed an ideal woman's measurements: 5 feet 5 inches in height, 27 inch waist, 34 inch bust, thighs 25 inches. The specificity of such a description would ensure that the vast majority of women would find one or more of their measurements didn't fit the ideal.[79] The message sent was reshape your body, because no matter what body you have, it is not what fashion dictates. Indeed, the goal of undergarments was to provide women with bodies that could best show off the fashions currently in style. Fashions were not being designed to fit "real" bodies, especially if they were overweight.

In the 1920 Spring/Summer catalogue, advertisements for Nemo Corsets illustrated the range of bodies that manufacturers catered to: "medium and tall stout figures," "full figures," "slight and medium figures," and "average figures." Once a woman had figured out what type or size of body she had, then she learned about the flaws of her body that each corset could offset. She could get a "Self-Reducing Corset for the Average Figure" to "reduce the abdomen" or a "Self-Reducing Model with Lasticurve Back" for the medium and tall stout figure to ensure that "the flesh [was] evenly spread." Others improved health through "lifting the abdominal organs." If you didn't need "abdominal reduction," perhaps you were "too heavy in hip and thigh."[80] For impatient women in the 1930s who didn't want to diet, there were reduction rubber girdles. But choosing a corset (or girdle) was not easy, and if the wrong one was worn it could be a fashion and personal disaster. Even women with average figures required help "to take care of surplus flesh across the hips," "to prevent flesh from bulging," and to control "the excess flesh in front of the thighs."[81]

Full corsetry was still popular in Eaton's catalogues in the 1940s. Targeting all sizes, the corset message was clear – get your body under control to look good in the fashions available. The proportional drawings for corsets at Eaton's provided nine choices: short, medium, and tall were the three categories, and within each category there were slender, average, and stout choices.[82] In this description, slender became a category all its own, which meant that anyone with an average figure would never really be able to approach the slender ideal. The average figure in this context had become a larger figure. Corsets for younger women (waists 24 to 30) were lightweight, but the firm-control corsets were designed for more developed women and offered inner panelling and boning. Another difference was that young girls in undergarments were depicted in drawings, whereas photographs were used for adult models.[83] The morality of showing girls in their underwear most likely prohibited the use of real children and teenage models. Worrisome, however, were the drawings of young girls that showed pointed and large breasts for their body size, and the catalogue offered girdles and corselets (from chest to thighs) to girls as young as eight years old. Nature seemed to be failing when even young women and girls needed help for their bodies.[84] If such girls needed an uplift, what did it say about attitudes towards the adult female body?

Foundation garments didn't change much in the 1950s, but nylon gained attention. It was a magical material "to give definition to the figure of a teen-ager ... to give control to the young matron ... and support to the more mature woman." Girdles for larger women provided the most control, and control was demanded no matter what the woman was doing. Wearing a girdle allowed a woman to show off her "natural" figure. As an advertisement for Warner's Girdle explained: "It's still you ... a more natural you!"[85] The reality of fashion made what was natural and artificial interchangeable. Undergarments introduced an Alice-in-Wonderland world. In the 1955 Eaton's catalogue, the "Magic Controller" was described as able to provide "waist control" and to "trim away unwanted rolls and bulges."[86] But where did the rolls and bulges go?

As had been the case for some time, the full body corsets in the 1960s tended to be for and modelled by an older woman with a "mature figure," and the lightweight bras and girdles by younger women.[87] New on the scene were Hanes' Panty Pair, consisting of underwear to provide control and hosiery that was kept up by folding the panty's cuff over the hose for a "smooth, flat, unbroken line from waist to toe." That had long been the goal – a smoothness to the body as opposed to bumps and bulges. Foundation garments continued to offer this illusion. For example, there was a niche market for the "Original Subtract ... as advertised in *Weight Watchers*" magazine. Designed for women on diets, it promised a good fit as you lost up to one or two sizes of weight. If you needed to look like you had lost weight without doing so, the Miss Mary/Lady Mary of Sweden had the corselette, brassiere, or girdle for you. The "after" "photograph" in advertisements showed a raised bust, a smooth line from there to the lower thighs, and made the body look at least two sizes smaller without having the flesh that was being rearranged appearing elsewhere. The figures also seemed distorted. In the "before" body visual, the head and neck were out of proportion to the large body but not on the more slender "after" body visual.[88] One corset advertisement in the 1974 catalogue assured its women readers that its "spandex reinforcement" worked for "the tummy, hips, thighs and derriere." For bust sizes to 52, there was a corselette that had an "inner belt, boned to provide good support for the abdomen ... [with] acetate and rubber leno weave elastic inserts at the side."[89] Manufacturers advertised the modern technology of body supports, which claimed to give the wearer a sense of success, feeling her body in control and looking slender.

There was an irony in the variety of categories, sizes, and changing fashions for women, because the depiction of women did not individualize them compared to the visuals for men. What was acceptable for women was clear – being slender and looking youthful. While a slim look for women was the norm throughout the sixty-year period, some decades seemed more taken with it than others. No woman was exempt. Focusing the slimming message on women more than on men resulted in a decline in the availability of clothing for women who were fat. Many women who were interviewed for this study commented on the limited available choice of clothing. Men's clothing was not as form-fitting as women's. Neither were men's body flaws as visible under the suits they wore. Consequently, the male ideal was easier to emulate. Larger women would not often see themselves in Eaton's catalogues, even though Eaton's offered large sizes. The models in such clothing just didn't look fat. Neither would the older and mature-figured woman see herself very often in the catalogues.

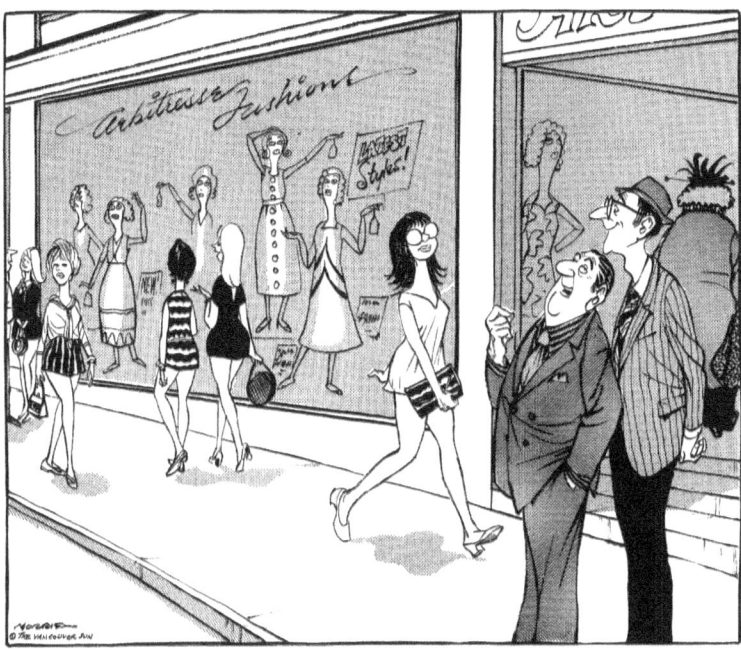

The image for young women had changed by the 1970s. Women wanted to be thin rather than slender. This 1970 cartoon portrays women with thin ankles, legs, and long necks, not unlike the fashion drawings for Eaton's catalogues from the 1920s. What was different in 1970 was that young women's clothes showed even more of the body than they had in the 1920s. The men in the cartoon, however, are still wearing suits that hide more than they reveal and have changed relatively little since the 1920s. Source: MsC 25-494, 1-1970-07-10, SFU Special Collections, Len Norris Collection, Simon Fraser University Library.

Conclusion

The unreality of the idealized body image experienced by most Canadians seemed designed to prompt a negative reaction to their own bodies. The products were designed (and still are) to change the appearance of bodies, to make them similar – slender and young. The examination of body image has emphasized the gendered nature of the past. It underlines, in part, what we long have known – that an idealized body for a woman was more significant in society than one for a man. Visuals and discussions of women's bodies were widespread, making appearance and womanhood a conventional pairing. The media and marketers were entranced by women's bodies, but the body they wanted was largely an abstraction, only possible through modification of a woman's actual shape. Men's bodies were viewed differently. Suits hid their bodies, allowing more latitude for both age and body shape. The suits and other clothes for men played down the slimming aspect of their clothes, while slimming and youthfulness dominated the descriptions of women's clothes. A natural-looking body became a fashion construct that dictated every woman needed to wear a corset or girdle and brassiere. The natural body needed assistance just to be. The support underwear for men to meet the male standard was not nearly as dominant or intrusive. Fat women to a greater extent than fat men were outliers, in terms of fashion. But for both fat men and women, the idealized body was a stigma. While body image from the media was a social and cultural construct, it was also one that medical experts used. Both had their normative measurements. Fat has been viewed as negative in culture, social life, and medicine in different ways and over time. Gender was a base in all three. What fat men and women thought concerning the advice given to them about their bodies and their clothes is the focus of the next chapter.

8 Narratives of Fat Canadians

"Who said fat ladies are jolly? They are usually miserable. Miserable enough to eat a little more of the wrong kind of food while they worry about being overweight."[1]

In the January/February 2013 issue of *The Walrus*, Katherine Ashenburg introduced readers to Terry Poulton, a sixty-eight-year-old woman whose life has revolved around her size. She was raised by a single mother who took a job when Poulton was about nine, leaving her to come from school to an empty home. There she comforted herself by overeating. Her weight increased, and she encountered the stigma that many fat Canadians experience: called a "bull moose" by a dancing teacher, rejected by boys, fired from a job for being too fat, and living with a man who introduced her not as someone important to him but as a "tenant." In trying to control her weight, Poulton followed the diet route, trying various diets including a liquid protein diet and injections of human chorionic gonadotropin (HCG) accompanied by a 500-calorie diet. What made her life positive was her work as a freelance writer for *Maclean's*, *Chatelaine*, and *Toronto Life*. In 1982, the editors at *Chatelaine* approached her to write about a weight-loss program using her own body as the focus. She agreed. Determined to be successful in losing weight, she cheated on her program – instead of going down to 1,200 calories a day as suggested, she ate less than 1,000 calories; and instead of exercising 45 minutes a day, she exercised twice as much. Wanting to be close to her fitness club, she moved, with the result that her "fiancé" quickly replaced her.

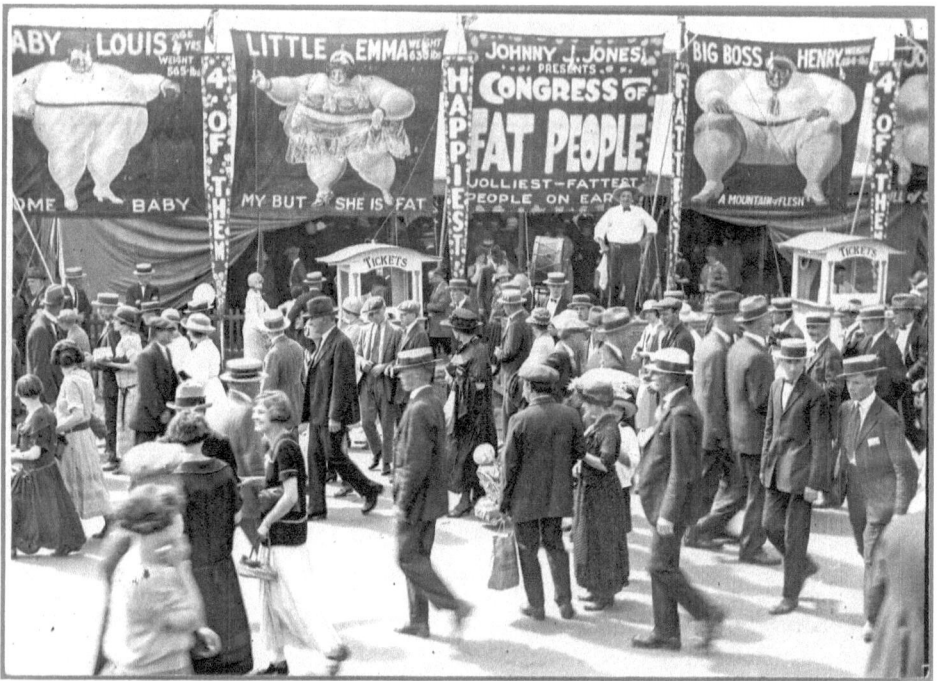

Fat people were often stigmatized. The midways highlighted people who were considered "freaks." In this photograph of the Midway Sideshow at the 1913 Canadian National Exhibition (CNE) in Toronto, the centre sign announces: "Johnny J. Jones presents Congress of Fat People, Jolliest – Fattest People on Earth." Source: William James Family fonds, 1244, Item 279F, City of Toronto Archives.

Losing weight was not easy, but *Chatelaine* didn't let Poulton tell her readers how difficult it actually was. And, as with so many dieters, her weight loss was regained. In 1985, a doctor suggested she have a stomach staple procedure, but that didn't work either. Nothing did. She became convinced that all her dieting had slowed her metabolism, a belief that some researchers also accept today. In 1996, she wrote *No Fat Chicks: How Women Are Brainwashed to Hate Their Bodies and Spend Their Money*. It was a response to her life and told how she eventually accepted her own body. She hoped that by reading her book other women, too, would reject the pressure to fit their bodies into a slender ideal.²

Only occasionally have the voices of those who self-identified as fat been heard in this study. Yet, such voices are important, for they offset the overwhelming opinions, speculations, and prejudices of those who have never been fat. If historians have worried about the appropriation of voices of those with limited power due to class, ethnicity or race, gender, sexual orientation, or age, surely we should be sensitive to those whose bodies were seen as overweight or obese. The voices in this chapter confirm some of the themes already presented in other chapters and challenge others.³ The voices describe their lives. The sources for these voices are twofold. The first are the advertisements and articles in magazines using the "before" and "after" snapshots of a life being fat and the transformed life after weight was lost. Usually, what was voiced was conformity, wanting to have a normal body, one that was not overly fat. These narratives were used by advertisers to sell a plethora of products and magazines to keep their readers engaged. The second source of voices came from thirty interviews. The difference between these voices and the published voices is that their narratives are more complex and more analytical about their lives.

Fat Narratives in the Popular Press

Advertising

While there were certainly lots of articles and advertisements on dieting in the 1920s and 1930s, the use of before and after narratives was relatively limited when compared to what followed. An early advertisement (1928) by Marmola prescription tablets showed a drawing of a slender woman looking at a photograph of her former weighty self. There was no testimony and no sense of a real visual narrative, only a fictional one.⁴ A February 1932 advertisement in *The Chatelaine* for Kruschen Salts contained testimony from Mrs P. (no address). At twenty-two, she weighed 163 pounds and was experiencing back and head pains as a consequence of her weight. After taking Kruschen Salts for six months, she had lost 19 pounds. Another advertisement in *Maclean's* for the salts emphasized a husband's weight loss to his wife's "delight." The salts were not a weight-loss product per se. They were to "assist the internal organs to perform their functions properly – to throw off each day the wastage and poisons that encumber the system."

Weight loss was a by-product.[5] These advertisements were precursors to later, popular before and after narratives.

In the 1940s, and in subsequent decades, marketers honed the technique of narrative testimonials. In the February 1942 issue of *Chatelaine*, an advertisement for the DuBarry Success course related the experience of Jeannette Bascobert, thirty-four and a mother of two children. "Once pretty, she was now overweight." The third person description of Bascobert was a distancing tactic that implied an objective observer. The theme of the advertisement was that underneath the fat of an overweight woman was a thinner pretty one, the underlying assumption being that a fat woman could not be pretty. Believing this notion, Bascobert decided to gain control of herself, "snap out of it," and follow the DuBarry course in her own home. The result was a loss of 20 pounds in six weeks. Two surface changes apparently accompanied weight loss – a better complexion and hair "glossy and alive." Even more important was Bascobert's new-found ability to sleep and wake up "refreshed." This part of the tale was a narrative to which many women could relate – the need for more energy to take care of a household and a growing family.[6] The narrative was the hook. It was enough – you didn't need details of what the DuBarry course actually was or what you had to do. Indeed, details were not supplied. Wasn't it enough to know that the course would transform you?

Vagueness about how weight loss worked was characteristic of other narratives, while the results were clear. In 1958, Catherine Ann Johnson, a voice student, revealed that by losing weight she *"WON A NEW LIFE."* Unlike Bascobert, Johnson had always been overweight and "unhappily" so. She had tried all sorts of diets, but they had failed her. Then she found the "Knox [Gelatine] Eat-and-Reduce Plan." It was a dietary grail, and it was "easy." She lost 39 pounds, now wore a size 14 dress rather than a size 20, and her singing voice was improving. She felt "hopeful" about her life and her future, all because of "balanced eating."[7] Of course, balanced eating was what the doctors, nutritionists, and educators had long advised, but in Johnson's narrative the product precipitated the change.

By the 1960s, Metrecal (a powder of skim milk and nutrients to be mixed with liquid) had entered the dieting market, and its advertisements also used the narrative appeal. Promises were one thing, but hearing from a person who had actually been successful was more believable, especially when that person was not a Hollywood starlet, for example, as in the advertisements for products such as Ayds.[8] Instead,

Colleen Dimson was someone to whom many Canadian women could relate. She was a young mother, married four and a half years, and during those years had put on weight. She was now faced with wanting to lose it. In her words: "It's nice to be slim." She heard about Metrecal and decided to try it. She ordered the "dietary powder" from her pharmacist and found that it worked for her without any significant interference in her life. It tasted "pleasant," "satisfied her hunger," and since she could use it as a substitute for other meals, it didn't interfere with "family meals." Significant messages emerged from this advertisement: Metrecal was purchased at the pharmacy, indicting it must be safe; the process of losing weight was conceptually easy; and it didn't impinge on the dieter's family to any notable extent.[9]

A common theme in many of these types of advertisements was the ease with which weight could be lost when taking the right product – be it Marmola pills, Kruschen Salts, the DuBarry Success course, the Knox Eat-and-Reduce Plan, or Metrecal. Ease was part of the consumer ideology, which existed at many levels of Canada's social classes. Ironically, while food consumerism may have caused the fat, diet product consumerism claimed the ability to easily solve the fat problems. The only agency required was to follow the instructions of how to use the product or keep to the diet plan. In using a narrative trope, the advertisements made their products familiar and their claims believable. It all seemed so easy.

Articles

More important than product advertisements were the narratives of women and men presented in featured articles. In *Chatelaine*, the narratives more often than not appeared in the April issue each year, when most of the articles on dieting were offered. This time frame corresponded to the trend in fashion advertisements, which sported lighter and more revealing clothes for summer. Having experienced winter weight gain and facing the prospect of wearing bathing attire and other skimpy clothes, readers were primed to take in the dieting message. Magazines knew what their readers craved, just as advertisers did.

In 1937, Nita Ward told *Chatelaine* readers about her efforts to lose 30 pounds over three months. Hers was a success story: she was "healthier" and "happier," and six years later she could say that her "old careless ways" had given way to "will power." She told a familiar tale of getting married, having a child, and putting on weight as a result. She wasn't really aware of the weight gain until her husband made a remark that made her look in a mirror with her clothes off. What she saw was disturbing and negative – "fat had congealed from the waist down." Once a glandular cause of her weight gain had been eliminated, her doctor suggested she take long walks and not eat rich food in hopes that this strategy would eliminate her bilious attacks and headaches, which were a cause of bad digestion. She lost some weight, but not until she went to a "physical culture teacher" did she lose significant weight. Her regime consisted of a liquid diet for two weeks, the purpose of which was to "rid the system of poisons," followed by a series of exercises at night and in the morning, dieting, and more exercise to harden her body. During the years afterwards, she maintained her exercises and her diet.[10] Her narrative was one of the few that gave a follow-up: she didn't regain weight.

While most of the before and after narratives were by women, some came from men. In the 15 February 1949 issue of *Maclean's*, James Bannerman, an author, critic, and broadcaster, wrote an article about his successful diet. His narrative was full of wry humour and self-analysis, compared to many such articles in *Chatelaine*. He noted for his readers that even before he began his diet, but after he had determined to go on one, he found that his perspective had changed. No longer did he have a niggling awareness of being overweight – he was now going to do something about it. He also challenged the image of the jolly fat man by letting his readers know that he, at least, had never been one of those. How could he be? Being fat meant never feeling really well, being tired every time he tried to do something, and feeling older than he was. He admitted that body image was important, and being fat meant he couldn't share the male dream of looking "dashing." He acknowledged that the actual dieting wasn't easy, but the result of his dieting was successful. Was he transformed? Not in the way women were. He felt better, he had more energy, and he felt "smug" about his achievement.[11] But he didn't seem to believe that he had been transformed.

In November 1952, *Chatelaine* introduced three women to its readers: Patsy O'Day, Blanche Kilpatrick, and Mildred Bennett. All three had been given makeovers, but Bennett's also consisted of significant weight loss. The author of Bennett's narrative was Rosemary Boxer, beauty and fashion editor. Many narratives used the third person point of view, with the author cast in the role of interpreter, the guarantor of truth and authenticity. At least that is one way of looking at it. Use of the third person also assured the magazine that the narrative would be concise and to the point. For readers, the lack of a constant first person voice might have lessened their connection to the person speaking, but it allowed them space (provided by the third person's view) to think about what had happened to the subject who was placed in a familiar frame. In this case, Bennett was an Ontario woman whose children had grown up and left home, leaving "the familiar pattern of family life suddenly shattered." Bennett had always been interested in fashion and had even put on shows for her church guild, so not surprisingly she thought of fashion again. "Every fashion show needs a 'matron' model – why not me!" She knew she had put on weight over the years of raising her family – she was now 170 pounds – but didn't know what to do about it. At this point, *Chatelaine* entered her life and essentially took on her weight as a project. She went on a "simple and nourishing diet," and after the weight loss, her makeover continued with a new haircut and cosmetic tips. As well, Bennett changed her clothes. "No more of those grandmotherish things for me!" Her final words in the article proclaimed: "I feel like a grey-haired Cinderella." That she was an older woman (her age was not divulged) made her story of interest. It sent the message to readers that it was never too late to lose weight, and life still had much to offer older women. Determined to change her life, Bennett took hold of it, albeit with help. She left a life of emptiness (children were gone) and boredom (little to keep her occupied). With the transformation of her body, she gained pride, confidence, and a sense of worth in her modelling career. She had made a "comeback" to life.[12] Her narrative was positive for older women.

Bob Blackburn did not look for a magic solution to his weight, but he told *Maclean's* readers in 1966 about his Drinking Man's Diet – eat and drink what you want, but just keep carbohydrates down to 60 grams a day. It worked for him, as he lost 40 pounds. The word he used to describe his new self was the same word that Bannerman used – "smug."[13] It was a gendered word, not found in the stories of women's weight loss. Indeed, most men's narratives saw their changes as prosaic. Body image seemed to be more significant for women, and for that reason the transformation narratives were all found in *Chatelaine*, while the prosaic ones to this date were in *Maclean's*.

By the 1960s, *Chatelaine* had perfected the script. One theme, however, was new – what the woman (and they were almost all women) generally ate for years before she decided to lose weight. Readers experienced a vicarious shock, as the amount eaten was often considerable. This new element placed the reader in a situation that was not as extreme as the woman telling her story, and gave the reader encouragement. If "such" a woman could get her act together, so could the reader.[14] In the April 1963 issue, Eveleen Dollery described "3 Dazzling Diet Successes." One was Maria Manshanden of Walkerton, Ontario. A farmer's wife, thirty-six and a mother of four, she had emigrated from Holland about nine years previously. Her weight was 275 pounds, and she was experiencing fatigue and weakness. There was no doubt about what had caused her weight gain – eating. For breakfast, she ate "5 slices of homemade bread, spread with homemade butter, cheese, cold sausage, jam, tea with cream and sugar." This meal was followed by a morning snack; lunch similar to her breakfast; another snack in the afternoon; a dinner of "potatoes, fried meats in butter, gravy made from drippings, vegetables with white sauce ... coffee or tea, cream and sugar, dessert, milk soup – milk and oatmeal"; and while watching TV, another snack. Her physician responded to her physical complaints by putting her on a diet of 1,000 calories. In seven months, she weighed 160 pounds. She didn't find the diet particularly difficult, and her way to avoid snacking was to write long letters and have a nap in the afternoon. She also took iron pills. When she reached 160 pounds, her doctor increased her food intake to 1,500 to 2,000 calories as a maintenance diet; at the time of publication, she had not regained a pound (of course not even a year had passed). The result was a "new beauty" for her.[15] Similar themes and narrative formats continued to be repeated. Somewhere in the narrative would be the shock of how much the woman weighed and why, the immediate prod that drove her to diet or to try dieting once again, and a description of the diet and the individual tricks she had devised to stay on the diet. The story then ended with a life transformed and fulfilled.[16] The descriptions of success emphasized the achievement made. Not just losing 5 or 10 pounds but more than 100 pounds was something readers could only imagine and feel relieved that they didn't need to face.

Willa Bodnar's story was a variation on the established script. After *Chatelaine* published a narrative of her weight loss of more than 100 pounds, she found herself slipping back, not able to keep to a balanced diet. She then looked to the Ayds Vitamins and Mineral Candy Reducing Plan to help her.[17] At that point, Bodnar spoke to *Chatelaine* readers through an Ayds advertisement. The distance between advertisement and article had narrowed. Her extended story went beyond the happy ending of weight loss to the issue of regaining weight. The magic solution was still there, providing ease of control over appetite, but underlying Bodnar's story was the suggestion that keeping weight off was an ongoing battle. But, unlike a battle, the tactics of dieting with Ayds were always successful if followed correctly and maintained.

The narratives in *Chatelaine* in the 1970s continued to follow the script: the trope of women who weighed too much, many of them since childhood or their teenage years; overate; felt they had no life being fat; got a wake-up call from a family member or friend; tried dieting to no avail; found a way of dieting by themselves or with the help of a physician or a dieting organization; kept to the diet through various means; and, at the end, lost weight and gained beauty and success.[18] The use of the extreme situation continued, allowing readers to revel in someone else's life, a life on the edge of carnivalesque weight. Eveleen Dollery told the story of Marla Donsky in "Take It Off! Take It Off!," an article that contained most of the standard script.[19] A five-foot-two-inch bride, Marla weighed 185 pounds, but very quickly put on weight and reached 215 pounds and a size 24. She found herself retreating from love, seldom engaged with others, and felt reluctant to leave the house. But her pattern as a fat child continued – her unhappiness led to more eating. When she finally decided to lose weight (suggesting that this is all she needed to do), she did so alone: no friends, no advice from a physician, and no weight-loss clubs – the latter becoming a choice of increasing numbers of women. She ate regularly and ate nutritious food, and she cut out most of her carbohydrates with the exception of the occasional potato at dinner. At the time the article was written, Donsky was "slim and attractive," weighing 119 pounds and wearing a size 9. When tempted to eat, she would look at a photograph of the person she had once been – a 215-pound woman wearing "a sacklike dress." Her narrative was a soap opera, with all the extreme feelings, isolation, and plot structure. Her redemption was even greater because of the dismal picture painted of her life as a fat woman.

A new development in the 1970s was men willing to expose their emotional reaction to their weight. In 1973, an article appeared in the *Financial Post* on Mike Crowe. Crowe, aged twenty-nine, remembered his childhood nickname: "Fatso." Because of his size, he didn't have a social life and had never had a girlfriend. A civil servant, he was lonely; when he was at home alone in his apartment, he ate "steadily" until he went to bed. He described his body as a "grotesque, lumbering 340 pounds." But he decided to do something about his body. After all, he assumed weight was something you could control, and by not doing so he felt he was "failing." He went to a physician, was given a diet card, and once on the diet, he recognized how much food he had been eating and what he needed to do to lose weight. He went on an extreme diet of 600 calories a day, compared to his usual 4,000 to 5,000 calories. Within a year, he was down to 200 pounds, although he didn't feel any better. But he decided to go to Europe, and there, for the first time, he "saw the world through thin eyes." He even went to bed with a "girl," the first time since he was seventeen. He regained some weight, but resumed his diet on returning to Canada and went down to 167 pounds, at which point he took a leave of absence from his job to enrol in law school. He still went on eating sprees. His obesity had damaged his circulation, and as a result, he experienced blind spells. He also felt cold all the time.[20] His is a rare narrative describing his continuing health problems after weight loss.

Two other narratives were quite different. The first was a 1957 article by CBC radio personality Byng Whitteker, which appeared in *Maclean's*. In the article, Whitteker acknowledged he was fat, but said he was happy as he was, and he was tired of hearing about the need for dieting. His blood pressure and other vital signs were healthy, his weight hadn't affected his social life, and he didn't stress about his size, which was more than many others could say about their own weight. He did see one negative aspect of his size: "I am a rather complex individual but sometimes I have the sensation of being enclosed by a walking stereotype. It gets monotonous."[21]

The second narrative appeared in the June 1961 *Chatelaine* article, "Who Says *Anyone* Can Lose Weight?" Ethel Gillingham wrote an impassioned response to the pressure on women to be "thin," pressure she had experienced herself. Gillingham was most upset by health experts attributing psychological problems as the cause of people being overweight. She was willing to acknowledge that it might be true in individual cases, but what frustrated her, as it did Whitteker, was the denial that someone could be happy and still be fat. Gillingham's article provided an outlet for the anger and frustration experienced by those trying to lose weight (or not).[22] Experts often acknowledged the reality that dieting didn't work; nevertheless, some form of dieting was all they could offer, and they placed the responsibility for failure to lose weight on the person who was on the diet. Dieting was a cycle with which many readers could identify, and having Gillingham express her annoyance was key to her article's appeal. For Gillingham, a life surrounded by guilt about the consequences of being fat was not a life. Indeed, her view of weight and the problems of being overweight

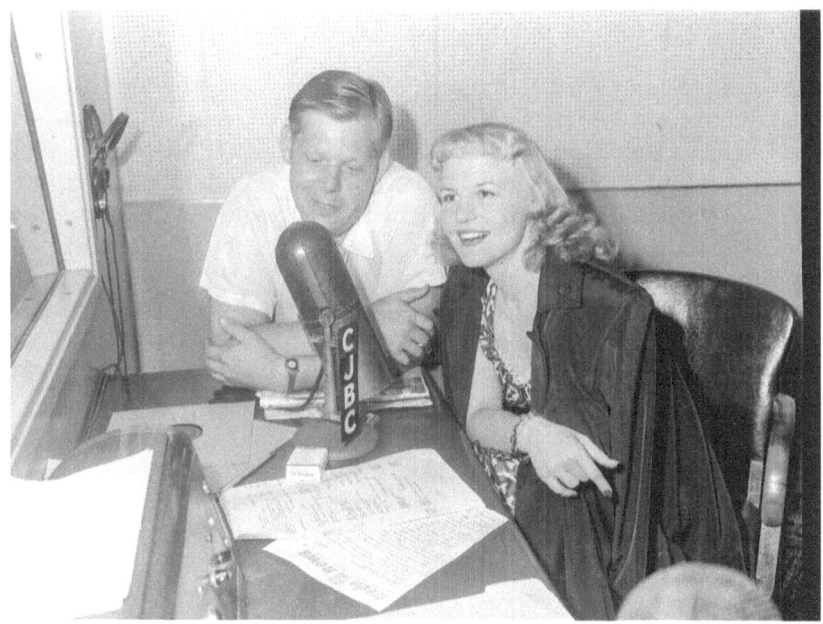

Radio broadcaster Byng Whitteker (Whittaker) admitted in an October 1957 *Maclean's* article that his body was big, perhaps fat, but he didn't bother about it. It was just him. This 1948 photograph shows Byng Whitteker and Peggy Lee at a CJBC microphone in Toronto. Obviously his weight didn't get in the way of his career. Source: Gilbert A. Milne; 10020074.jpg, Archives of Ontario.

tended to be quite holistic and explained with wit, sarcasm, and a sense of truth based in common sense, which originated in personal experience and observation.

The before and after scripts did not suggest the emotional complexity Gillingham astutely describes. Rather, the narratives were about dichotomized lives before and after weight loss – more extreme for women than for men. Such a dichotomy does not appear in the interviews. Rather, the direct voices of memory are charged with emotional tension, a sense of childhood warped by others' views, feeling betrayed by their bodies, and an anger on the part of some at having lived with the consequences of not being "normal" with no access to any antidote.

Interviews

Fat narratives published in the media are often shaped by the needs or interests of the advertisers, the individual author writing the article, or the magazine publishing it. Interviewing is influenced, if not directed, by the interviewer's perspective, which limits the authenticity of the voices of those interviewed.[23] Nevertheless, interviews remain the best way to explore how those who were or are fat see themselves and perceive the world around them and their place in it. Thirty interviews form the source for this section, featuring five men and twenty-five women.[24] Of the thirty, three were born in the 1930s, seven in the 1940s, eleven in the 1950s, eight in the 1960s, and one in the 1970s. Because of the 1980 cut-off date for this study, many of the memories concerned experiences as children, adolescents, and young adults. Those interviewed lived in places ranging from British Columbia to Ontario; most were Canadian born. Some were well off, most seemed financially comfortable, and others had and still have trouble making ends meet. Some grew up in farming communities or small towns, but most lived in urban areas. Two were raised in single-parent families. Three women were molested during their childhood, and another was a victim of family violence. Whether such experiences were a factor in weight gain would lend itself to a psychological analysis if that were the focus for the interview. Certainly, these women were vulnerable, and being overweight exacerbated their sense of vulnerability. Despite the differences, the vast majority of interviewees were white and had been able-bodied as children, although a few had had serious illnesses or health problems.[25] Unlike the fat narratives presented in weight-loss columns and features, the interviewees were less optimistic about their ability to lose weight.

Early Years Families

Unlike some of the recent literature that addresses obesity, the narratives contained no evidence that the birth weight of the interviewees was linked to later obesity. The majority were normal in birth weight. Four deemed themselves heavy at birth, ranging from 8 pounds to 11 pounds. Some didn't know their birth weight because they had been adopted. Neither was there a strong link between infant feeding and future obesity. Few mentioned being breastfed, presumably because most were born when breastfeeding was on the decline. Five did have stories about their feeding. For example, Stephanie's adopted parents put her on a formula that contained evaporated milk and karo syrup (corn syrup). She was not sure how the formula was constituted, but as an adult she saw in the formula the beginning of her weight problem, deeming herself as an infant "drinking fat and sugar." As a newborn, Nina didn't seem to eat at all. Her mother was an older mother (early forties) and didn't have enough milk to breastfeed, so the hospital tried Nina on formula, and she rejected it. As a result, hospital officials told her mother to take Nina home and get her christened, because there was nothing they could do – her baby was going to die. Living in a rural area, however, Nina's parents had neighbours with a dairy farm who offered them unpasteurised whole milk, which Nina was able to take and thrive on. Jane's mother was unable to breastfeed, although Jane thought she probably had tried. In thinking back on it, Jane speculated on "how much anxiety about food got stirred up right at the very very beginning." For these women, infant feeding experiences were the potential beginnings of their future weight. The fact that their infant eating stories existed reflected their interest in understanding the trajectory their lives took and perhaps explaining why they put on weight. They identified infancy as worthy of attention, just as physicians in the later decades of the period covered by this study did, and as present-day researchers do.

Heredity as a cause of obesity has long been a contentious issue in the literature on obesity. While acknowledging its influence, physicians were ambivalent as to whether obesity ran in families or certain eating habits did. Not surprisingly, the majority of people interviewed had a strong sense of the former. At least two-thirds of them were very aware of who in their family was fat, in part because relatives who were big provided children with a sense of why they, too, were heavy. Just as parents' weight made their fat child felt less alone, having a sibling who was big did so even more. For those with a sibling who wasn't overweight, a sense of "why him or her" and "not me" could appear. More than a third of respondents had a sibling who didn't have a weight problem. Grace recalled that her "skinny" brother was able to eat whatever he wanted – so much so that her mother bought special food for him such as Coke or cookies, which were off limits to Grace and her sister. Fatness also runs in families because of learned eating habits. Whether born in the 1930s or in the 1960s, respondents remembered the family eating dinner together.

Compared to today, food choices for dinner in the past were limited. For the main meal of the day, potatoes and meat dominated (usually beef or pork, and less often chicken).[26] A few mentioned eating fish, rice, or pasta. For immigrant families, food would vary from the anglo norm. For example, Olive's meals often included Hungarian specialties. For Leona, who lived in the North, meals could include deer, moose, or beaver meat. Some families simply liked variety in food. Tammy's response to questions about the quality of food in her family was representative of a good number of the interviewees: "I always tell everybody, the food was lousy really. My mother was a lousy cook, god rest her soul. And my father came from Scotland … no cuisine there, that I can see. We had, everyday, meat, potatoes, and some other overcooked vegetable. Like a holy triangle." Several interviewees reported that once a week, usually on Sundays, their families ate a more elaborate meal. Other than remembering the overcooked food served, most remarked on the limited number of vegetables in childhood meals. Those who remembered fresh vegetables lived in farm families. Otherwise, canned or frozen vegetables were prevalent. Despite the emphasis nutritionists put on eating vegetables, vegetables did not seem to be a significant part of the meals. Salads were even rarer. In the memories of interviewees, breakfast did not seem to be a significant meal. Lunches were most often sandwiches and/or soup, something quick so the children could get back to school. When the schools were too far away to eat at home, as were most high schools, children and teenagers took their lunches, usually sandwiches. There was not very much variety.

Fruits were available, mostly apples followed by bananas, oranges, and berries. Canned fruit was common, and some remembered their families canning fruit. When questioned about desserts, about half recalled having had some kind of dessert every day. Eleven described specific desserts for special occasions such as birthdays and Sunday/Saturday meals. Eating desserts, whether at mealtime or other times, was a contested issue for children who were fat. Lucy remembered that dessert was available at dinner, but her mother controlled whether she could have any or not. Like Grace, her brother was "skinny" and could have dessert, but Lucy was usually limited to fruit. However, when she and her mother were out together, her mother often encouraged her to have a treat in which her mother would join her. Looking back, Lucy noted that there was no consistency to her mother's message. Doris remembered that in her family "there was always desserts … [M]y mother had a wicked sweet tooth … [and] it was always … available." But Doris found that frustrating because of her weight.

Snacks and treats were, by their very nature, memorable. Those interviewed had strong memories of going out for ice cream or buying their own penny candy. Julie probably had more treats than most since her mother worked at restaurants so they ate out often. She would also go to the restaurant after school and be given pie or ice cream. Rose remembered receiving candies and cookies as a reward for being good, a habit that weight experts have criticized. Aileen's father brought home candy bars for her sweet tooth; it seemed to have been a way of showing love, something that nutritionists frowned upon as well. Tammy estimated that she drank a 6-ounce bottle of Coke with her friends every day after school. For her, that was rationing it. Nina claimed she drank much more than what Tammy remembered.[27] In addition to treats, snacks filled the gap between school and dinner, and between dinner and bedtime. The litany of what some children ate was far removed from the snacks nutritionists were advocating. Laura remembered often eating cereal or cake after school and toast or cereal before bed. Grace ate chips, popcorn, or cookies before bed.

Not all the interviewees had parents who were lenient about food. Nevertheless, as children and/or teens, they were ingenious in finding ways to satisfy their hunger and sweet tooth. Grace remembered that she was too short to reach the cookies at home, but she could reach the package of Tang in which she would put her finger and then lick the powder off.[28] Lucy learned how to become a "secret" eater; if her mother had baked a cake, she would remove the icing from the bottom of the cake where it wasn't noticeable. Olive would hide a jar of peanut butter in her room; she loved eating peanut butter, but her Hungarian parents thought it disgusting. A number of interviewees recalled stealing money to buy sweets. Grace stole from her blind grandmother and bought chips, chocolate, or McDonald's sundaes. All those youths were showing their agency, something that many adults, including practitioners, didn't see.

Sometimes the family's economic situation determined eating habits. The Depression dictated Alice's eating as a child. She remembered sometimes having meals of only bread and milk with some brown sugar for several days at a time. When eggs were not needed for market, her family would eat mostly eggs. For Nina, eating had no limits when she was growing up. Her mother ran a boarding house to support both of them, and as a result, food was plentiful. "Two or three pieces of pie if you wanted it." When asked what her mother's concern was, her answer was poignant: "Her concern was … money, and keeping a roof over our heads." Connie's mother, a single mom, had come from war-torn Europe after World War II. Although Connie had issues with her mother and the food she piled on her plate, Connie realized it was her mother's own experience of deprivation that led to it. Connie also admitted the meals served were healthy, and her mother was a good cook.[29]

Other factors, too, determined food habits. Leona's father was not always home for days due to his work, and when he was away, her mother made what was easy for her or food that her father didn't like. At times, eating was fraught with tension and very much a contested act. Leona's eating was complicated because she was unable to taste food. She chose food by smell and texture, which meant she could eat almost anything if she put enough ketchup on it. Her father, however, didn't seem to understand her disability. One night, he was determined she would eat potatoes, which she hated, and forced her to eat them nevertheless; she ended up being sick over the kitchen table. Irene, Leona's sister, remembered the dinner battlefield because of Leona's problem and their father wanting to control his children and have them finish their meals.

Despite the efforts of nutritionists, educators, and advertisers to educate Canadians about nutrition, some of those interviewed claimed they didn't know very much about it when they were growing up. Experts giving advice had to contend with family habits as well as the desires of children to fit in with their peers, food being very much cultural and sometimes age related. William didn't recall his parents discussing nutrition, but he did get some instruction in health class at school. He also remembered his doctor giving him a sheet on food groups, but mostly, he learned through "osmosis" from TV, the Canada Food Guide, advertisements, and articles. What emerged from the interviews was a disconnect between the nutritional advice literature and how people actually ate.

Social Life

Most of the interviewees remembered unkind acts linked to their weight. Eight of them clearly recalled being teased at school because of their weight. While details about her younger years were vague for Laura, she was adamant that she hated school and mentioned that her older sister looked out for her. "I know that she used to beat a lot of people up because they were picking on me." Leona remembered school children calling her "Fatty, fatty, two by four." For Rose, the teasing reached into university. Even what seemed normal at the time could make children conscious about their weight, for example, having children weighed at school and making the weight public to other students.[30] Teachers could also be the source of anguish by mentioning a child's or adolescent's weight. Randy had strong memories of his gym teacher constantly pushing him to climb the ropes, even when he knew that he couldn't do it; the result: "All it did was tear down my self-worth even more."

There were many sources of teasing, name calling, and hurtful acts. For some who had obese parent(s), childhood was protected and weight was often not an issue. For others, family members were a source of teasing. Leona remembered her father's favourite greeting to her: "How's my little Miss Piggy?" One day, Grace's brother brought some friends home to see the dogs his mother was breeding. Before they came in, however, he asked Grace if she could go to her room when they arrived. "I just don't want them to see you."[31] Strangers, too, left a mark. Lucy remembered going to see a movie wearing a purple shirt and having some people in the line make reference to "moo in purple." Incidents of hurt were not easily forgotten.

Worse than teasing and hurtful comments was physical violence. Sasha experienced sitting on an eraser full of pins placed on her school chair by a classmate. There was no way she could get the pins out; consequently, she had to walk up to the front of the room and show the teacher what had happened, embarrassing herself in front of her peers. Grace remembered being beaten up in grades 5 and 6. Professor Carla Rice interviewed a woman who recalled boys waiting for her on her way home from grade school and spitting all over her.[32] Randy saw himself as an "easy target." In the 1970s, the high school bully followed him and, in Randy's words, "grabbed me by the throat, pulled me in and I got kneed[ed] in the spine, on the coccyx. And literally, my legs went numb and I went to the ground, then the guy laughed at me and walked away." When Randy told his mother, she had little sympathy and told him to fight back. The physical terrorizing occurred so often that Randy saw himself as a person for "people to abuse." Only rarely did youth fight back. Sylvie was big, and she knew that boys didn't like fat girls who fought back. While fighting a popular boy whom she could beat, she attracted other boys who took his place when he tired. "I [eventually] got exhausted. Then they all started pounding me. So they were putting me in my place."[33] Violence against fat youths is still going on.[34]

Such incidents had long-lasting effects. The pain they caused can still be heard in the memories of those interviewed. Stephanie: "It was hard ... I hated school. Hated school"; Laura: "I actually quit high school in grade 10, I hated it. I hated it ... I hated being the fat person in schools"; Aileen: "I didn't want to go to school ... [K]ids can be so cruel." Grace looked back at her experiences at school and remembered it "was sooo hurtful." She remembered asking someone at home: "'Why? What did I do to them?' Not recognizing that I'm different visually." When asked whether he was unhappy at school, William replied: "Oh god yes." Irene looked back on her childhood and explained: "I had no self-esteem at all ... I just deserved to be beaten up." This comment came from a woman who as a pre-adolescent had been repeatedly sexually molested.

Not all memories were bad, but the pleasant ones were more sporadic – a kindness here, a kindness there. A few interviewees fondly remembered compliments: a dance instructor told Doris that she was "the lightest person I've ever danced with"; a customer referred to Mary as "pleasingly plump," and a friend called her "an appetizing little woman." Sasha recalled a friend of her father's who always treated her well. He owned a large size clothing store, and he liked big women. Jane remembered the meeting of eyes with a man in Algeria and feeling attractive because men in Algeria liked large women.

The isolation of anyone who is different can be wearing. Friends, however, can provide a sense of safety and different models to emulate. Aileen recalled a Polish girl who was a friend – they were both fat. The girl's whole family was overweight, and her friend was happy and confident. But her parents learned about violence between Aileen's parents and forbade their daughter to have anything to do with Aileen. Nina couldn't bring many friends home because of her father's violence during his epileptic episodes. But one good friend pointed out to Nina that at least it wasn't her father's fault – her friend's father was an alcoholic. Nina thus learned that she wasn't alone and the situation with her father could have been much worse. While Grace was unhappy at high school, she was popular and involved in all sorts of activities, albeit not with an "in" group. For some, good friends came later in life. For Heather and Jane, it was within the Large as Life self-help group. Not all friendships were supportive or healthy. Rose remembered her "friends" were people who accepted her for what she was willing to do (have sex and drink) and not for who she was. Her behaviour may have been self-destructive, but it was her way of creating social contact.

Similarly, Connie felt that her stealing money from her mother and treating her friends with it was a condition of their friendship.

The years around puberty, when sexual attraction to others begins, can be traumatic for most young people, but more so for those who are heavy. Too often, acceptance by their friends didn't carry over into the dating world. Laura remembered it "wasn't cool to date a fat chick." Doris remembered that when she was dating her husband-to-be (the only man she had dated), his mother said to him: "Why do you want to marry her? Somebody that's that big and that fat. All she's going to do is bring you down. And all you're going to do is look after her all your life and she's not going to be able to work." The sad irony was that the opposite happened. After the birth of their daughter, her husband decided he didn't want to work and had what Doris referred to as "supposedly ... breakdowns." She ended up taking care of him. Jane recalled an incident when she was twenty, wearing a raincoat and meeting a "guy" who was attractive. They seemed to be getting along well, and she sensed a "real attraction" between them. And then he said something like: "'Well, what do you look like? Take your rain coat off.' So I took my rain coat off and his face just went into a mask of disgust and revulsion. Horrible. Horrible. It made me very very angry for many many years." Most of those interviewed who were willing to talk about relationships were or had been married. Nina's and Lucy's descriptions of their marriages suggested that being fat was something that should be discussed or at least acknowledged. Even in the happy relationships, the fatness of one partner somehow needed to be accepted – it wasn't just there, part of the package like bad eyesight or being shorter than the norm. Even when the non-fat person seemed oblivious of his or her partner's fatness, the fat partner wasn't. For those whose relationships were not supportive, their weight seemed to be an issue, or at least they believed it was. With some partners, the support was not there when the other partner did lose weight. Nina went to Taking Off Pounds Sensibly (TOPS) after 1980, but when she lost weight she noted that her husband "sabotaged everything. He didn't like me thin because other people were talking to me."[35]

One of the strongest themes raised about growing up fat was the difficulty finding clothing, a problem that Eaton's catalogues reflected in the past and that still exists in other catalogues, although to a lesser degree.[36] For the interviewees, clothing was an ongoing issue, but particularly so for prepubescents and adolescents. For girls, clothes were part of the teenage culture, a sign of their youth and power as young women.[37] Looking back on her childhood, Laura considered the only positive aspect of being fat was that she never had hand-me-down clothing, since no one had clothes big enough to fit her. But it was difficult to find new clothes in age-appropriate styles. For example, Laura wanted girl's jeans but they didn't fit her, so she bought a pair in the men's shop. Leona described finally finding some jeans, even though they were too small for her. Determined, she managed to put them on, albeit with her "belly overhang." Nicole remembered crying because she couldn't find a decent dress for her grade 8 celebration.

Few stores offered clothing in large sizes, and those that did were in larger cities. Pennington's catered to large women, but the clothes were styled for older women. Laura preferred shopping out of the Sears catalogue from the women's and half-size clothing. While the styles may have been a bit better than Pennington's, they still were not designed with children or adolescents in mind. Randy had memories of going to Bi-Ways, Zellers, and George Richards for jeans. He hated shopping at Budds in Kitchener, Ontario, even though it had a husky section. "Everything that I had was husky ... husky shirts, husky pants, husky suits. I hated the word 'husky.'" Shopping in the United States was feasible for those who lived close to the border and could afford to get there. There was more choice in good quality clothes for large people and larger sizes than were available in most of Canada. One solution to the clothing problem was to sew your own clothing. Having mothers or grandmothers who could sew was an advantage. Boys seldom had home-made clothes, in part because sewing a daughter's clothing was something of a norm for many mothers.

For some of the interviewees, the lack of appropriate clothing wasn't important when they were children. Julie remembered not being interested in clothes; as long as she had a T-shirt and jeans she was happy, but for most other clothing she was fraught with frustration. Mary noted that "the clothing issue ... never went away. Never ever, ever, ever." Jane's experience was no different – clothes shopping was "just awful." In university, she told a professor that she was "going to start a large liberation movement" to raise the issue of clothing for big women. She eventually published an article in a Vancouver newspaper about what it was like to shop for large sizes, and as a result, received many supportive calls. She had touched something with which many big women could identify. But, while other fat women could understand the clothing issue, some women were not supportive. Entering into a fitness club, Jane overheard a discussion concerning her complaints about not being able to find "decent" clothes that fit her. One of the group remarked, "Well, why would anybody in a size 20 want nice clothes?"

Weight Causes and Treatments

Those interviewed could be quite blunt about the cause of their weight.[38] Some admitted that they ate too much. Laura had a mother and a grandmother who tried to limit what she ate, but neighbours who loved to eat would invite Laura over to have lunch with them. They told her mother, "Look at her, she's hungry, look at her. She loves the food. Let her eat." Some simply had a hankering for sweets or other fattening foods. Many of those interviewed tried to understand when they began to be fat, just as health professionals did. For Heather, being fat was always a part of her life; she could not remember a time when she had not been overweight. Randy was a thin child up until age three when his tonsils were removed. At that point, he started gaining weight, and by the time he started school, he was the "chunkiest" child in class. Stephanie thought the age of six was crucial for her – the year when she and her best friend started to follow her friend's mother's happy-eating behaviour. But she also noted that her candy fixation appeared after she was abused by a neighbour.

Many interviewees were specific about the impact of puberty, not necessarily as the cause of their fatness, but as the time when their awareness of it emerged. Others pointed to weight gain during pregnancy and not being able to lose it. Indeed, their weight increased with every pregnancy.[39] None of the women could remember any physician being concerned about their weight gain during pregnancy. For Frank, weight gain was linked to the death of his father. At that point, Frank stopped swimming and doing regular exercise. Others, like Mary, just pointed to a life too busy and stressful, in her case having two children, getting a BA, MA, and PhD as a mature student, and working many sessional teaching jobs. Before she knew it, she weighed 200 pounds. Pressure was constant, and eating relieved it somewhat. Still others pointed to unhappiness, illness, boredom, or taking drugs. For most, the problem with putting on weight was their inability to lose it or keep it off.

Since most of those interviewed became fat while living at home, their family situation was frequently the key. Certainly, medical experts were often willing to blame the parents (usually mothers) for any problems children were having. Most parents of the interviewees were aware that their child was overweight, although most didn't know what to do about it except to cut back on their child's food consumption. One mother queried if she should do anything other than give her child unconditional love. Others just ignored the issue. The focus for Tammy's parents was on her younger brother who was thin and didn't eat well. Tammy was doing what children were supposed to do: eat what was placed in front of them so they would be healthy. The thin child who didn't eat was the problem child. Nina, who helped her mother in their boarding house, remembered her mother doing little about her weight and, indeed, taking her out for fries. Looking back, Nina sees that eating fries together was a special time when mother and daughter were able to get out of the house and be with each other. Money was tight, and fries were affordable and a treat for both of them. Other parents were more proactive. Some encouraged their kids to eat less or to go on a diet, but such children saw their parents as trying to control them. Most parents talked to their children about their weight, which for many children was more like nagging than concern. For Stephanie, the talk her father had with her was simply hurtful. Children knew their parents were worried, but somehow the blame for the child's weight seemed to be placed on the child: being told what to eat, what not to eat, or refusing to let them eat certain foods.

Physicians didn't loom large for most of those interviewed until well into adulthood. For some, however, their doctors participated in the family dialogue on weight and did so in various ways. Laura's mother took her to a doctor when she was only six months old, and the doctor told Laura's mother her child was fine. Nevertheless, the mother continued to "drag" Laura from doctor to doctor looking for an answer to her weight. Most doctors didn't make a big deal about an infant's or young child's weight other than to mention the weight based on a visual assessment or a weight measurement. Some provided nutrition literature for dieting, or simply gave their opinion of the diets the patients had created for themselves. When Leona's parents took her to a doctor, he told them to stop her from eating peanut butter sandwiches.

From the perspective of those who sought help, not all practitioners showed respect to fat patients or to their parents (usually the mother) if the patient was underage.[40] A physician in St Catharines told Jane's parents: "She's not overweight, she's gross." Or at least that was what Jane remembered overhearing. Doris recalled doctors when she was a child in the 1950s: "They spoke to you like you were a fungus that they didn't want in their office or whatever." Neither does Doris believe that anything has changed. In later life, Randy rejected his doctor blaming his weight for his diabetes and was appalled by the doctor's suggestion that he have his jaw wired shut so he could lose some weight. He admitted that weight was probably a factor in some of his health problems, but felt the physician at least should have considered his body shape before he began a rant. Terry Poulton recalled having had an internal examination during which the doctor made the comment that examining her was like working "through all her upholstery," referring to her fat.[41] Nurses, too, were not always sympathetic.[42]

Of all the methods of losing weight, dieting held pride of place in medicine and with people who wanted to lose weight. The "treatment" was an emotional rollercoaster: the determination to lose weight, the effort to do so, the success in doing so and the euphoria that came with it, the difficulty in maintaining stability, and then the discouragement of regaining weight. As noted in chapter six, the medical literature on dieting did not endorse dieting for children and teens; a shift from non-nutritional to nutritional eating was all that was prescribed. Nevertheless, many of the interviews indicate that a number of interviewees were exposed to dieting when they were young. While most didn't go to practitioners, Julie did. In 1976, when Julie was fourteen, her grandmother's physician wanted to put her on a liquid protein diet. She weighted 175 pounds at the time. Her physician monitored her blood over the dieting period; in the fourth week, when Julie went for her blood check, her physician took her off the diet – a number of people in America had died on the same diet.[43] Although Julie had lost 40 pounds, her physician did not advise any more dieting experiences. She was to eat what she had been eating before going on the liquid diet. Three months after stopping the diet, she was in the hospital with blood poisoning and a bladder infection, and her kidneys began to shut down, all of which she blamed on the liquid protein diet. At the age of sixteen, Olive went to Dr Vitou's clinic in Port Royal, Quebec. At the clinic she received acupuncture, and was told not to eat during the day but to eat meat and some vegetables just before bed. Dr Vitou ran the clinic out of her home, and Olive remembered her as a "really scary woman, gruff." Even though she lost 45 to 50 pounds, Olive had dizzy spells and noted that Dr Vitou did not believe in vitamin pills. Looking back on her experience, Olive concluded: "These things cannot be good for you. Like they can't be. No how." Doris, too, was under the surveillance of experts. In the early 1960s, she entered the Toronto General Hospital for weight loss under the supervision of Dr Calvin Ezrin, author of *Your Fat Can Make You Thin*. Put on a 500-calorie diet, she was basically living on water and vitamin pills for the first seven weeks. She lost weight, but was also getting weaker since the hospital workers kept her in bed. As a result, in the fifth week they let her have some jello, and by the seventh week she had put on 25 pounds. Not accepting that she was putting on weight while still on the planned diet except for the jello, the doctors were convinced that food was being sneaked to her, despite her denials and those of her parents. Unwilling to believe her, they preferred to hold on to their faith in dieting.

Jane had behavioural therapy. While a student at McGill, she became a subject for Professor Ernest Poser who was looking for volunteers for an experiment he was running. To give her an adverse reaction to eating chocolate chip cookies, she was asked to drink something "vile" every time she ate a cookie. It certainly worked for the short time, but not for the long term. But then, she admitted, nothing she tried worked. "I'm just not disciplined enough. I'm too independent and anti-authoritarian to stick" to diet programs.

At least one-third of those interviewed had tried drugs to help them lose weight.[44] When she was in grade 8, Stephanie took prescribed amphetamines of some kind for what she thought was a full year. They didn't help her lose weight, and the only reason she stayed on the amphetamines was for her parents, who wanted her to keep trying to lose weight. Doris was a teenager when she tried diet pills to suppress her appetite. She first took them in her early teens in the mid-1950s and then in her late teens. They bothered her sleeping, but otherwise they had no real effect, even though she took them for six to seven months. Olive also tried diet pills, but hers were not prescribed. A friend's father who was a physician prescribed them to his daughter and Olive tried them – she liked the idea of taking a pill and not being hungry. Whatever she took didn't work.

Hypnosis was another treatment involving an expert. Laura, William, and Olive each saw hypnotists. Laura was taken to a physician for hypnosis by her stepfather. At the end of the appointment, the physician complained that Laura was the "most insolent" child he had ever dealt with. Laura remembered her stepfather saying, "'This guy is wacked,' because I was the furthest thing from the insolent child." Her interpretation was that the doctor was unable to hypnotize her and put the blame on her. William saw a hypnotist, but it was unclear if he actually underwent hypnosis. The hypnotist did suggest he go on a liquid diet for three weeks – the liquid could be anything, even milkshakes. The logic of the diet was unclear to William. When Olive was seventeen or eighteen, she was sent to a hypnotist. She found the experience "very bad," believing that the "guy tried to take advantage of me physically."

Less formal treatments were more popular. In 1969, at age twelve, Irene went on a diet with her father who wanted to lose weight. The diet of choice was the Stillman diet, which advocated eating high levels of protein and avoiding carbohydrates. Irene loved the diet, meat being among her favourite foods. But the diet was not healthy, and she was convinced that both she and her father developed health problems because of it. Rose went on a diet overseen by her mother between grades 7 and 8. For Rose, the dieting was wonderful because it meant her mother paid attention to her; at the same time she also lost 20 to 25 pounds. Part of the diet was Metrecal in milk for breakfast and lunch, followed by a normal dinner meal. For Rose, the diet was worth it – at its end she could get into blue jeans and she "felt pretty sexy." But, as with others, the weight didn't stay off. More eccentric diets were tried. Mary remembered following the grapefruit diet when she was sixteen. Grace and Aileen tried the banana diet. Tammy had her own way of losing weight – smoking and drinking black coffee, a habit she had developed before high school. William tried fasting, the "stupidest" effort at weight loss he ever tried; without medical supervision, he just took in water (not even broth) and did so for eighteen to nineteen days. Towards the end of the fast, he experienced hallucinations.

Many interviewees tried some type of formal group weight-loss program at some point in their lives. Of the weight-loss groups, Weight Watchers by far led the list, with five individuals having taken the organizations's program before 1980, followed by TOPS with two, and Calorie Counters with one. Frank was vehement about not joining a weight-loss group: "I can't stand this baring my soul in groups ... no, no. I'm too busy." Two more of the five men interviewed similarly rejected group programs. As one study of men in weight-loss groups in Scotland noted, men are more likely to watch their partners attend and then follow the program at home.[45] Being in a weight-loss program reveals men's vulnerability. While the supportive and safe environment of weight-loss groups was part of their attraction for women, some details were worrisome. Lucy went to Weight Watchers in 1980 at age ten, but even before that, at age eight, she went to a woman who helped people in her community lose weight. Looking back at being on a diet as a child, Lucy sees it is something a child shouldn't have to do. Certainly, it raises questions of how a weight-loss program designed for adult women (or even for adolescents) could be safe for a growing child.[46] In her preteens, Laura attended Calorie Counters in the local church basement and remembered how much she hated being weighed in front of others. In her teens, she joined Weight Watchers. Fat camps were more positive for Olive, Jane, and Connie. They enjoyed getting away and being in an environment that seemed happy and safe for them. Fat camps weren't popular in Canada in the literature on childhood obesity, probably because of the cost.[47] Whether camps or weight-loss organizations, attending them is a form of public "coming out," a public acceptance that one is fat.[48]

Not everyone was interested in traditional or even eccentric dieting. Julie claimed she was allergic to almost anything "medication wise," which made her "gun-shy" about diets. Others simply cut down on portions or altered what they ate or drank. Tina determined her problem was when she ate during the day. She tried to save her cravings for the morning; while it seemed to help her lose weight, the evenings became very long and, in her words, the "food call[ed]" her.

Contrary to the image of fat children as lazy, many of the interviewees remembered being quite active during their childhood: riding their bicycles, walking, playing street sports, and/or working on the farm. Fewer were involved in organized exercise or sports, perhaps because team sports required being picked for a team and fat children didn't have a reputation for being physically able. Some took up exercise as part of a weight-loss plan, while others simply did not like physical activity after a certain age or couldn't remember ever liking it or being encouraged to like it. For Irene, physical sport was uncomfortable. As she asked, who wants to fall in winter on a hard surface and who wants to do activity in the summer with its mosquitoes and heat? In any event, at sixteen she was diagnosed with arthritis and that ended any attempt she was willing to make. For those who remembered being active, it seemed associated with a certain period in their lives, rather than an ongoing lifestyle.[49] Only Mary, born in 1934, characterized her life as "very active." For the interviewees, exercise wasn't a significant weight-loss treatment.

Among the interviewees, it is clear that some tried more than one treatment. For example, Doris went on a 500-calorie diet in a hospital and also used a drug to help while on a different diet; William tried fasting and went to a hypnotist; Laura saw a hypnotist and was a member of Calorie Counters and Weight Watchers; Jane went to a fat camp and later tried behaviour therapy; and Olive went to a hypnotist, tried a clinic which gave her a weird diet and acupuncture, tried the fat camp, and used a non-prescribed drug. None of these treatments worked.

Conclusion

What emerges from the interviewees is how aware they were of their weight as young children or adolescents. Some became aware of their weight in traumatic ways: the taunts of "friends"; clothing that wouldn't fit; the efforts of their parents to keep their weight down; and sometimes by being taken to a physician, a visit that could only indicate that something was wrong with them. Once faced with the notion that they were fat, it was difficult for them not to find confirmation of it among their families, their friends, their peers, and strangers. Those who were interviewed articulated the causes of their being overweight only after years of thinking about it. They acknowledged eating was a joy for them, but eating didn't seem sufficient as an explanation. For many, puberty was a turning point, especially for girls; pregnancy was another factor for women. What all agreed upon was that once the weight was gained, it was difficult to lose.

Very few lost weight by dieting. For most, as soon as the diet was over, weight was regained and eventually a new diet tried. The damage caused by the up and down of weight is hard to imagine. Neither were other forms of weight loss any better. Weight-loss programs such as Weight Watchers had some success, but not with those interviewed. Life simply intervened. Neither did drugs work. Indeed, giving powerful drugs to the young is worrisome. Exercise was never a weight-loss program, only an adjunct to dieting, and for most of the interviewees exercise didn't seem to be something they did, at least not when they were adolescents or adults. The sedentary society was too strong to resist, and lives as lived did not offer the time for much exercise. Weight-loss surgery was not a choice for these individuals before 1980.

These fat narratives underline the actions and settings in which people learned about their fatness and how they were reminded of being fat.[50] Allyson Mitchell has noted that the experiences of fat children and adolescents "fly in the face of dominant perceptions and representations of 'home as haven.'" In particular, she points out that for children, mothers loom.[51] While true, there was also a significant mention of fathers in the interviews for this project. The father could be the figure who taught the child that eating too much was not acceptable; some fathers encouraged the eating, others disciplined to control eating, and some reminded their children of their fatness. For many of those interviewed who had had a long life of being fat, memories revolved around how to be fat – memories of dealing with such day-to-day issues as how to choose clothing and where to get it, as well as of coping with systemic difficulties such as physical pain and emotional trauma. It involved being under surveillance and also being invisible.[52]

Underlying the discrimination and hostility of society towards those who were and are heavier than the norm is the centrality of body image. For many of those interviewed, "normal" sized people seemed incapable of relating to them. Rose noted that those around her refer to "the weight" she is carrying as if it is not part of her. Body image also affects how you feel about yourself. Poor body image resulting in prolonged low self-esteem is not easy to overcome. Nina remembered that by age seven she had been told she was fat so often that she believed "nobody would want me." As Olive observed, you can't have self-esteem if everyone seems to be judging you in a negative way.

Epilogue

"History is not merely a project of fact-retrieval ... but also a set of complex processes of selection, interpretation, and even creative intervention – processes set in motion by, among other things, one's personal encounter with the archive ... and the pressure of the contemporary moment on one's reading of what is to be found there."[1]

When people ask me about the past and the present with respect to obesity, the word that always comes to me is "quagmire": a quagmire for those who are fat; for practitioners who want to help patients who come to them asking how to lose weight; for scholars in the humanities and social sciences who often see in the literature on obesity the blaming of individuals for their weight without putting them in a social context; for scientists who often see their nuanced research and conclusions distorted in media headlines; and for those in the media who have to wend their way through literature that is often contradictory. Questions about obesity seem to lead to more questions. The problems of measurements, statistics, and concepts that were recognized as problematic in the past are still with us. Almost any view of obesity – its risks, its causes, and its treatments – can be challenged and is being challenged. Even the concept of normality is unclear. Disputes reflect a lack of consensus on how obesity was and is seen. Is it a disease, an illness, a condition, or is it only a fat body? Is it something that a person can't control, or is it the result of a person's behaviour, or is it just how the person is? Does it even depend on the individual, or is it caused by the modern obesogenic environment? Indeed, underlying much of the obesity literature is a sense of unease with the society in which we live, a belief in an earlier time when Canadians were fit and slender, a time that gets rosier the farther removed we are from it.

The conviction that eating too much was the major cause of obesity seemed obvious in the past and the treatment simple – don't eat so much. Eating, however, is complicated. How do people see eating, and how important are family dynamics in eating? Blaming mothers was dominant in the nutritional literature on infants, children, and teens, and it still is.[2] Yet, seldom were mothers' voices heard. Why is that? Some interviewees blamed their mothers for not instilling a nutritional way of eating when they were children; some acknowledged resenting and subverting mothers' attempts to control what they ate. As explained in chapter one, however, most mothers have long been doing their best to provide proper nutrition for their children, often at risk to their own health. Other interviewees recognized the challenges of mothers (and fathers) and the complexity of their own families and their eating habits. As a society, we don't like to blame children for being obese, and we should not blame them (or not entirely), but we believe someone else has to be blamed. Heredity can lessen blame, but even that can focus on the mother. A recent study suggested that a mother's early puberty is linked to an early puberty in her children and obesity in childhood or adulthood, as if the mother could control when she reached puberty. A more recent study in Canada focused on women who were significantly obese and then underwent weight-loss surgery. Their infants born before the surgery had genes connected to obesity-related diseases, but infants born after the surgery had genes that behaved differently, making their risk for obesity less than that of siblings born before the mother's surgery.[3]

The history of obesity illuminates the past complexity and contentiousness surrounding what to eat, how much, the statistics of weight, and the understanding of each of them. Little has changed. We are still trying to figure out what to eat and what not to eat. As noted in chapter one, most Canadians do not eat the recommended servings of fruits and vegetables each day. Yet, most Canadians think they eat well.[4] Part of that confidence comes from the use of stand-alone vitamins and minerals. But experts have long noted that the best way to get the nutrients we need is through food. Recently, a study (again) found that stand-alone vitamins and minerals have "no measurable health benefits" if you are already healthy.[5] But it isn't easy to know what food to eat. For example, the International Agency for Research on Cancer (IARC), an agency of the World Health Organization (WHO), classified "consumption of processed meat as 'carcinogenic to humans' and consumption of red meat as 'probably carcinogenic to humans.'" But what does this mean? In the press release, there was a risk estimate attributed to the IARC Working Group, yet the agency didn't estimate the risk of each of the agents they listed as carcinogenic. Even if the press release had not mentioned a risk estimate, it is not clear that the press or most people would understand the work of IARC. The statement "gives you an idea about the strength of evidence that [a specific agent] causes cancer but it doesn't give you any clue about how much you need to be exposed [to the agent] to get cancer."[6] Even if you did understand what IARC was claiming, how would you change your eating habits?

Advice given to Canadians changed from generation to generation, whether the advice was about eating, nutrition, dieting, or exercise. Small wonder Canadians never seemed to be able to keep up with the advice being offered. What advice should we follow? A recent book challenges what we have been taught about milk, generally seen as a superior food for calcium. Another book argues that saturated fat is not bad and that a low-fat diet is not as healthy as many made it out to be.[7] At least one reviewer is critical of both arguments,[8] and there are certainly individuals who are not able to lose weight on a low-fat diet. Dr Yoni Freedhoff, medical director of the Bariatric Medical Institute, Ottawa, points out that low-fat diets only seem to make an individual hungry, whereas fat does satiate hunger.[9] But what is new? During the period 1920 to 1980, trends in dieting often went from low-fat to high-fat dieting. It seems high-fat eating is in vogue today. But it isn't the only aspect. At the moment, sugar is deemed to be the cause of the obesity and diabetes epidemic – maybe. The author of *The Case Against Sugar* also sees sugar "linked" to hypertension, some cancers, and even dementia.[10]

We don't always understand how decisions are made about how much weight is good or bad for us. For example, in 1995, the WHO Obesity Task Force lowered the body mass index (BMI) at which individuals would be considered obese. The task force was funded by Abbott Laboratories; at the time, Abbott Laboratories manufactured an obesity drug and diet products, certainly a conflict of interest that many would see as problematic if they had known.[11] As in the past, practitioners today generally agree a balance of food is best for health. Their advice to dieters is to limit the size of food portions and to make sure the variety of foods are balanced to provide nutrients for health. Even more, obesity experts are now accepting that a dieter doesn't need to achieve an "average" weight to be healthy:[12] it is acknowledged that a healthy spectrum of weight is quite broad. However, the goal for too many Canadians is still a limited spectrum of weight driven by the desire to meet a specific body image. That is the area where the fatness advocates and fat studies are significant.

Being healthy has generally meant being fit, and being fit was deemed attractive. In the rhetoric of the cause and treatment of obesity, exercise was included. But the rhetoric on fitness seldom went beyond the idea. Practitioners in the past were not enamoured by exercise, either as a cause of obesity because Canadian didn't exercise enough, or as a treatment. Yet, there are significant studies demonstrating that people with high BMIs who are fit live longer than people who have "normal" BMIs but who aren't fit. It doesn't mean that high BMI people don't have other risks. But people who have "normal" BMI can have health risks too.[13] A recent study on exercise by the London School of Economics found moderate exercise – brisk walking – is the best; people who were moderate in their exercise rather than vigorous, had lower BMIs and were generally healthier. But British Columbia's Dr Brett Belchetz looked at the study and concluded that while moderate exercise was best for women, it wasn't for men under fifty. For them, vigorous exercise was best.[14] Although exercise helps, how fitness is achieved is not something that most health experts are taught. Certainly, it was not something that seemed to be part of medical treatment. Indeed, there is much connected to obesity about which most doctors have little expertise. Past physicians couldn't keep up to date with new developments. Christopher Labos, cardiologist and epidemiologist at the McGill University Health Centre, describes the same concern today. In his words, "New doctors are often told that five years after medical school half of what they learn will be proven wrong."[15] Dr Gilles Plourde and Denis Prud'homme, in their 2012 article "Managing Obesity in Adults in Primary Care," reflect another concern, one they have in common with their past colleagues: practitioners today generally don't know how to deal with their obese patients. Looking at several studies, it would seem that 45 per cent of physicians don't feel able to help their obese patients. According to another study, only 49 per cent of overweight or obese patients are given advice for weight loss – 50 per cent of those are advised to diet, and 41 per cent to increase their exercise.[16]

The complexity and contentiousness of all these factors simply makes it difficult for practitioners and lay people to know how best to deal with obesity or being fat. Studies of and attitudes towards obesity have emphasized the negativity of fatness. Or is it that the stigma placed on fatness has made obesity negative? We expect medicine to be a science and that science will lead us to the best practice. Science through medicine was an actor in the history of obesity, although how it was used and understood was at times problematic. If we still don't understand science and seldom read it, we learn about it through the media. Statistics are at the core of understanding science in a modern society; yet, too often, we don't understand statistics either. For example, many of us don't seem to understand the language of correlation (link, associate, and risk) or cause and effect, and the differences between them. Without some understanding of scientific methodology, it is difficult to evaluate the information science provides. Also, medicine often has to function in areas of scientific uncertainty, where the scientific research may suggest courses of action but does not demonstrate their efficacy. This situation is very much the case with obesity.

Fatness can be a stressful condition for many. The lives of the interviewees after 1980 were still full of pain about how they had been treated in the past and how they are still treated today. Too many find their physicians unable to see them as individuals who are more than their weight. But physicians are not alone. Stephanie described the discrimination she experiences in the workplace as a result of being fat. Having lived in the United States, she found such discrimination stronger in Canada. Laura has a sense of people always judging her and making assumptions about her because of her weight, for instance thinking that she is less intelligent because she is fat. Nina has noticed shifts in how people respond to weight. When she was fat, hardly anyone held a door open for her or greeted her; when she lost weight, both happened. Thus, civilities of life are withheld from those who are fat. As Randy put it, however, "A sandwich doesn't judge you."

Notes on Sources

"Any leftover of the past can be considered a source. It might well be a document ... but it might also be a building, a piece of art or an ephemeral object ... Sources only become historical evidence, however, when they are interpreted by the historian to make sense of the past. The answers they provide will very much depend on the sorts of questions historians are asking ... This is why it makes little sense to ask if something is 'good historical evidence', without knowing what evidence it's supposed to provide."[1]

The major primary sources for *Fighting Fat* are Canadian medical journals. They varied from provincial to national journals, and during the years between 1920 and 1980 more than 100 journals were published. Some were narrow in focus, for example, the *Canadian Cancer Conferences*. The ones I chose had the most readers and were more general in what they published, including journals on public health. The public health journals, themselves, offered advice not only to professional practitioners, but also to those who were interested in the health of the society as a whole. National journals published more on obesity than regional journals, although nutrition was of significance in both of them. While the focus is largely on English Canada, I looked at *L'Union Médicale du Canada* (*UMC*) as a foil to the English journals to see whether the French literature was different or similar. That journal began in 1872; in 1938, l'Association des médecins de l'Amérique du Nord merged its bulletin with it, making *UMC* "the" French-Canadian medical journal. I also used William Osler's *The Principles and Practice of Medicine* in all its editions from 1893 to 1980 as a way of tracing some of the shifts in the perception of obesity from the perspective of a general text that was popular in Canada.

Medical journals are rich sources for illuminating debates within medicine, the changing nature of treatments for any specific disease or condition, the problems that different treatments caused patients, and what was happening in faculties of medicine throughout the country. Physicians who were members of those faculties and who also practised within hospitals were the elite in medicine, and many wrote articles that were published in the journals. That doesn't mean that general practitioners were ignored. Often the most interesting articles were written by those who were at the front line of taking care of Canadians in cities, towns, and rural areas. Such articles described the author's patients and their health concerns, and how the physician-author reacted to those patients. The reviews of work being done outside Canada and the reprinting of some articles published in other countries kept Canadian practitioners up to date and reminded them that they were members of a wider medical "fraternity" beyond Canada's borders. Journals and their contents remind historians about the range of practitioners that existed.

One of the research problems for a history of obesity is that medical journals did not have a lot of practitioners' narratives that talked about seeing and treating patients who were obese. Those narratives seem to appear in discussions that took place around surveys of nutrition and at times when weight was a health concern. Public health periodicals, however, were especially useful, since they encouraged Canadians to take care of themselves. They were full of literature on nutrition, what a healthy weight was, and the need for Canadians to exercise. Nutrition was especially important since it embraced the concern about malnourishment, which later led to seeing too much weight as a problem. The public health literature often addressed Canadians directly, as did nurses, nutritionists and dietitians, practitioners, and public health experts. *The Canadian Nurse* also contained significant articles on nutrition and obesity, issues nurses saw in their work in public health. Results of different surveys of Canadians' weight were published in the journals. Generally, the surveys appeared to reach a consensus, but the details could be different. For example, surveys varied based on where they were done, who was being surveyed, and how the survey was conducted, something the reader should keep in mind. The surveys and the statistics on weight generated had problems, as statistics today still do.[2]

In examining medical journals from over the years, the increasing numbers of advertisements for appetite suppressants became obvious. Historians have long used advertisements to access the past and discussed their advantages and disadvantages. As Jackson Lears notes, advertisements "signify a certain vision of the good life," with products advertised having a "symbolic" purpose as well as a "utilitarian" one.[3] In the twentieth century, subliminal tactics were used in some advertisements (or what some people would describe as "depth psychology"). Theorists also refer to the "gaze," the point of view that "often expresses attitudes of which the viewer may not be conscious."[4] Medical advertisements for appetite suppressants provide historians with an insight into the goals practitioners set for their patients, the changing nature of treatment, the way in which the patient-doctor relationship was seen, the continuation of physician education, and the influence of advertisements within medicine.[5]

Generally, advertisements are composed of two parts: images and text. Drawings, cartoons, and photographs are the hooks to get physicians to look further and read details about the specific drug being advertised. Sometimes, the visual components are stylized, and at other times highly representative. Some advertisements are much more sophisticated than others in terms of the amount of text offered and the detail of the visuals. Those in the *Canadian Medical Association Journal* (*CMAJ*), for example, were generally more informative and visually attractive than those in *The Canadian Doctor*, although the same advertisement was sometimes placed in both journals. Some drug companies advertised in particular journals, perhaps due to a matter of cost, although the main pharmaceutical companies tended to advertise in the major journals. The drugs advertised in *UMC* were often from France and from major pharmaceutical companies outside of France.

What emerges from the advertisements is how many pharmaceutical diet drugs were available, how many advertisements were produced for these products, and how often the advertisements were repeated. The advertisements began to have a notable presence in the late 1940s, increased in number throughout the 1950s and 1960s, and then decreased in the 1970s. The decline in the number of advertisements in the 1970s did not necessarily reflect a decline in the popularity of diet aids, but rather the consolidation of the market, with fewer products dominating it. Despite the growing relationship between Canadian medical journals and some of the major pharmaceutical companies, Canadian content in the advertisements was limited. Most of the pharmaceutical companies were based in the United States or elsewhere. Occasionally, Canadian content appeared through a reference to a Canadian study that supported the advertised drug or a vague comment about obesity being a problem in Canada.[6] Advertisements for obesity drugs are a significant historical source. They are predicated on the power of science and the willingness of practitioners to prescribe drugs. But that power was only significant if drugs were available, if physicians judged them useful, and if the wider population believed in their efficacy. All three conditions came together in the postwar years and beyond. The text of the advertisements, the part that "pushed" a specific pharmaceutical, tried to develop a comfort zone through the expression of shared values between the drug companies and the physicians. The ads directly engaged the practitioner by presenting one side of a dialogue, while the practitioner's reaction to the advertisement became the other side. The goal for the companies was to create a partnership with physicians. Nonetheless, the dialogue was one sided and didactic, providing physicians with information about a drug's safety and efficacy to encourage its use.

Popular magazines provided Canadians with an awareness of many subjects, including health. Some of the authors published by the magazines wrote in a casual, conversational tone so that they became a "friend." At times, the author addressing the readers was a physician or nurse. And those readers were numerous. By 1932, *Chatelaine* had 150,000 paid subscribers; by 1938, the number had increased to 200,000; and by 1940, it had reached 260,000.[7] By the late 1960s, 24.6 per cent of English-Canadian adults read *Maclean's* and 23.2 per cent read *Chatelaine*. More specifically, *Chatelaine* was a mass audience magazine, reaching 37 per cent of all households in Canada. Its readers were largely married, female (although approximately 25 per cent were men), and the readership reflected the economic status of the general population.[8] In addition to *Chatelaine* and *Maclean's*, I examined the *Canadian Home Journal* until it was absorbed by *Chatelaine* in 1958. Periodical bibliographies helped find specific articles on obesity in other magazines.

Popular magazines had the ability to communicate with Canadians through articles, stories, and advertisements. In return, topics such as nutrition, health, diets, fashions, and body image helped bring in readership. The selling of specific products was clear in magazine advertisements. As Judith Williamson describes in her book *Decoding Advertisements*: "The technique of advertising is to correlate feelings, moods or attributes to tangible objects, linking possible *un*attainable things with those that *are* attainable, and thus reassuring us that the former are within reach." In buying a product you are, in part, also buying something that you can't purchase – contentment, perhaps even happiness.[9]

In recent years, historians of consumerism have emphasized the agency of the consumer.[10] No longer can we assume a direct connection between product advertisement and product purchase. Potential consumers read advertisements through their own perspectives, and they react to them in different ways – feeling annoyed by them, ignoring them, rejecting them, and possibly accepting them. But if there is no automatic cause and effect between product presentation and a sale, there is certainly influence. *Chatelaine's* content was 50 per cent advertisements by the late 1960s. While the potential consumers could reject specific advertisements, half a magazine's worth of messages is difficult to ignore.[11]

The "before" and "after" articles and advertisements about losing weight, whether featuring women or men, introduced a Cinderella trope for women and a somewhat less obvious Prince Charming trope for men. The before photographs and drawings of a person who was fat, mostly women rather than men, emphasized poor posture and the lack of fashion sense, both in clothes and hairstyle. The after picture was usually a confident, active, and happy-looking woman, whose fashion sense sent out a message of success. These narratives, many of which purported to include the voices of persons transformed, were marketing tools to sell a product and/or a magazine. Their numbers reflect a side of consumerism that appealed to the insecurity of readers about their bodies or a sense of voyeurism about someone else's life. Even the fictional stories could tell readers how to see people who were fat. Major characters in the stories were seldom fat.

Another media used in this study was the catalogues of Eaton's department stores. Eaton's catered to both the urban and rural market, and to the "lower, middle-class and upper-working-class." By the 1930s, Eaton's controlled 58 per cent of department store sales and more than 7 per cent of all retail sales in Canada. While Donica Belisle in her excellent study of Eaton's argues that Eaton's "perpetuated specific ethnic, race, and class hierarchies in Canada," she also points to the economic broadness and ethnicities of Eaton's customers.[12] Certainly, the catalogues appealed to Canadians as a practical way to shop, but for some, flipping through the pages also provided entertainment. The catalogues were available twice a year and mailed to households free of charge, at least for past customers.

The catalogues offered departments full of household items and appliances, but clothing dominated. Because of that domination, the catalogues were an incredibly rich source. Both the visuals and the texts about clothes lend themselves to historical analysis about body image(s), including fat bodies. The historian can therefore determine how those images were gendered, how they differed according to age (and to a lesser extent class), and how the clothes changed over time.[13] In the early years, images tended to be drawn, but reader demand, in part, increased the use of photographs in the catalogues. By 1940, most of the women's and men's fashions were depicted with photographs.[14] Whether shown in photographs or drawings of models, the fashions represented little that was radical. Looking at the clothing reveals that the silhouettes of fashion were much more mercurial for women than for men. For both, however, the silhouette was an illusion – the main measurements could only be chest, waist, and hips, and not all of them were used. Beyond depicting an illusion, the way in which the advertising text discussed the fashions of the day and how they could help minimize body flaws not only reinforced the existence of an idealized body standard, but also exposed which aspects of the body were problematic and in which individuals. While sizing varied, it also reflected the standardization of bodies. Eaton's sizing was not the only one available, and even using Eaton's measurements was problematic, as there was no guarantee that a size at one point in time was equivalent in measurements to the same size at another time. The variety of sizes made it difficult for anyone to "know" their size, making shopping stressful. That is why Eaton's often inserted measurement charts in their catalogues to help their customers. In that way, customers learned how their bodies were seen by clothing manufacturers.[15]

Catalogues have limitations as historical sources. Looking at the visuals and reading the texts make the purpose of the catalogues clear: selling clothes. The visuals were also selling a fantasy; as time passed, that fantasy became more and more difficult for most women to approach, compared to men. The catalogues could entice Canadians to buy, but what was not within their purview was the emotional toll exacted on women who were larger than the norm trying to find fashions that would fit well and look good on them. Advertisements for suits for men allowed more body types to be covered comfortably, or at least that was what was promoted. Of course, the clothing in the catalogues tell us what was available, not necessarily what was purchased.[16] But, as with any historical source, the insight into what was available is significant.

The last major source for *Fighting Fat* is thirty interviews with Canadians who self-defined themselves as significantly fat before 1980. Their voices provided a sense of the emotional turmoil caused by being fat in a society that was hostile to it. Those interviewed were recruited from various sources: articles in the media; friends; weight-loss programs, where the project was presented and members asked to consider being interviewed; respondents to notices on specific websites; and through the snowball effect. Unlike the before and after narratives analysed here, there was no common script of how those interviewed lived their lives, although there were many commonalities. What emerged were varying problems the interviewees faced, some of which the professional and popular literature did not emphasize. The interviews also gave rise to multiple themes not touched in the medical and dieting literature, and only hinted at in the before and after scripts. The interviews, more than any source, "fleshed" out the lives of people who just happened to be heavier than others.

Using interviews as historical sources has problems, and historians have spent time addressing them, especially in recent years in the field of memory studies. A major concern is the dependence on what is remembered, and privileging it over what may have occurred but is not remembered. As we remember, we refashion our lives to fit a coherent narrative, a narrative that makes "sense."[17] Those who offer their memories for examination do so for many reasons: some may see the larger project behind the interview as significant; others need to have their experiences told and validated; still others welcome a chance to re-examine their lives; and certain of them offer their stories to provide an opportunity for others to learn from their experiences. As a result, their expectations of the interview may be quite different from that of the researcher. The interviewer may also have a variety of reasons for doing the project in the first place, and the dangers of appropriating the voice of an individual being interviewed looms large. But any historical source has its own advantages and disadvantages. For this project, the voices of those who considered themselves fat may have limitations: Do they remember their early years accurately? Are they glossing over the role their weight played in their lives? Or are they exaggerating that role? Nonetheless, not hearing those voices would have limited a study about obesity. Especially limited would be the voices of fat children. While Mona Gleason, in her book *Small Matters: Canadian Children in Sickness and Health*, recognizes the problems of an adult's childhood memories, she argues that "oral histories [of adults about their childhood] do invite different questions about the past, illuminating overlooked, ignored, and silenced perspectives."[18] The voices of adults examining their lives from childhood and their lives into adulthood provide a sense of the emotional affect of being fat and how it shifted over their lives.

Journal Abbreviations

BCMJ	British Columbia Medical Journal
CAHPER	Canadian Association of Health, Physical Education and Recreation Journal
CC	Canadian Consumer
CCJ	Canadian Congress Journal
CD	The Canadian Doctor (became Canadian Doctor in November 1960)
CFP	Canadian Family Physician
CHJ	Canadian Home Journal
CHW	Canada's Health & Welfare
CJP	Canadian Journal of Psychology
CJPH	Canadian Journal of Public Health
CLNH	Canada Lancet and National Hygiene
CLP	The Canada Lancet and Practitioner
CM	The Canadian Magazine
CMAJ	Canadian Medical Association Journal
CN	The Canadian Nurse
CPAJ	Canadian Psychiatric Association Journal
CPHJ	Canadian Public Health Journal
CSMJ	Canadian Services Medical Journal
CW	Canadian Welfare
DMJ	Dalhousie Medical Journal
JAMA	Journal of the American Medical Association
JHE	The Journal of Home Economics
ManMR	Manitoba Medical Review
MMAR	Manitoba Medical Association Review
MMC	Modern Medicine of Canada

MSJ	Medical Services Journal Canada
NSMB	The Nova Scotia Medical Bulletin
OMR	Ontario Medical Review (Ontario Medical Association Bulletin to 1949)
PHJ	The Public Health Journal
UMC	L'Union Médicale du Canada

Notes

Introduction

1 From "Wit's End," *Health* 42, no. 4 (Winter 1977): 26.
2 Christopher E. Forth has argued that the upper class in early nineteenth century England was beginning to see a slender silhouette as important. At the same time, "a large belly still symbolized prestige." Christopher E. Forth, *Masculinity in the Modern West: Gender, Civilization and the Body* (New York, NY; Basingstoke, UK: Palgrave Macmillan, 2008), 101.
3 Nic Clarke, *Unwanted Warriors: The Rejected Volunteers of the Canadian Expeditionary Force* (Vancouver, BC: UBC Press, 2015) showed that at the beginning of World War I the military had high standards for fitness, but by the end of the war the standard was lower.
4 See Alana J. Hermiston, "'If It's Good for You, It's Good for the Nation!' The Moral Regulation of Nutrition in Canada, 1930–1945" (PhD diss., Carleton University, 2005). For details on the Depression, see Lara Campbell, *Respectable Citizens: Gender, Family, and Unemployment in Ontario's Great Depression* (Toronto: University of Toronto Press, 2009); Eric Strikwerda, *The Wages of Relief: Cities and the Unemployed in Prairie Canada, 1929–39* (Edmonton, AB: Athabasca University Press, 2010).
5 W. Bruce MacKinnon, "Poor Health – Our Silent Saboteur," *Maclean's* 56, no. 2 (15 January 1943): 14.
6 On Prince Philip, see Manfred Jager, "CASS Grows Bigger – But It's All Muscle, No Flab," *CMAJ* 106, no. 10 (20 May 1972): 1119. For a comment from the minister of state, fitness, and amateur sport on the Canadian Home Fitness Test, see Iona Campagnolo, "To the Editor," *CMAJ* 118, no. 7 (8 April 1978): 769–70, https://www.ncbi.nlm.nih.gov/pmc/articles/PMC1818175/.

7 For references to "epidemic," see the following study, which examines the language employed by the American media on obesity: Abigail C. Saguy and Rene Almeling, "Fat in the Fire? Science, the News Media, and the 'Obesity Epidemic,'" *Sociological Forum* 23, no. 1 (March 2008): 53–83. For an analysis of the use of the word "epidemic," see Sander L. Gilman, *Fat: A Cultural History of Obesity* (Cambridge: Polity Press, 2008), 18–19. The word "epidemic" is used so pervasively that the discourse on it has become a study in and of itself. See Bronwen Meredith Vivien Williams, "The 'Epidemic of Obesity' in the Public Media: A Discourse Analysis" (MSc thesis, University of Toronto, 2006). For the WHO, see "Controlling the Global Obesity Epidemic," in Nutrition Topics, World Health Organization website, http://www.who.int/nutrition/topics/obesity/en/. For use of the term "pandemic," see Peter T. Katzmarzyk, "The Canadian Obesity Epidemic, 1985–1998," *CMAJ* 166, no. 8 (16 April 2002): 1039.

8 For reference to the thirty health problems, see Kelly D. Brownell, *Food Fight: The Inside Story of the Food Industry, American's Obesity Crisis and What We Can Do About It* (New York, Chicago: McGraw-Hill, 2004), 43. For a list of problems caused by obesity, see Katzmarzyk, "The Canadian Obesity Epidemic, 1985–1998," 1039; Christel Le Petit and Jean-Marie Berthelot, "Obesity: A Growing Issue," in *Healthy Today, Healthy Tomorrow? Findings from the National Population Health Survey*, Statistics Canada series 1, no. 3 (Ottawa: Statistics Canada, 2005), 2, http://www.statcan.gc.ca/pub/82-618-m/82-618-m2005003-eng.htm. See also Bruce A. Reeder et al., "Obesity and Its Relation to Cardiovascular Disease Risk Factors in Canadian Adults," *CMAJ* 146, no. 11 (1 June 1992): 2009–19; Peter T. Katzmarzyk and Christopher I. Ardern, "Overweight and Obesity Mortality Trends in Canada, 1985–2000," *CJPH* 95, no. 1 (January–February 2004): 16–20; Kim D. Raine, *Overweight and Obesity in Canada: A Population Health Perspective* (Ottawa: Canadian Institute for Health Information, 2004). For obesity's effect on dementia, see Hans Krueger et al., *The Health Impact of Smoking and Obesity and What to Do About It* (Toronto: University of Toronto Press, 2007), 19. For a discussion of obesity as a disease, see Annemarie Jutel, "Doctor's Orders: Diagnosis, Medical Authority, and the Exploitation of the Fat Body," in *Biopolitics and the "Obesity Epidemic": Governing Bodies*, ed. Jan Wright and Valerie Harwood (New York: Routledge, 2009), 60–77. For obesity as a mental disease, see Nora D. Volkow and Charles P. O'Brien, "Issues for DSM-V: Should Obesity Be Included as a Brain Disorder?" *American Journal of Psychiatry* 164, no. 5 (May 2007): 708–9, accessed 1 January 2015, http://ajp.psychiatryonline.org/doi/full/10.1176/ajp.2007.164.5.708. Dr Bailey has seen fatty livers in her practice.

9 Peter T. Katzmarzyk and Ian Janssen, "The Economic Costs Associated with Physical Inactivity and Obesity in Canada: An Update," *Canadian Journal of Applied Physiology* 29, no. 1 (2004): 90–1; Robert Preidt, "Cost of Obesity Approaching $30 Billion a Year," *Healthday: News for Healthier Living*, 11 January 2011, accessed 2 February 2011, https://consumer.healthday.com/public-health-information-30/health-cost-news-348/cost-of-obesity-approaching-300-billion-a-year-648708.html.
10 Mark Schlesinger, "Weighting for Godot," *Journal of Health Politics, Policy and Law* 30, no. 5 (October 2005): 787.
11 Dominique La Haye, "Group Calls On Feds to Impose a Sugar Tax," QMI Agency, 3 February 2011, accessed 7 February 2011, http://www.saultthisweek.com/2011/02/03/group-calls-on-feds-to-impose-a-sugar-tax-8; Aaron Derfel, "The War Against Obesity," *Montreal Gazette*, 26 March 2011, accessed 9 August 2011, https://www.pressreader.com/canada/montreal-gazette/20110326/292590353334364; André Picard, "'Fat Tax' Idea Gets Mixed Reviews," *Globe and Mail*, 25 July 2001, A3; CTV.ca News Staff, "New Research Links Soft Drinks to Type 2 Diabetes," *CTVNews.ca*, 27 October 2010, accessed 28 October 2010, https://www.ctvnews.ca/new-research-links-soft-drinks-to-type-2-diabetes-1.567678. For the Fraser Institute, see quote in Michael Gard, *The End of the Obesity Epidemic* (London: Routledge, 2011), 127.
12 World Health Organization, "Obesity and Overweight," Fact Sheet no. 311, updated October 2017, http://www.who.int/mediacentre/factsheets/fs311/en/.
13 Tanya Navaneelan and Teresa Janz, "Adjusting the Scales: Obesity in the Canadian Population after Correcting for Respondent Bias," Statistics Canada Catalogue no. 82-624-X, accessed 11 November 2015, http://www.statcan.gc.ca/pub/82-624-x/2014001/article/11922-eng.htm. For statistics on the slowing rate of gain, see Heather M. Orpana, Mark S. Tremblay, and Philippe Finès, Statistics Canada, *Trends in Weight Change among Canadian Adults: Evidence from the 1996/1997 to 2004/2005 National Population Health Survey* (Ottawa: Ministry of Industry, 2006), 10; Organisation for Economic Co-operation and Development (OECD), "Obesity and the Economics of Prevention: Fit Not Fat, Key Facts – Canada, Update 2012," 21 February 2012, accessed 15 March 2013, http://www.oecd.org/els/health-systems/49712071.pdf. For Indigenous children's obesity rates, see Active Healthy Kids Canada, *Older But Not Wiser: Canada's Future at Risk – Canada's Report Card on Physical Activity for Children & Youth* (Toronto: Active Healthy Kids Canada, 2007), 3, http://dvqdas9jty7g6.cloudfront.net/archivedreportcards/full-english-report-card-2007.pdf; Scott A.

Lear et al., "Appropriateness of Current Thresholds for Obesity-Related Measures among Aboriginal People," *CMAJ* 177, no. 12 (4 December 2007): 1499. For obesity rates among low-income people, see Le Petit and Berthelot, "Obesity: A Growing Issue," 5; Elaine M. Power, "Determinants of Healthy Eating among Low-Income Canadians," *CJPH* 96, s.3 (July/August, 2005): S37. For gender, age, and location, see Orpana, Tremblay, and Finès, *Trends in Weight Change*. For a critical look at the statistics in the twenty-first century, see Michael Gard, "Hearing Noises and Noticing Silence: Toward a Critical Engagement with Canadian Body Weight Statistics," in *Obesity in Canada: Critical Perspectives*, ed. Jenny Ellison, Deborah McPhail, and Wendy Mitchinson (Toronto: University of Toronto, 2016), 44–6. See page 48 for Gard's view of the obesity statistics among Indigenous peoples.

14 For ads for fattening food, see Laurette Dubé, "Advertising and Food Preferences," in *Contemporary Challenges in Food and Food Services Marketing: Proceedings from Health and Pleasure at the Table*, ed. L. Dubé et al. (Montreal: Université de Montréal, 1995), 151; for more on advertising, see Karl Moore and Laurette Dubé, "Mea Culpa: We Marketers Helped Make Your Kids Fat," *Globe and Mail*, 13 August 2003, A11. For ingredients of processed food, see Michael Moss, *Salt Sugar Fat: How the Food Giants Hooked Us* (New York: Randon House, 2013). For the effect of eating in fast food places, see Raine, *Overweight and Obesity in Canada*, 24–6. For the decline of home cooking and the rise of pre-prepared food, see Michael Pollan, *Cooked: A Natural History of Transformation* (New York: Penguin Books, 2013), 3, 192.

15 For statistics on Canadians eating out, see Krueger et al., *The Health Impact of Smoking and Obesity*, 185. In a 2004 Gallup poll, 40 per cent of Canadians claimed they had daily family dinners, and 40 per cent more said they had them four to six times a week. Compare this rate with the 28 per cent of Americans who ate daily dinners with family. Nathalie Cooke, "Home Cooking: The Stories Canadian Cookbooks Have to Tell," in *What's to Eat: Entrées in Canadian Food History*, ed. Nathalie Cooke (Montreal, Kingston: McGill-Queen's University Press, 2009), 230.

16 Le Petit and Berthelot, "Obesity: A Growing Issue," 5; Mark Bittman, "Is Junk Food Really Cheaper," *New York Times*, 24 September 2011, accessed 10 October 2011, http://www.nytimes.com/2011/09/25/opinion/sunday/is-junk-food-really-cheaper.html.

17 For nutrition in school curricula, see Raine, *Overweight and Obesity in Canada*, 45. For mothers and nutrition, see Hermiston, "If It's Good for You, It's Good For the Nation!," 149.

18 For a US perspective, see April Michelle Herndon, *Fat Blame: How the War on Obesity Victimizes Women and Children* (Lawrence: University Press of Kansas, 2014).
19 For poor food, see Thomas F. Pawick, *The End of Food: How the Food Industry Is Destroying Our Food Supply – And What You Can Do About It* (Vancouver, Toronto: Greystone Books, 2006); see also Anthony Winson, *The Industrial Diet: The Degradation of Food and the Struggle for Healthy Eating* (New York: New York University Press, 2014). For high-fructose corn syrup, see Morgan Spurlock, *Don't Eat This Book: Fast Food and the Supersizing of America* (New York: Berkeley Publishing Group, 2005), 97. On the rise of corn, see Michael Pollan, *The Omnivore's Dilemma: A Natural History of Four Meals* (New York: Penguin Books, 2006), 62–3, 93, 95.
20 CBC-TV, "It Takes Guts," *The Nature of Things*, season 2015–2016, episode 3, 29 October 2015, http://www.cbc.ca/player/play/2678011123.
21 For the percentage of sedentary Canadians, see Krueger et al., *The Health Impact of Smoking and Obesity*, 9. Concern about children is reflected in James Sallis, "Can We Modify the Social Environment of Children and Youth to Overcome the Physical Activity Deficit?" in *Presentation and Poster Abstracts from the International Conference on Physical Activity and Obesity in Children* (Toronto: International Conference, 24–7 June, 2007), 22. For information on schools in Canada, see Raine, *Overweight and Obesity in Canada*, 28.
22 For social contagion, see Clay A. Johnson, *The Information Diet: A Case for Conscious Consumption* (Sebastopol, CA: O'Reilly Media Inc., 2012), 119. For genetic modification, see Sam Savage, "Study: Alternative Causes of Weight Gain," *RedOrbit*, 25 November 2010, http://www.redorbit.com/news/health/1956476/study_alternative_causes_of_weight_gain. For man-made chemicals, see CBC-TV, "Programmed to Be Fat?" *The Nature of Things*, season 2011–2012, episode 9, 12 January 2012, accessed 27 March 2017, http://watch.cbc.ca/theanatureaofathings/season-51/programmedatoabeafat/38e815a-009e2482f21. For modernity, see Jane Dixon and Dorothy H. Broom, eds., *The Seven Deadly Sins of Obesity: How the Modern World Is Making Us Fat* (Sydney, AU: University of New South Wales Press, 2007), 2; Natalie Boero, *Killer Fat: Media, Medicine, and Morals in the American "Obesity Epidemic"* (New Brunswick, NJ: Rutgers University Press, 2013), 4.
23 See "Body Image and Clothing in Eaton's" in chapter 7 of this volume.
24 Neil Seeman and Patrick Luciani, *XXL: Obesity and the Limits of Shame* (Toronto: University of Toronto Press, 2011), 106–14, chapter 4, "Healthy Living Vouchers."

25 For the thrifty gene hypothesis, see Jennifer Poudrier, "The Geneticization of Aboriginal Diabetes and Obesity: Adding Another Scene to the Story of the Thrifty Gene," in *Obesity in Canada*, ed. Jenny Ellison, Deborah McPhail, and Wendy Mitchinson (Toronto: University of Toronto Press, 2016), 122–47. The article examines the thrifty gene hypothesis and shows how it is racism.
26 For obesity as hardwired, see Greg Critser, *Fat Land: How Americans Became the Fattest People in the World* (Boston, New York: Mariner Books, 2004), 40. For more on this view, see Anne Scott Beller, *Fat & Thin: A Natural History of Obesity* (New York: Farrar, Straus and Giroux, 1977); Brownell, *Food Fight*, 5–6.
27 Elizabeth Kolbert, "XXXL: Why Are We So Fat?" *The New Yorker*, 20 July 2009, accessed 17 July 2009, https://www.newyorker.com/magazine/2009/07/20/xxxl.
28 For the set-point hypothesis, see Glenn A. Gaesser, *Big Fat Lies: The Truth about Your Weight and Your Health* (New York: Fawcett Columbine, 1996), 26, 81. For an example of set-point, see Katherine Ashenburg, "Critical Mass," *The Walrus*, January/February 2013, 33. For a history of set-point, see also Gary Taubes, *Good Calories, Bad Calories: Challenging the Conventional Wisdom on Diet, Weight Control, and Disease* (New York: Alfred A. Knopf, 2007), 298, 428. Taubes doesn't support the set-point theory.
29 For gender and ethnicity, see Harvey Levenstein, *Revolution at the Table: The Transformation of the American Diet* (Berkeley: University of California Press, 2003), 12, 103, 176–7. For heredity, see Claude Bouchard, "Is There a Biological Basis for the Obesity Epidemic?" in *Presentation and Poster Abstracts from the International Conference on Physical Activity and Obesity in Children* (Toronto: International Conference, 24–7 June, 2007), 16. For bitter tasters, see International Conference on Physical Activity and Obesity in Children, Toronto, 24–7 June 2007, information from the audience participation. For being sensitive to fat, see Julie Wan, "Fat Might Be the Sixth Basic Taste," *The Washington Post*, 4 June 2012, https://www.washingtonpost.com/national/health-science/fat-might-be-the-sixth-basic-taste/2012/06/04/gJQAt218DV_story.html?utm_term=.943fcb26a55b.
30 Denise Mann, "New Genes Linked to Obesity, Belly Fat," *WebMD*, 11 October 2010, accessed 8 November 2010, https://www.webmd.com/diet/news/20101011/new-genes-linked-to-obesity-belly-fat#1. For viewing genes as the significant cause of obesity, see Philip A. Wood, *How Fat Works* (Cambridge, MA: Harvard University Press, 2006), 193.

31 For the first range, see Brownell, *Food Fight*, 23; for the second, see Seeman and Luciani, *XXL*, 41.
32 Quoted in Mann, "New Genes Linked to Obesity, Belly Fat." For the virus, see Daniel J. NeNoon, "Obesity Virus: More, Bigger Fat Cells," *WebMD*, 20 August 2007, accessed 21 November 2011, http://www.webmd.com/diet/news/20070820/obesity-virus-more-bigger-fat-cells; "Obesity 'May Be Linked to Virus,'" *BBC News*, 21 August 2007, accessed 21 November 2017, http://news.bbc.co.uk/2/hi/health/6956543.stm. For a perspective on infection as the cause of obesity, see Gilman, *Fat*, 22–4.
33 For criticism of feminists, see Marcia Millman, *Such a Pretty Face: Being Fat in America* (New York and London: W.W. Norton & Company, 1980), 93; Leanne Joanisse, "Reducing and Revisioning the Body: Women's Experiences of Weight Loss Surgery" (PhD diss., McMaster University, 2003), 74. For a more in-depth discussion of feminism and fat, see Abigail Saguy, "Why Fat Is a Feminist Issue," *Sex Roles* 66 (2012): 600–7. For women and fat as natural, see Cecilia Harley, "Letting Ourselves Go: Making Room for the Fat Body in Feminist Scholarship," in *Bodies Out of Bounds: Fatness and Transgression*, ed. Jana Evans Braziel and Kathleen LeBesco (Berkeley: University of California Press, 2001), 67–8; J. Eric Oliver, *Fat Politics: The Real Story Behind America's Obesity Epidemic* (New York: Oxford University Press, 2006), 83.
34 Lisa Schoenfielder and Barb Wieser, eds., *Shadow on a Tightrope: Writings by Women on Fat Oppression* (San Francisco: Spinsters/Aunt Lute, 1983).
35 See Braziel and LeBesco, *Bodies Out of Bounds*; Esther Rothblum and Sondra Solovay, eds., *The Fat Studies Reader* (New York: New York University Press, 2009), 2. This book has six parts: "What Is Fat Studies? The Social and Historical Construction of Fatness"; "Fat Studies in Health and Medicine"; "Fatness as Social Inequality"; "Size-ism in Popular Culture and Literature"; "Embodying and Embracing Fatness"; and "Starting the Revolution."
36 Rothblum and Solovay, *The Fat Studies Reader*, 2.
37 Elena Levy-Navarro, ed., *Historicizing Fat in Anglo-American Culture* (Columbus: Ohio State University Press, 2010), 2–3. See also Tamara Beauboeuf-Lafontant, "Strong and Large Black Women? Exploring Relationships between Deviant Womanhood and Weight," *Gender & Society* 17, no. 1 (2003): 111–21.
38 Kathleen LeBesco, *Revolting Bodies? The Struggle to Redefine Fat Identity* (Amherst, MA: University of Massachusetts Press, 2004), 6.
39 Samantha Murray, *The "Fat" Female Body* (New York: Palgrave Macmillan, 2008), 27.

40 Cat Pausé, Jackie Wykes, and Samantha Murray, eds., *Queering Fat Embodiment* (Surrey, UK: Ashgate, 2014), 1, 10.
41 Robyn Longhurst, "Queering Body Size and Shape: Performativity, the Closet, Shame and Orientation," in Pausé, Wykes, and Murray, *Queering Fat Embodiment*, 13, 14.
42 Stefanie A. Jones, "The Performance of Fat: The Spectre Outside the House of Desire," in Pausé, Wykes, and Murray, *Queering Fat Embodiment*, 33.
43 Allyson Mitchell, "Corporeographies of Size: Fat Women in Urban Spaces" (PhD diss., York University, 2016), iv, 3. See also Allyson Mitchell, "Pissed Off," in *Fat: An Anthropology of an Obsession*, ed. Don Kulick and Anne Meneley (New York: Penguin, 2005): 211–26.
44 For HerSize, see Jenny Ellison, "From 'FU' to 'Be Yourself': Fat Activisms in Canada," in Ellison, McPhail, and Mitchinson, *Obesity in Canada*, 303; Carla Rice, *Becoming Women: The Embodied Self in Image Culture* (Toronto: University of Toronto, 2014), 4–6. Rice has written many other articles on fatness: Carla Rice, "How Big Girls Become Fat Girls: The Cultural Production of Problem Eating and Physical Inactivity," in *Critical Feminist Approaches to Eating Dis/Orders*, ed. Helen Malson and Maree Burns (New York: Routledge, 2009), 97–109; Carla Rice, "Becoming 'The Fat Girl': Acquisition of an Unfit Identity," *Women's Studies International Forum* 30, no. 2 (2007): 158–74, https://doi.org/10.1016/j.wsif.2007.01.001; Carla Rice, "Revisioning Fat: From Enforcing Norms to Exploring Possibilities Unique to Different Bodies," in Ellison, McPhail, and Mitchinson, *Obesity in Canada*, 419–39.
45 Kathleen LeBesco, "On Fatness and Fluidity: A Meditation," in Pausé, Wykes, and Murray, *Queering Fat Embodiment*, 49, 55; LeBesco, *Revolting Bodies?*
46 Canadian Obesity Network (website), http://www.obesitynetwork.ca; Jenny Ellison, Deborah McPhail, and Wendy Mitchinson, "Introduction," in Ellison, McPhail, and Mitchinson, *Obesity in Canada*, 4.
47 Darlene McNaughton and Cynthia Smith, "Diabesity, or the 'Twin Epidemics': Reflections on the Iatrogenic Consequences of Stigmatizing Lifestyle to Reduce the Incidence of Diabetes Mellitus in Canada," in Ellison, McPhail, and Mitchinson, *Obesity in Canada*, 134; Rice, "Revisioning Fat," 426.
48 Ellison, McPhail, and Mitchinson, *Obesity in Canada*. For other literature, see John Evans et al., *Education, Disordered Eating and Obesity Discourse: Fat Fabrications* (London and New York: Routledge, 2008); Paul Campos,

The Obesity Myth (New York: Gotham Books, 2004); Wright and Harwood, eds., *Biopolitics and the "Obesity Epidemic"*; Abigail C. Saguy, *What's Wrong with Fat?* (Oxford and New York: Oxford University Press, 2013); Boero, *Killer Fat*; Gaesser, *Big Fat Lies*; Oliver, *Fat Politics*; Lee Monaghan, *Men and the War on Obesity: A Sociological Study* (New York: Routledge, 2008).

49 For anchoring to weight, see Dan Gardner, *Risk: The Science and Politics of Fear* (Toronto: McClelland & Stewart, 2008), 42. For the change in the United States, see Campos, *The Obesity Myth*, 122.

50 Gard, "Hearing Noises and Noticing Silence," 48, 39. Canada's lag in collecting obesity statistics is discussed in Elise Paradis, "'Obesity' as Process: The Medicalization of Fatness by Canadian Researchers, 1971–2010," in Ellison, McPhail, and Mitchinson, *Obesity in Canada*, 79.

51 For the view that some extra weight is not harmful, see Harvey A. Levenstein, *Paradox of Plenty: A Social History of Eating in Modern America*, rev. ed. (Berkeley, Los Angeles, London: University of California Press, 2003), 249–50. For problems with dieting, see "Children and Weight: The Dilemmas," *Body Positive®: Boosting Body Image at Any Weight* (website), accessed 30 March 2009, http://www.bodypositive.com/childwt.htm. On the efficacy of dieting, see Kelly Crowe, "Obesity Research Confirms Long-Term Weight Loss Is Almost Impossible," *CBC News*, 4 June 2014, accessed 12 June 2014, http://www.cbc.ca/news/health/obesity-research-confirms-long-term-weight-loss-almost-impossible-1.2663585. For exercise, see Jesse Singal, "Going from Extremely Lazy to Pretty Lazy Could Be Lifesaving," *NYMAG.com*, Science of Us, 14 January 2015, accessed 21 January 2015, http://nymag.com/scienceofus/2015/01/sorta-lazy-is-much-healthier-than-extremely-lazy.html. For Canada, see Kate Lunau, "Don't Just Sit There," *Maclean's* 126, no. 1 (14 January 2013): 55. This article points out that movement not exercise is what is needed. For a discussion on whether overweight people can be healthy, see Peter Janiszewski, "Can You Be Both Obese and Healthy?" *Scientific American* blog, 18 January 2011, accessed 2 February 2011, https://blogs.scientificamerican.com/guest-blog/can-you-be-both-obese-and-healthy/. For a definition of health, see Jonathan M. Metz and Anna Kirkland, eds., *Against Health: How Health Become the New Morality* (New York: New York University Press, 2010), especially the essay by Lauren Berlant, "Risky Bigness: On Obesity, Eating, and the Ambiguity of 'Health,'" 26–39.

52 Avner Offer notes that there is a dispute about the danger of being overweight, but argues that being overweight is not benign. Avner Offer,

"Body Weight and Self-Control in the United States and Britain since the 1950s," *Social History of Medicine* 14, no. 1 (2001): 80.

53 For the racism inherent in these concepts, see Jennifer Poudrier, "The Geneticization of Aboriginal Diabetes and Obesity: Adding Another Scene to the Story of the Thrifty Gene," *Canadian Review of Sociology and Anthropology* 44, no. 2 (2007): 237–61; Margery Fee, "Racializing Narratives: Obesity, Diabetes and the 'Aboriginal' Thrifty Genotype," *Social Science & Medicine* 62 (2006): 2988–97. It is interesting to note that just before geneticist James Neel, the originator of the thrifty gene concept, refuted his theory, researchers were beginning to refer to it. Taubes, *Good Calories, Bad Calories*, 245.

54 For the social factors, see Michael Gard, "Understanding Obesity by Understanding Desire," in Malson and Burns, *Critical Feminist Approaches to Eating Dis/orders*, 39.

55 For set-point, see Gaesser, *Big Fat Lies*, 26, 81. For support for set-point, see Ashenburg, "Critical Mass," 33. For a history of set-point, see also Taubes, *Good Calories, Bad Calories*, 298, 428. Taubes does not subscribe to the set-point theory.

56 See McNaughton and Smith, "Diabesity, or the 'Twin Epidemics,'" 122–47.

57 Campos, *The Obesity Myth*, 20, 27, 32. For the media and the BMI, see Laura Jakul, *The Effect of Anti-Obesity Media on Body Image and Antifat Attitudes* (Winnipeg: University of Manitoba, 2005), 83. For criticism of the BMI, see Bethan Evans, "'Gluttony or Sloth': Critical Geographies of Bodies and Morality in (Anti)Obesity Policy," *Area* 38, no. 3 (2006): 262. For the power of the BMI, see Michael L. Power and Jay Schulkin, *The Evolution of Obesity* (Baltimore, MD: John Hopkins University Press, 2009), 17. For problems of defining obesity and measuring, see Evans et al., *Education, Disordered Eating and Obesity Discourse*, 41. For problems of the BMI, see Raine, *Overweight and Obesity in Canada*, 3. For the gender bias, see Kristen Bell and Darlene McNaughton, "Feminism and the Invisible Fat Man," *Body & Society* 13, no. 1 (2007): 126.

58 Campos, *The Obesity Myth*, ix; Jan Wright, "Biopower, Biopedagogies and the Obesity Epidemic," in Wright and Harwood, *Biopolitics and the "Obesity Epidemic,"* 4–5.

59 For an excellent explanation of moral panic, see Moss Edward Norman, "Living in the Shadow of an 'Obesity Epidemic': The Discursive Construction of Boys and Their Bodies" (PhD diss., University of Toronto, 2009), 11, fn 9. For social construction, see Ian Hacking, *The Social Construction of What?* (Cambridge, MA: Harvard University Press, 1999); Krista K. Barker, "The Social Construction of Illness: Medicalization

and Contested Illness," in *Handbook of Medical Sociology*, 6th ed., ed. Chloe Bird et al. (Nashville, TN: Vanderbilt University Press, 2010), 147–62. For modern dislike of fat, see Oliver, *Fat Politics*, 6; Women's Health Clinic, *Women, Weight and Power: Weighing Women's Presence in the World* (Winnipeg, MB: Women's Health Clinic, 2012), http://womenshealthclinic.org/wp-content/uploads/2013/10/WHC-Women-Weight-and-Power.pdf?x88868. *Women, Weight and Power* is based on the content of an interactive workshop delivered at the Women's Worlds Conference held in Ottawa, Ontario, in July 2011.

60 For a discussion of the diet industry benefitting from obesity, see Jane Ogden, *Fat Chance! The Myth of Dieting Explained* (London: Routledge, 1992). On blaming the pharmaceutical and medical interests as complicit in the panic about obesity, see Oliver, *Fat Politics*, x; Alicia Mundy, *Dispensing with the Truth: The Victims, the Drug Companies, and the Dramatic Story Behind the Battle over Fen-Phen* (New York: St Martin's Press, 2001), 42. For a discussion of media bias, see Williams, "The 'Epidemic of Obesity' in the Public Media," 16.

61 Michael Gard and Jan Wright, *The Obesity Epidemic: Science, Morality and Ideology* (London and New York: Routledge, 2005), 2, 9, 38, 45–6.

62 Offer, "Body Weight and Self-Control," 79–106; D. Haslam, "Obesity: A Medical History," *Obesity Reviews* 8, suppl. 1 (2007): 31–6; Laura Fraser, "The Inner Corset: A Brief History of Fat in the United States," in Rothblum and Solovay, *The Fat Studies Reader*, 11–14; Jesse Berrett, "Feeding the Organization Men: Diet and Masculinity in Postwar America," *Journal of Social History* 30, no. 4 (Summer 1997): 805–25; Richard Klein, *Eat Fat* (New York: Pantheon Books, 1996), 126–31; David Haslam and Fiona Haslam, *Fat, Gluttony and Sloth: Obesity in Literature, Art and Medicine* (Liverpool: Liverpool University Press, 2009); Roberta J. Park, "Historical Reflections on Diet, Exercise, and Obesity: The Recurring Need to 'Put Words into Action,'" *Canadian Bulletin of Medical History* 28, no. 2 (2011): 383–401; Levenstein, *Revolution at the Table*; Jane Nicholas, "'I Was a 555-Pound Freak': The Self, Freakery, and Sexuality in Celesta 'Dolly Dimples' Geyer's *Diet or Die*," *Journal of the Canadian Historical Association* 21, no. 1 (2010): 83–107; Sander L. Gilman, *Obesity: The Biography* (Oxford: Oxford University Press, 2010); Katharina Vester, "Regime Change: Gender, Class, and the Invention of Dieting in Post-Bellum America," *Journal of Social History* 44, no. 1 (Fall 2010): 39–70; Elena Levy-Navarro, "Fattening Queer History: Where Does Fat History Go from Here?" in Rothblum and Solovay, *The Fat Studies Reader*, 15–22; Joyce Huff, "A 'Horror of Corpulence': Interrogating Bantigism and

Mid-Nineteenth-Century Fat-Phobia," in Braziel and LeBesco, *Bodies Out of Bounds*, 39–59; Kerry Segrave, *Obesity in America, 1850–1939: A History of Social Attitudes and Treatment* (Jefferson, NC: McFarland & Co., 2008); Christopher E. Forth, "Fat, Desire and Disgust in the Colonial Imagination," *History Workshop Journal* 73, no. 1 (Spring 2012): 211–39; Georges Vigarello, *The Metamorphoses of Fat: A History of Obesity*, trans. C. Jon Delogu (New York: Columbia University Press, 2013).

63   For hostility, see Annemarie Jutel, "Weight Health: The Moral Burden of Obesity," *Social Semiotics* 15, no. 2 (2005): 122; Peter N. Stearns, *Battleground of Desire: The Struggle for Self-Control in Modern America* (New York: New York University Press, 1999), 24; Christopher E. Forth, "Melting Moments: The Greasy Sources of Modern Perceptions of Fat," *Cultural History* 1, no. 1 (2012): 85.

64   Levenstein, *Revolution at the Table*, 13; Braziel and LeBesco, *Bodies Out of Bounds*, 2.

65   Hillel Schwartz, *Never Satisfied: A Cultural History of Diets, Fantasies and Fat* (London: Collier Macmillan Publishers, 1986), 45; Amy Erdman Farrell, *Fat Shame: Stigma and the Fat Body in American Culture* (New York: New York University Press, 2011).

66   For Stearns's work, see Peter N. Stearns, *Fat History: Bodies and Beauty in the Modern West*, rev. ed. (New York: New York University Press, 2002), xiii (ideal), xv (snacking), 72; Peter N. Stearns, "Fat in America," in *Cultures of the Abdomen: Diet, Digestion, and Fat in the Modern World*, ed. Christopher E. Forth and Ana Carden-Coyne (New York: Palgrave Macmillan, 2005), 239–40, 246, 251 (leading world). For French culture and eating habits, see Claude Grignon and Christian Grignon, "Long-Term Trends in Food Consumption: A French Portrait," *Food and Foodways* 8, no. 3 (1999): 151–74; Claude Grignon, "Rule, Fashion, Work: The Social Genesis of the Contemporary French Pattern of Meals," *Food and Foodways* 6, nos. 3–4 (1996): 205–41. For smoking and its limit on metabolism, see James M. Rippe and Weight Watchers, *Weight Loss That Lasts: Break Through the 10 Big Diet Myths* (Hoboken, NJ: John Wiley & Sons, 2005), 125. Although Stearns described the United States as having the highest prevelance of obesity, it actually ranked twelfth on the obesity scale in 2016. Most likely he was thinking of the United States as ranking first among Western countries. See "Country Comparison: Obesity – Adult Prevalence Rate," *The World Factbook 2017* (Washington: Central Intelligence Agency, 2017), https://www.cia.gov/library/publications/the-world-factbook/rankorder/2228rank.html.

67 Stearns, *Fat History*, 74, 100. For seeing women as experiencing more stigma, see Norman, "Living in the Shadow of an 'Obesity Epidemic'"; Monaghan, *Men and the War on Obesity*.
68 Levenstein, *Revolution at the Table*, 8, 42–3. See also Levenstein, *Paradox of Plenty*, 114; Margaret Willson, "Indulgence," in Kulick and Meneley, *Fat: An Anthropology of an Obsession*, 160.
69 Sander L. Gilman, *Fat Boys: A Slim Book* (Lincoln, NB: University of Nebraska, 2004); Gilman, *Fat: A Cultural History of Obesity*; Sander L. Gilman, *Obesity: The Biography* (Oxford: Oxford University Press, 2010).
70 Gilman, *Fat Boys*, 11.
71 Gilman, *Fat: A Cultural History of Obesity*, 3.
72 For Ellison's works, see Jenny Ellison, "Large as Life: Self-Acceptance and the Fat Body in Canada, 1977–2000" (PhD diss., York University, 2010), 7, for a list of the groups; Ellison, "From 'FU' to 'Be Yourself,'" 294, 312, for the comments on Canada. See also Jenny Ellison, "'Stop Postponing Your Life Until You Lose Weight and Start Living Now': Vancouver's Large as Life Action Group, 1979–1985," *Journal of the Canadian Historical Association* 18, no. 1 (2007): 241–65; Jenny Ellison, "Weighting In: The 'Evidence of Experience' and Canadian Fat Women's Activism," *Canadian Bulletin of Medical History* 30, no. 1 (2013); 55–76. In 2016, Ellison was one of the three editors of *Obesity in Canada*.
73 Deborah McPhail, "Canada Weighs In: Gender, Race and the Making of 'Obesity,' 1945–1970" (PhD diss., York University, 2009), iv, 2, 42; Deborah McPhail, "What to Do with the 'Tubby Hubby'? 'Obesity,' the Crisis of Masculinity, and the Nuclear Family in Early Cold War Canada," *Antipode* 41, no. 5 (2009): 1021–50; Deborah McPhail, "'This is the Face of Obesity': Race, Class, Gender, and the Feminization of Fat," chapter 1 in *Contours of the Nation: Making Obesity and Imagining Canada, 1945–1970* (Toronto: University of Toronto Press, 2017), 25–52.
74 John Cranfield, Kris Inwood, and J. Andrew Ross, "Before the Obesity Epidemic: The Body Mass Index of Canadians in the First and Second World War," *Canadian Bulletin of Medical History* 32, no. 2 (2015): 319–35; Peter T. Katzmarzyk, "The Canadian Obesity Epidemic: An Historical Perspective," *Obesity Research* 10, no. 7 (July 2002): 666–74. See also M.S. Tremblay, P.T. Katzmarzyk, and J.D. Willms, "Temporal Trends in Overweight and Obesity in Canada, 1981–1996," *International Journal of Obesity* 26 (2002): 538–43; Katzmarzyk and Ardern, "Overweight and Obesity Mortality Trends in Canada," 16–20.

75 For the significance of place for health, see Erika Dyck and Christopher Fletcher, eds., *Locating Health: Historical and Anthropological Investigations of Health and Place* (London: Pickering & Chatto, 2011).
76 Some scholars have inquired about the methodology I employed while researching and writing *Fighting Fat*. A methodology is defined as "a body of methods used in a particularly branch of activity" (*Canadian Oxford Dictionary*, 2002). In my view, a single methodology is inadequate for the context of this book; I have therefore drawn on a variety of methodologies in order to effectively explore the many different themes and branches discussed in the book. For decades, historians have used identities related to class, race (ethnicity), and gender. Over time, other identities have been added: sexuality, ability, age, and embodiment. All these identities are relevant to the history of obesity. Even more than these elements, however, weight is significant in this context. Other methodologies have also been applied. For example, I have made use of discourses within medicine, such as healthism. Tropes are part of the discourse in magazine stories, and the linguistic turn and the affective turn are helpful in understanding the stigmatizing of people who are fat. I also utilized personal narrative (Carla Rice) to give fat people a voice.
77 Joanne Entwistle, "Fashion and the Fleshy Body: Dress as Embodied Practice," *Fashion Theory* 4, no. 3 (2000): 335.
78 See Forth and Carden-Coyne, *Cultures of the Abdomen*; Christopher E. Forth and Ivan Crozier, "Introduction: Parts, Wholes and People," in *Body Parts: Critical Explorations in Corporeality*, ed. Christopher E. Forth and Ivan Crozier (Lanham, MD.: Lexington Books, 2005), 1–16; Jan Purnis, "The Stomach and Early Modern Emotion," *University of Toronto Quarterly* 79, no. 2 (Spring 2010): 800–18.
79 For the meaning of obesity, see Kelly D. Brownell and Albert J. Stunkard, "Physical Activity in the Development and Control of Obesity," in *Obesity*, ed. Albert J. Stunkard (Philadelphia: W.B. Saunders Company, 1980), 300. For dislike of the word "obesity," see Marilyn Wann, "Foreword: Fat Studies: An Invitation to Revolution," in Rothblum and Solovay, *The Fat Studies Reader*, xii–xiii.
80 Boero, *Killer Fat*, 9. David Healy's book *The Creation of Pharmacology* (Cambridge, MA: Harvard University Press, 2002) notes how measurements and randomized clinical trials have shifted the way in which we view the normal with respect to a psychiatric agenda. Much of his concern can also be seen in how we look at and treat obesity. See chapter 8, "Democracy," 334–90.

81 Deborah Lupton, "Risk as Moral Danger: The Social and Political Functions of Risk Discourse in Public Health," *International Journal of Health Services* 23, no. 3 (1993): 433.
82 Norman, "Living in the Shadow of an 'Obesity Epidemic,'" 21. Norman is working on Michel Foucault's concept of biopower.
83 Robert Crawford, "Healthism and the Medicalization of Everyday Life," *International Journal of Health Services* 10, no. 3 (1980): 365–88, especially 378; see also M. Shea and Natalie Beausoleil, "Breaking Down 'Healthism': Barriers to Health and Fitness as Identified by Immigrant Youth in St John's, NL, Canada," *Sport, Education and Society* 17, no. 3 (January 2012): 97–112; Juliann Cheek, "Healthism: A New Conservatism?" *Qualitative Heath Research* 18, no. 7 (July 2008): 974–82.
84 Kathleen Woodward, *Statistical Panic: Cultural Politics and Poetics of the Emotions* (Durham, NC: Duke University Press, 2009), 8, 31.
85 For literature on the affective turn, see Athena Antanasiou, Pothiti Hantzaroula, and Kostas Yannakopoulos, "Towards a New Epistemology: The 'Affective Turn,'" *Historein* 8 (2008): 5–16; Patricia Ticento Coleman and Jean Halley, eds., *The Affective Turn: Theorizing the Social* (Durham, NC: Duke University Press, 2008); Marlene Goldman and Jill Matus, "Introduction," in "Models of Mind and Consciousness," ed. Marlene Goldman and Jill Matus, special issue, *University of Toronto Quarterly* 79, no. 2 (2010): 615–31; Imogen Tyler, "Methodological Fatigue and the Politics of the Affective Turn," *Feminist Media Studies* 8, no. 1 (1977): 43–65; and Rebecca Wanzo, "Against Proper Affective Objects," *American Quarterly* 61, no. 4 (2009): 967–78.
86 For example, see Steve Penfold, *The Donut: A Canadian History* (Toronto: University of Toronto Press, 2008); Dorothy Duncan, *Canadians at the Table: Food, Fellowship, and Folklore: A Culinary History of Canada* (Toronto: Dundurn Press, 2006); Carole Ferguson and Margaret Fraser, *A Century of Canadian Home Cooking: 1900 through the '90s* (Scarborough, ON: Prentice Hall Canada, 1992); Jo Marie Powers and Anita Stewart, eds., *Northern Bounty: A Celebration of Canadian Cuisine* (Toronto: Random House Canada, 1995); Jo Marie Powers, ed., *Buon Appetito! Italian Foodways in Ontario* (Willowdale, ON: Ontario Historical Society, 2000); Elizabeth Driver, *Culinary Landmarks: A Bibliography of Canadian Cookbooks, 1825–1949* (Toronto: University of Toronto Press, 2008); Thelma Barer-Stein, *You Eat What You Are: A Study of Canadian Ethnic Food Traditions* (Toronto: McClelland & Stewart, 1979); Cooke, *What's to Eat?*; Meribeth Clow, Dorothy Duncan, and Glenn J. Lockwood, eds., *Consuming Passions, Papers Presented at the 101st Annual Conference of the Ontario Historical Society, 1989*

(Willowdale, ON: The Ontario Historical Society, 1990); Franca Iacovetta, Vareriе J. Korinek, and Marlene Epp, eds., *Edible Histories, Cultural Politics: Towards a Canadian Food History* (Toronto: University of Toronto Press, 2013); Edmund Searles, "Food and the Making of Modern Inuit Identities," *Food and Foodways* 10 (2002): 55–78.

87 Shannon Stettner and Tracy Penny Light, "The Politics of Reproductive Health History: Visible, Audible, and Consequential," *Canadian Bulletin of Medical History* 31, no. 2 (2014): 10.

88 Ian Mosby, "Administering Colonial Science: Nutrition Research and Human Biomedical Experimentation in Aboriginal Communities Residential Schools, 1942–1952," *Histoire sociale/Social History* 46, no. 91 (May 2013): 145–72.

Chapter 1

1 George Orwell paraphrased by Leon Rappoport, *How We Eat: Appetite, Culture and the Psychology of Food* (Toronto: ECW Press, 2003), 42. The quotation in the title of this chapter is taken from "Food," *CLP* 65, no. 2 (August 1925): 55.

2 For fruit and vegetables, see Laura Jakul, "The Effect of Anti-Obesity Media on Body Image and Antifat Attitudes" (MA thesis, University of Manitoba, 2005), 28.

3 For the federal level, see Aleck Samuel Ostry, *Nutrition Policy in Canada, 1870 to 1939* (Vancouver, BC: UBC Press, 2006); Alana J. Hermiston, "'If It's Good for You, It's Good for the Nation!' The Moral Regulation of Nutrition in Canada, 1930–1945" (PhD diss., Carleton University, 2005); Ian Mosby, *Food Will Win the War: The Politics, Culture, and Science on Canada's Home Front* (Vancouver, BC: UBC Press, 2014). For the provincial level, see Tara D. Corless, "'Lunch Boxes on the March': Women, Family-Feeding, and the Nova Scotia Nutritition Programme, 1935–1959" (MA thesis, Dalhousie, Saint Mary's, and Mount Saint Vincent Universities, 1998); Gail Lush, "Nutrition, Health Education, and Dietary Reform: Gendering the 'New Science' in Northern Newfoundland and Labrador, 1893–1928" (MA thesis, Memorial University, 2008); Caroline Durand, *Nourrir la machine humaine: Nutrition et alimentation au Québec, 1860–1945* (Montreal and Kingston: McGill-Queen's University Press, 2015); Caroline Durand, "Patates, pain, et lard salé valaient-ils mieux que céréales, bacon et boeuf haché? La diète quotidienne et la santé au Québec, 1861–1941," *Canadian Bulletin of Medical History* 32, no. 2 (2015): 275–6. For nutritional policy and Indigenous people, see Krista Walters, "'A National Priority': Nutrition

Canada's *Survey* and the Discipining of Aboriginal Bodies, 1964–1975," in *Edible Histories, Cultural Politics: Towards a Canadian Food History*, ed. Franca Iacovetta, Valerie J. Korinek, and Marlene Epp (Toronto: University of Toronto Press, 2012), 433–51.

4 Beverly Soloway, "'mus co shee': Indigenous Plant Foods and Horticultural Imperialism in the Canadian Sub-Arctic," *Canadian Bulletin of Medical History* 32, no. 2 (2015): 253–73.

5 For composition of food, see L.B. Pett, C.A. Morrell, and F.W. Hanley, "The Development of Dietary Standards," *CJPH* 36, no. 6 (June 1945): 233. See also Harmke Kamminga and Andrew Cunningham, "Introduction: The Science and Culture of Nutrition, 1840–1940," in *The Science and Culture of Nutrition, 1940–1940*, ed. Harmke Kamminga and Andrew Cunningham (Amsterdam: Rodopi, 1995), 10. For legislation, see Ostry, *Nutrition Policy in Canada*, 6, 17–18, 61 (quote on the 1911 act on page 17). In the United States, malnutrition of children was also a significant issue. See A.R. Ruis, "'Children with Half-Starved Bodies' and the Assessment of Malnutrition in the United States, 1890–1950," *Bulletin of the History of Medicine* 87, no. 2 (Fall 2013): 378–406.

6 For an emphasis on vitamins, see Virginia Lea, "Eating Off Weight," *CM* 72, no. 4 (October 1929): 42. For vitamin D, see Sir Arbuthnot Lane, "Says Short Skirt Good for Health," *Maclean's* 42, no. 14 (15 July 1929): 24. See also John R. Murlin, "The Need of Further Investigation of the Effect of Commercial and Household Processes on the Vitamine Content of Foods," *JHE* 13, no. 9 (September 1921): 389–95; Katharine Blunt, "The Present Status of Vitamines," *JHE* 13, no. 3 (March 1921): 97–119. For a history of vitamins, see Rima D. Apple, *Vitamania: Vitamins in American Culture* (New Brunswick, NJ: Rutgers University Press, 1996).

7 For lack of knowledge among doctors, see Beryl Knox, "Public Health Nurse as an Organizer in a Rural Community," *CN* 17, no. 6 (June 1921): 344. For discussions, see Bernard Fantus, "What We Eat and Why," *CLP* 64, no. 4 (April 1925): 177–84; "The Importance of the Mineral Elements in the Diet," *CMAJ* 14, no. 12 (December 1924): 1220–2; Milton Bridges, "The Physician and Modern Dietetics," *CMAJ* 34, no. 6 (June 1936): 659–63; *CMAJ* 37, no. 3 (September 1937): 309, advertisement for Fellow's Syrup; Lennox G. Bell, "Protein Requirements in Normal Nutrition," *CMAJ* 38, no. 4 (April 1938): 387.

8 For various foods, see "Brown Bread and Butter," *CLNH* 62, no. 5 (May 1924): 171–2. For margarine history in Canada, see Caroline Lieffers, "'A Wholesome Article of Food': Rhetoric of Health and Nation in Canada's Oleomargarine Debates, 1917–1924," *Canadian Bulletin of Medical History*

32, no. 2 (2015): 337–62. For margarine history in the United States, see Bee Wilson, *Swindled: The Dark History of Food Fraud, from Poisoned Candy to Counterfeit Coffee* (Princeton, NJ: Princeton University Press, 2008), 167–74. For an excellent book on white bread, see Aaron Bobrow-Strain, *White Bread: A Social History of the Store-Bought Loaf* (Boston: Beacon Press, 2012). For milk, see Arthur G. Clark, "'Of Mice and Men' – and Milk!," *Maclean's* 33, no. 8 (1 May 1920): 35; William Fleming French, "Our Food and Our Future," *Maclean's* 34, no.13 (1 July 1921): 66; Emma D. Scott, "Are You Neglecting the Big Four," *Chatelaine* 2, no. 6 (June 1929): 26. For a different take on milk today, see Alissa Hamilton, *Got Milked: What You Don't Know about Dairy, the Truth about Calcium, and Why You'll Thrive without Milk* (New York: HarperCollins, 2015). On Stefansson, see "They Thrive on All-Meat Diet," *Maclean's* 42, no. 17 (1 September 1929): 40, reprint. For the results of eating well, see Phyllis Warner, "Eating for Health," *CM* 71 (April 1929): 22; Susan Yager, *The Hundred Year Diet: America's Voracious Appetite for Losing Weight* (New York: Rodale Inc., 2010), 63, 66.

9 For sugar, see Sister Irene Marie, "Health Preservation through Adequate Diet," *CN* 25, no. 4 (April 1929): 177; "Sugar-Saturated, Vitamin-Starved America," *CLP* 72, no. 5 (May 1929): 195. For the present concern about eating sugar, see "Lower Sugar Intake to Less Than 5% of Daily Calories, WHO Says," *CBC News*, 5 March 2014, accessed 7 January 2016, http://www.cbc.ca/news/health/lower-sugar-intake-to-less-than-5-of-daily-calories-who-says-1.2560639. For fat, see F.H. Whetmore, "Remarks on Deficiency Diseases," *CMAJ* 12, no. 12 (December 1922): 875.

10 For canning, see Elizabeth Robinson Scovil, "Importance of Green Vegetables," *CN* 16, no. 9 (September 1920): 547. For refining flour, see Ester L. Kinney, "A Few Facts about Vitamins," *CN* 18, no. 10 (October 1922): 609; and Ester Kinney, "White Whole Wheat Bread?" *CN* 21, no. 7 (July 1925): 361. For shelf life, see A. Bruce Macullum, "Some Practical Considerations about the Vitamins," *CN* 21, no. 9 (September 1925): 454.

11 For any class, see Chas. S. Macdougall, "Malnutrition in Children of School Age," *PHJ* 16, no. 1 (January 1925): 26. For poverty, see Edmund S. Grant, "Are Economic Conditions Effecting [sic] Our Children's Teeth?" *Health* 1, no. 2 (June 1933): 9; Margaret S. McCready, "Considerations of Nutrition in Relief Work IV – Relief Allowances in Ontario," *CPHJ* 24, no. 5 (May 1933): 216–21; E.W. McHenry, "Dietary Standards," *CPHJ* 24, no. 7 (July 1933): 308–15. On ignorance, poverty, and disease, see H. Medovy, "The Malnourished Child," *CN* 27, no. 3 (March 1931): 118. For poverty and ignorance, see Editorial, "Nutrition: A Nutritional Problem," *CPHJ* 30, no. 1 (January 1939): 60.

12 On national legislation, see Ostry, *Nutrition Policy in Canada*, 58, 61; J.J. Heagerty, "What to Eat," *Health* 1, no. 3 (October 1933): 10; L.I. Pugsley, "The Administration and Development of Federal Statutes on Food and Drugs in Canada," *MSJ* 23, no. 3 (March 1967): 387–449; Aleck Ostry et al., "The Establishment of a National System of Food in Canada," *CJPH* 94, no. 4 (July–August, 2003): 266. For response to the League, see Hermiston, "If It's Good for You, It's Good for the Nation!," 59 (quote), 64. For a critique of the report, see also Corless, "Lunch Boxes on the March," 40. For the role of the League of Nations, see James Vernon, *Hunger: A Modern History* (Cambridge, MA: The Belknap Press of Harvard University Press, 2007), 129.

13 For Marsh, see Corless, "Lunch Boxes on the March," 41. For women's groups, see Hermiston, "If It's Good for You, It's Good for the Nation!," 64–7. Some of the groups interested in nutrition included the Visiting Homemakers Association, the Canadian Dietetic Association, the Canadian Home Economics Association, and the YMCA. For the CCN, see Ostry, *Nutrition Policy in Canada*, 80, 99, 105.

14 Government of Canada, "Canada's Food Guides from 1942 to 1992," 5 February 2007, accessed 22 September 2014, https://www.canada.ca/en/health-canada/services/food-nutrition/canada-food-guide/background-food-guide/canada-food-guides-1942-1992.html. See also Ian Mosby, "Making and Breaking Canada's Food Rules: Science, the State, and the Government of Nutrition, 1942–1949," in Iacovetta, Korinek, and Epp, *Edible Histories*, 409–32. For the quote, see *CHW* 4, no. 2 (November 1948): n.p., which appears under the heading "Malnutrition: The Problem of Distribution and Utilization of Food 3. Food Habits in Canada." For problems following the rules, see Corless, "Lunch Boxes on the March," 82.

15 For Simpson's quote, see News Brief, "The Fitness of Future Citizens," *CD* 7, no. 7 (July 1941): 59. For girls and women working, see Hiram McCann, "Canada's Faulty Diet Is Adolf Hitler's Ally," *Saturday Night* 56, no. 40 (14 June 1941): 8. On war and feeding the army, see Helen G. Campbell, "Vitamins for Victory," *Maclean's* 54, no. 18 (15 September 1941): 67–9; Charlene D. Elliott, "Big Persons, Small Voices: On Governance, Obesity, and the Narrative of the Failed Citizen," *Journal of Canadian Studies* 41, no. 3 (Fall 2007): 137. Elliott noted that Hillel Schwartz made the same point about the situation in the United States. See Hillel Schwartz, *Never Satisfied: A Cultural History of Diets, Fantasies and Fat* (London: Collier Macmillan Publishers, 1986). For the families of those serving, see Marion Harlow, "Improving Nutrition via the Family Budget," *CPHJ* 32, no. 6 (September 1941): 460.

16 For the women, see Mosby, *Food Will Win the War*, 91–6, 172–3, 179, 206. For regulations, see Pugsley, "The Administration and Development of Federal Statutes on Food and Drugs in Canada," 387–449, (on vitamins, 414); Ostry et al., "The Establishment of a National System of Food in Canada," 266.
17 Editorial, "Two Forgotten Aspects of Nutrition," *CJPH* 36, no. 9 (September 1945): 374; E.W. McHenry, "Food in Canada," *Health* (January/February 1948): 22; John O'Neill, "Scientists Now Turn to Theory Fat Person Is Undernourished," *Saturday Night* (3 May 1949), n.p. For obesity, see also W.W. Baker, "Battle of the Bulges," *Maclean's* 59, no. 16 (15 August 1946): 38.
18 L.B. Pett, "Nutrition," *Health* 17, no. 2 (March/April 1949): 10.
19 For gullible, see D.S. McEwan, "Factors and Fancies about Food," *CN* 36, no. 1 (January 1940): 21–2; McHenry, "Food in Canada," 15; Helen G. Campbell, "Food Foolishness," *Chatelaine* 16, no. 1 (January 1943): 40. On the value of the potato, see Rica McLean Farquharson, "Startling Recruit Revelations," *CHJ* 38, no. 9 (February 1942): 24.
20 For Dominion, see Barry E.C. Boothman, "Mammoth Market: The Transformation of Food Retailing in Canada, 1946–1965," *Journal of Historical Research in Marketing* 3, no. 3 (2011): 294, accessed 16 July 2012, http://www.emeraldinsight.com/toc/jhrm/3/3.
21 For fat, see Peter H. Nash, "Health...and the Businessman," *Health* 24, no. 5 (September–October 1956): 10. For anaemia, see Lorraine Miller, "The Staff Studies Nutrition," *CN* 46, no. 10 (October 1950): 810.
22 Miller, "The Staff Studies Nutrition," 810. "Food Habits of New Canadians," *CN* 55, no. 10 (October 1959): 945. For more on foodways of immigrants and Canadians, see Franca Iacovetta, "Food Acts and Cultural Politics: Women and the Gendered Dialectics of Culinary Pluralism at the International Institute of Toronto, 1950s–1960s," in Iacovetta, Korinek, and Epp, *Edible Histories*, 359–84.
23 Jennifer Hough Evans, "Turning 'Space' into 'Place' with Food: Immigrant Women's Food Narratives in Post-1945 North Bay, Ontario," *Ontario History* 157, no. 2 (Autumn 2014): 214–34, quote 219. See also Marlene Epp, "Eating Across Borders: Reading Immigrant Cookbooks," *Histoire sociale / Social History* 48, no. 96 (May 2015): 45–65.
24 "People Have Reasons for Eating What They Do," *CHW* 12, no. 4 (April 1957): n.p., "Food and People," supplement no. 34.
25 On eating fat, see J.A.F. Stevenson, "Trends in Nutrition," *CSMJ* 12 (April 1956): 360. For consumerism, see Harvey Levenstein, *Paradox of Plenty: A Social History of Eating in Modern America*, rev. ed. (Berkeley: University of

California Press, 2003), 107–10. For convenient foods, see "Meals Off the Shelf," *Chatelaine* 28, no. 2 (February 1955): 18–20, 33; Alan Phillips, "Is This Your Heart's Worst Enemy?" *Maclean's* 68, no. 25 (10 December 1955): 121. High fats included meat and sweets.

26 For obesity malnutrition, see Gordon E. Wride, "Canada's Unmet Needs in Health Care," *CHW* 11, no. 9 (November 1956): 5; E. Gordon Young, "An Appraisal of Canadian Nutriture," *Canadian Bulletin on Nutrition* 3, no. 1 (July 1953): 24; W.A. Cochrane, "Nutritional Excess in Infancy and Childhood," *CMAJ* 81, no. 6 (15 September 1959): 454. For the United Nations, see L. Bradley Pett, "How Many Calories?" *CMAJ* 75, no. 3 (1 August 1956): 241. For Canada's rank, see "We Live in an Unequal World," *CHW* 12, no. 4 (April 1957): n.p., "Food and People," supplement no. 34. For Quebec eating, see "L'appareil digestif ne résiste pas aux excès de table: La température au temps des fêtes," *UMC* 80, no. 1 (janvier 1951): 140; "Soyez sobres dans le boire et le manger pendant les fêtes," *UMC* 84, no. 1 (janvier 1955): 108.

27 For McLaren, see Sheila Kieran, "Why Diets Fail," *Chatelaine* 39, no. 12 (December 1966): 18. For E.W. McHenry, see Rosamond H. Ross, "Review of *Foods without Fads* by E.W. McHenry," *CN* 57, no. 8 (August 1961): 764.

28 For the Canada Food Guide, see "'Rules' Changed to Canada's Food Guide," *Health* 30, no. 1 (February 1962): 40; J.E. Monagle, "Canada's Food Guide: A Route to Health," *Health* 30, no. 5 (October 1962): 18, 28. For the Ontario manual, see "Diet Manual Available," *CN* 60, no. 6 (June 1964): 551.

29 "Recommended Intake of Protein," *CMAJ* 102, no. 12 (10 June 1970): 1406; Marjorie Harris, "The Great Nutrition Game," *Maclean's* 82, no. 4 (April 1969): 77, 79.

30 "Fabricated Food: A Risk to Future Generations' Health," *Montreal Gazette* (from *Chicago Tribune*), 20 February 1980, 29.

31 Extracts from a General Foods booklet in "What to Know about Weight Control," *Health* 39, no. 2 (Summer 1973): 21. For beef, see Alison Cunliffe, "Ottawa Wants Us to Trim the Fat," *Toronto Star* (10 November 1977), A7. For a different view of fat, see Nina Teicholz, *The Big Fat Surprise: Why Butter and Cheese Belong in a Healthy Diet* (Toronto: Simon & Schuster Canada, 2015).

32 For drinks, etc., see Bonnie Cornell, "Shortages on the Table," *Chatelaine* 47, no. 6 (June 1974): 16.

33 For the belief that income doesn't matter, see "Eating Better for Less: The Food Prices Review Board Report on Nutritional Costs," *CC* 5 (August 1975): 1. See also Earl Damude, "Unfit Canadians," *Chatelaine* 47, no. 2 (February 1974): 12. On store locations, see "What Price Nutrition?" *CW*

51 (May/June 1975): 20. For ignorance as the cause of poor nutrition, see A.W. Myers and Danièle Kroetsch, "The Influence of Family Income on Food Consumption Patterns and Nutrient Intake in Canada," *CJPH* 69, no. 3 (May/June 1978): 220.

34 Adrienne Pitt, "Lunchtime at School," *CC* 6 (October 1976): 29; Linda Diener, "School Vending Machines," *CC* 6 (October 1976): 37; Beverly Reichert, "Food and You," *Health* 39, no. 4 (Winter 1973/74): 22; Cunliffe, "Ottawa Wants Us to Trim the Fat," A7. In 1977, new nutrition recommendations were made by the Department of National Health and Welfare. T.K. Murray and Jesse Rae, "Nutrition Recommendations for Canadians," *CMAJ* 120, no. 9 (19 May 1979): 1241–2.

35 E.W. McHenry, "The Relation of Income to Diet Quality," *CPHJ* 23, no. 6 (June 1932): 296.

36 Franz Boas, "The Growth of Toronto Children," chapter 34 in *Report of the Commissioner of Education for the Year 1896–97*, vol. 2, US Bureau of Education (Washington: Government Printing Office, 1898), 1543. For early surveillance of students, see Norah Lillian Lewis, "Advising the Parents: Child Rearing in British Columbia during the Inter-War Years" (PhD diss., University of British Columbia, 1980), 4.

37 Alan Brown and G. Albert Davis, "The Prevalence of Malnutrition in the Public School Children of Toronto," *CMAJ* 11, no. 2 (February 1921): 124–6.

38 William Fleming French, "Making Children Healthy," *Maclean's* 34, no. 18 (15 October 1921): 57.

39 John W.S. McCullough, "Are You Sure of Their Health," *Chatelaine* 3, no. 12 (December 1930): 9.

40 For the 1937 study, see E.W. McHenry, "Nutrition in Toronto," *CPHJ* 30, no. 1 (January 1939): 6–7; for further analysis of this study, see E.W. McHenry, "Nutrition in Canada," *CPHJ* 30, no. 1 (September 1939): 431–4. For Marsh, see Julie Guard, "The Politics of Milk: Canadian Housewives Organize in the 1930s," in Iacovetta, Korinek, and Epp, *Edible Histories*, 278.

41 For descriptions of the four city survey, see Mosby, *Food Will Win the War*, 25–6, 171–2; Ostry, *Nutrition Policy in Canada*, 82, 109.

42 For the Edmonton survey, see George Hunter and L. Bradley Pett, "A Dietary Survey in Edmonton," *CPHJ* 32, no. 5 (May 1941): 259–65. For another study, see H. Siemens, "A Survey of Nutrition in the Public Schools of the Lamont Health District, Lamont, Alberta," *CPHJ* 31, no. 1 (January 1940): 42.

43 "Nutrition," *ManMR* 23, no. 1 (January 1943): 22.

44 For the 1953 national survey, see L.B. Pett, "A National Weight-Health Survey," *CJPH* 43, no. 11 (November 1952): 487. For the report, see L.B. Pett

and G.F. Ogilvie, "The Report on Canadian Average Weights, Heights, and Skinfolds," *Canadian Bulletin on Nutrition* 5, no. 1 (September 1957): 1–81 (quote, 44).
45 G.H. Beaton, "Nutritional Status of Canadians – An Unknown Entity," *CJPH* 61, no. 3 (May/June 1970): 194; Gerald Waring, "Journal Article Influences Decision for Massive Nutritional Survey," *CMAJ* 102, no. 2 (31 January 1970): 219; Una Abrahamson, "What's Your Nutrition IQ?" *Chatelaine* 44, no. 3 (March 1971): 16; Carole Peacock, "Nutrition Canada: A Progress Report," *CHW* 25, no. 4 (January–February 1971): 7.
46 For nutrient deficiency, see "What Price Nutrition?," 20; Cornell, "Shortages on the Table," 16. For the numbers, see Z.I. Sabry, "The Cost of Malnutrition in Canada," *CJPH* 66, no. 4 (July/August 1975): 291. The total cholesterol level was used to determine whether a person had high blood cholesterol, which was deemed a risk for heart attacks; not until the 1970s and 1980s was cholesterol divided into HDL and LDL cholesterol, which were seen as different from each other. For iron deficiency in teenage girls and much of the population, see Melvin Lee, "Nutrition Canada Survey – A Review," *BCMJ* 16, no. 3 (March 1974): 70. The survey determined that the Inuit population generally did not experience iron deficiency. For deficiencies affecting Indigenous people, see Lee, "Nutrition Canada Survey," 70, 71. For overweight numbers, see Z.I. Sabry et al., "Nutrition Canada – A National Nutrition Survey," *Nutrition Reviews* 32, no. 4 (April 1974): 108. For a discussion of vitamins for circumpolar peoples, see R.J. Shephard and A. Rode, *The Health and Consequences of 'Modernization': Evidence from Circumpolar Peoples* (Cambridge: Cambridge University Press, 1996), 28, 97.
47 Z.I. Sabry, "Nutrition in Canada," *CJPH* 65, no. 4 (September/October 1974): 343; L. Bradley Pett, "Letter to the Editor," *CJPH* 66, no. 2 (March/April 1975): 165; L. Pett, "Canadian Nutrition around 1950," *CJPH* 63, no. 2 (March/April 1972): 161.
48 Canadian Museum of History, "Maternal and Infant Mortality," in *Making Medicare: The History of Health Care in Canada, 1914–2007*, online exhibiton, accessed 21 October 2016, http://www.historymuseum.ca/cmc/exhibitions/hist/medicare/medic-1c05e.shtml.
49 Esther Kinney, "Why the Whole Wheat Bread?" *CN* 21, no. 7 (July 1925): 362.
50 For descriptions of the four city surveys, see Mosby, *Food Will Win the War*, 25–6, 171–2; Ostry, *Nutrition Policy in Canada*, 82, 109; F.W. Gershaw, "Diet and Health," *CCJ* 21, no. 8 (August 1942): 80–1. For CCN, see Mosby, *Food Will Win the War*, 29–30, 41, 176, 182, 190–2.

51 E.W. McHenry, Ruth Crawford, and Lillian Barber, "The Heights and Weights of a Canadian Group," *CPHJ* 38, no. 9 (September 1947): 438.
52 Sidney Margolius, "Lady, You're Starving Yourself," *Maclean's* 64, no. 2 (15 January 1951): 20. For an article that focused on and gave advice about how to avoid the increasing cost of food, see Sidney Margolius, "Ten Ways to Save Money on Food," *Maclean's* 65, no. 1 (1 January 1952): 10–11, 46–7.
53 Sabry et al., "Nutrition Canada," 109.
54 For the "troublesome condition," see Alan Brown, *The Normal Child: Its Care and Feeding* (Toronto: F.D. Goodchild Company Publishers, 1923), 145.
55 For the 1934 survey, see J.T. Phair, "Survey of Health Habits among School Age Children," *CPHJ* 25, no. 8 (August 1934): 382–3.
56 John McCullough, "Doctor, He Won't Eat!" *Chatelaine* 10, no. 2 (February 1937): 61. See also Anne Elizabeth Wilson, "Schools for the Home-Maker," *Maclean's* 40, no. 22 (15 November 1927): 64. For the clinics, see F.W. Tidmarsh, "Malnutrition," *CN* 20, no. 1 (January 1924): 779.
57 For calories needed, see Elizabeth Robinson Scovil, "The Food of Children," *CN* 17, no. 8 (August 1921): 297. For teen girls, see Charles E. Snelling, "No Excuse for Dietary Anaemia," *Health* 6, no. 4 (December 1938): 92. For coaxing, see Helen G. Campbell, "Feeding the Teens," *Maclean's* 50, no. 8 (15 April 1937): 78.
58 Tidmarsh, "Malnutrition," 426. For reprint of the article, see *CN* 20, no. 1 (January 1924): 777–9. See also French, "Making Children Healthy," 57, for the lack on discipline in children. Mona Gleason has looked at children's agency in the past. Mona Gleason, "Avoiding the Agency Trap: Caveats for Historians of Children, Youth, and Education," *History of Education* 45, no. 4 (2016): 446–59.
59 J.T. Phair, "Some Observations on the Diet of Children of School Age," *CPHJ* 21, no. 12 (December 1930): 623–4.
60 Mildred D. Goodeve, "Nutrition and Health of the School Child," *Health* 3, no. 3 (September 1935): 54; McCullough, "Doctor, He Won't Eat!," 61.
61 For Hattie, see Leslie Baker, "A Visitation of Providence: Public Health and Eugenic Reform in the Wake of the Halifax Disaster," *Canadian Bulletin of Medical History* 31, no. 1 (2014): 105. For Brantford, see C.C. Alexander and Will L. Hutton, "Nutritional Studies in Brantford, Ontario," *CPHJ* 23, no. 12 (December 1932): 579.
62 [Name withheld], "'I Am a Canadian Mother,'" [open letter to *Chatelaine* reproduced in article form] *Chatelaine* 6, no. 4 (April 1933): 18, 74. For mothers' reaction to the rise in milk prices, see Julie Guard, "The Politics of Milk: Militant Toronto Housewives Organize in the 1930s" (paper

presented at the Annual Meeting of the Canadian Historical Association, Vancouver, BC, June 2008).
63 Hunter and Pett, "A Dietary Survey in Edmonton," 259–65.
64 Gordon Young, "A Dietary Survey in Halifax," *CPHJ* 32, no. 5 (May 1941): 237. For the Quebec study, see J. Ernest Sylvestre et Honoré Nadeau, "Enquête sur l'alimentation habituelle des familles de petit-salariés dans la ville de Québec," *CPHJ* 32, no. 5 (May 1941): 241–50. For the Toronto study, see Jean M. Patterson and E.W. McHenry, "A Dietary Investigation in Toronto Families Having Annual Income between $1,500 and $2,400," *CPHJ* 32, no. 5 (May 1941): 251–8. For the study as a whole, see *CN* 38, no. 10 (October 1942): 771. For blaming mothers, see Ostry, *Nutrition Policy in Canada*, 85.
65 L.B. Pett, "Food Makes a Difference," *CPHJ* 33, no. 12 (December 1942): 568.
66 Elizabeth Chant Robertson, "Feeding Diffculties," *Chatelaine* 16, no. 10 (October 1943): 87.
67 Alton Goldbloom, *The Care of the Child*, 4th ed. (Toronto: Longmans, Green and Co., 1945), 187–8. For children, see *ManMR* 21, no. 10 (October, 1941): 191, advertisement for Abbott vitamins.
68 Joan Phillips, "Teen-Age Eating for Good Health and Good Looks," *CHJ* 41, no. 5 (September 1944): 38, 40.
69 For girls, see Kate Holliday, "Hollwood Designs for the Teens," *Chatelaine* 22, no. 1 (January 1949): 48–9. For the teen boys' image, see the story by Dorothy Thomas, "Sweet Summer," *CHJ* 38, no. 7 (December 1941): 8–9, 34, 36, 38; and Christopher J. Greig, "The Idea of Boyhood in Postwar Ontario, 1945–1960" (PhD diss., University of Western Ontario, 2008), 17, 119–21.
70 Ian Mosby, "The Gender of Calories: Nutrition, Domesticity and Canada's 'Manpower' Crisis, 1939–1948" (paper present at the Annual Meeting of the Canadian Historical Association, Vancouver, BC, June 2008), 13.
71 G.T. Haig, "Suppose Tommy Won't Eat," *CJPH* 44, no. 1 (January 1953): 18.
72 M.T. Doyle, M.C. Cahoon, and E.W. McHenry, "The Consumption of Recommended Foods by Children in Relation to Sex, the Use of Sweet Foods, and Employment of Mothers," *CJPH* 44, no. 7 (July 1953): 150–62. See also Mary T. Doyle, "The Nutrition of the School Child," *NSMB* 34, no. 1 (1955): 12–15.
73 R.H. Johnson, "What Mothers Should Know about Child Feeding," *Health* 23, no. 3 (May/June 1955): 6.
74 "Quebec School Children Suffer from Malnutrition," *CN* 65, no. 10 (October 1969): 19.

75 *Chatelaine* 36, no. 5 (May, 1963): 9–10, advertisement for Swift franks.
76 Canada, Department of National Health and Welfare, Nutrition Division, *Healthful Eating* (Ottawa: Department of National Health and Welfare, 1963), 17.
77 Elizabeth Chant Robertson, "Does Your Teen-ager Get the Right Food?" *Chatelaine* 29, no. 10 (October 1956): 128–9; Elizabeth Chant Robertson, "The Tragedy of the Fat Child," *Chatelaine* 31, no. 1 (January 1958): 46; Elizabeth Chant Robertson, "Food and Fitness," *Health* 33, no. 6 (June 1965): 29; Donna M. Baxter, "Food, Nutrition and Good Health," *ManMR* 46, no. 4 (April 1966): 269.
78 Catherine Sinclair, "'Picky' Eaters," *Chatelaine* 43, no. 12 (December 1970): 74.
79 For the quote and mothers working, see "Nutrition's Vital Role in Health Maintenance," *Health* 42, no. 2 (Summer 1976): 18, based on a speech by Lewis E. Lloyd, dean of the Faculty of Home Economics, University of Manitoba. For mother blaming, see Naomi Mallovy, "Good Food Habits Last a Lifetime," *Chatelaine* 46, no. 6 (June 1973): 97.
80 J. E. Dubé, "L'hygiène au Séminaire de Joliette," *UMC* 49, no. 3 (mars 1920): 112. For concern about the health issues of overeating, see Romeo Boucher, "Augmentation de la pression artérielle chez les gens normaux," *UMC* 53, no. 1 (janvier 1924): 10–13; F.M. Jones, "Health Hazards of Executives," *OMR* 6, no. 4 (August 1949): 90; Joan Phillips, "Busy Business People Need Wisely-Balanced Meals," *CHJ* 46, no. 12 (April 1950): 42
81 For the 1940s, see George S.Young, "How to Grow Old Successfully," *Health* 15, no. 3 (May–June 1947): 8; and J.-H. Lapointe, "La nutrition chez le vieillard," *UMC* 76, no. 4 (avril 1947): 413–21. For the 1950s, see Sidney Katz, "A Report on Eating," *Maclean's* 68, no. 12 (11 June 1955): 91; Dr René Rolland, "La Société médicale de Montréal," *UMC* 84, no. 6 (juin 1955): 717, notice of the symposium sur la gériatrie; and E.W. McHenry, "Nutrition for Older People," *CSMJ* 12 (March 1956): 199. For the 1960s, see J.E. Monagle, "Food Habits of Seniors," *CJPH* 58, no. 5 (May 1967): 205; also in the 1960s, see E.W. McHenry "Nutrition and Older People," *CJPH* 51, no. 3 (March 1960): 101–4. For after the National Survey, see Mike Grenby, "Living to Eat: Nutrition for Senior Citizens," *CN* 73, no. 4 (April 1977): 42; Doris Gillis, "Seniors: A Target for Nutrition Education." *CN* 76, no. 7 (July/August 1980): 28.
82 Earl Damude, "Eat Less, Live Longer," *Chatelaine* 52, no. 11 (November 1979): 14; *UMC* 99, no. 4 (avril 1970): 606, advertisement for Winstrol.
83 Hugh Shewell, *'Enough to Keep Them Alive': Indian Welfare in Canada, 1873–1965* (Toronto: University of Toronto Press, 2004), 330.

84 Ian Mosby, "Administering Colonial Science: Nutrition Research and Human Biomedical Experimentation in Aboriginal Communities and Residential Schools, 1942–1952," *Histoire sociale/ Social History* 46, no. 91 (May 2013): 145–72, quote 171. M.W. Partington and Norma Roberts, "The Heights and Weights of Indian and Eskimo School Children on James Bay and Hudson Bay," *CMAJ* 100, no. 11 (15 March 1969): 506; O. Schaefer, "Pre-and-Post-Natal Growth Acceleration and Increased Sugar Consumption," *CMAJ* 103, no. 10 (7 November 1970): 1059, 1066.

85 Mosby, "Administering Colonial Science"; Krista Walters, "'A National Priority': Food, Diet and Aboriginal Nutrition in Canada's Northwest, 1965–85" (paper presented at the Annual Meeting of the Canadian Historical Association, Vancouver, BC, June 2008), 21. For a negative view of such education, see Deborah McPhail, "'The White Man's Burden'? Obesity and Colonialism in the Developing North," chapter 4 in *Contours of the Nation: Making Obesity and Imagining Canada, 1945–1970* (Toronto: University of Toronto Press, 2017), 101–33.

86 University of British Columbia, First Nations and Indigenous Studies, "The White Paper 1969," indigenousfoundations.arts.ubc.ca, 2009, accessed 25 October 2016, http://indigenousfoundations.arts.ubc.ca/the_white_paper_1969/. For the text of the white paper, see Canada, Indian and Northern Affairs, *Statement of the Government of Canada on Indian Policy* (Ottawa: Department of Indian and Northern Affairs, 1969), http://epe.lac-bac.gc.ca/100/200/301/inac-ainc/indian_policy-e/cp1969_e.pdf.

87 Walters, "A National Priority," 7, 14, 19, 23, 27, 28, 38, 55; Gaile P. Noble, "Social Considerations in Northern Health Care," *CN* 74, no. 9 (October 1978): 16, 18.

88 See Deborah McPhail, "Indigenous People's Clinical Encounters with Obesity: A Conversation with Barry Lavallee," in *Obesity in Canada: Critical Perspectives*, ed. Jenny Ellison, Deborah McPhail, and Wendy Mitchinson (Toronto: University of Toronto Press, 2016), 175–84.

89 Hermiston, "If It's Good for You, It's Good for the Nation!," 89.

90 *CMAJ* 11, no. 12 (December 1921): 970, advertisement for Frosst's Blaud Capsules; *UMC* 53, no. 1 (janvier 1924): xxxv, advertisement for Ovaltine.

91 *Maclean's* 36, no. 8 (15 April 1923): 73, advertisement for FORCE; *Maclean's* 36, no. 10 (15 May 1923): 58, advertisement for FORCE. For value, see *CHJ* 16, no. 10 (February 1920): 28, advertisement for Purity Flour; *Maclean's* 33, no. 2 (1 February 1920): 71, advertisement for Quaker Oats.

92 For McCoy's Cod Liver Extract Tablets, see the description for men, *Maclean's* 39, no. 13 (1 July 1926): 46, advertisement; for women, see *Maclean's* 40, no. 19 (1 October 1927): 60, advertisement.

93 *Health* 2, no. 1 (March 1934): 17, advertisement for Ovaltine; *Health* 2, no. 3 (October 1934): 58, advertisement for Neilson's.
94 Hermiston, "If It's Good for You, It's Good for the Nation!," 124; *Maclean's* 55, no. 24 (15 December 1942): 25, advertisement with Elsie. Borden's was very astute in connecting their ads to the war effort. *UMC* 71, no. 10 (octobre 1942): 1131, advertisement for Borden's "Silver Cow." For Fleischmann's Yeast, see *Maclean's* 53, no. 4 (15 February 1940): 23, advertisement; and *CHJ* 45, no. 9 (January 1949): 32, advertisement.
95 For quote, see *CMAJ* 51, no. 5 (November 1944): 485, advertisement for Alphamin. For Abbott's advertisements, see *ManMR* 25, no. 9 (September 1945): 384; *ManMR* 27, no. 10 (October 1947): 600; *ManMR* 27, no. 3 (March 1947): 181.
96 For products and doctors, see *CD* 13, no. 6 (June 1947): 20, advertisement for Heinz; *CN* 45, no. 11 (November 1949): 807, advertisement for Heinz.
97 *CN* 55, no. 6 (June 1959): 545, advertisement for Farmer's Wife.
98 Alton Goldbloom, "The One Doctor in Four Talks Back," *Maclean's* 73, no. 25 (3 December 1960): 26; for Quebec eating, see "Canadian Quirks," *CN* 65, no. 2 (February 1969): 30; *UMC* 91, no. 11 (novembre 1962): 96, advertisement for Fleischmann oil. Corn oil didn't contain much saturated fat; saturated fats were believed to be a risk for heart attacks. For the history of the criticism of saturated fat, see Teicholz, *The Big Fat Surprise*. For Carnation, see *Chatelaine* 41, no. 9 (September 1968): 9, advertisement for Carnation Instant Breakfast. For Nutri-Bio, see Sidney Katz, "The Rose World of Nutri-Bio," *Maclean's* 75, no. 15 (28 July 1962): 36.
99 For example, Scott, "Are You Neglecting the Big Four," 26; French, "Our Food and Our Future," 65–6; Brown, *The Normal Child*, 36, 147, 149, 152–3, 156–9, 162. For welfare councils, see Alice MacKay, "Caring for the Children," *Maclean's* 41, no. 16 (15 August 1928): 63. For child hygiene, see "News Section," *CM* 12, no. 3 (March 1921): 141.
100 David Smith and Malcolm Nicolson, "Nutrition, Education, Ignorance and Income: A Twentieth-Century Debate," in Kamminga and Cunningham, *The Science and Culture of Nutrition*, 311.
101 For ads and institutions, see Marion Harlow, "Nutrition in the Health Mosaic," *CN* 35, no. 7 (July 1939): 370. For the Red Cross, see Margaret S. McCready, "Better Nutrition for All," *Health* 5, no. 3 (September 1937): 64, 82–3. For VON, see Marjorie Bell, "Nutrition Work with the Victorian Order of Nurses," *CN* 16, no. 10 (October 1930): 550. For others, see Hermiston, "If It's Good for You, It's Good for the Nation!," 72–3.

102 For Montreal, see Adélard Groulx, "La campagne d'alimentation à Montréal," *UMC* 72, no. 8 (août 1943): 926. For public service announcements, see *UMC* 72, no. 5 (mai 1943): 616–17, advertisement on healthy eating. For a listing of efforts in Quebec, see N. Laporte, "L'examen physique de l'enfant et la recherche de la dénutition," *UMC* 72, no. 6 (juin 1943): 670–81; and for New Brunswick Department of Health, see Florence Swan, "Rural School Lunch Program," *CN* 49, no. 9 (September 1953): 704. For films, see "The Internal Triangle," *CHW* 3, no. 10 (July 1948): 7; "Why Won't Tommy Eat?" *CHW* 4, no. 11 (November 1948): 2. For schools, see J.-A. Baudouin, "L'enseignement de l'hygiène dans les écoles de langue anglaise au Canada," *UMC* 72, no. 5 (mai 1943): 505–31; Jules Gilbert, "Technique de l'enseignement de l'hygiène alimentaire," *UMC* 75, no. 9 (septembre 1946): 1083–6. For lunch programs, see H. Ruth Crawford, "Nutrition Education and the Public Health Nurse," *CN* 43, no. 4 (April 1947): 272. For more on school lunches, see Helen G. Campbell, "Lessons in Lunches," *Chatelaine* 18, no. 2 (February 1945): 57–8, 71. For schools teaching how to eat properly through lunch programs, see Roma Amyot, "L'enseignement de l'hygiène dans les écoles élémentaires," *UMC* 75, no. 9 (septembre 1946): 1008.

103 Janet March, "Know Nutrition Values and Meals Will Be Appetizing and Good," *Saturday Night* 61, no. 2 (15 September 1945): 28.

104 "Should Vitamin D Be Given Only to Infants?" *NSMB* 23, no. 1 (1944): 32.

105 For vitamin K, see D.S. McEwan, "Facts and Fancies about Food," *CN* 36, no.1 (January 1940): 23. The decade opened with scientists aware of the existence of over twenty vitamins. Apple, *Vitamania*, 4.

106 For criticism of doctors, see Nan O'Garvock, "Low Cost Special Diets," *CN* 39, no. 2 (February 1943): 123.

107 "Canada's Enriched Bread – A Nutritional Insurance," *CN* 46, no. 5 (May 1953): 372.

108 On food fads, see Corinne Trerice, "Foods Fads at Face Value," *Health* 23, no. 5 (September–October 1955): 14; A. Corinne Trerice, "Food Faddism," *CAHPER* 19, no. 9 (May 1954): 21–3. For a fad, see Hauser's system. James Edgar, "Look What Gayelord's Got Us Eating," *Maclean's* 64, no. 4 (15 February 1951): 17. For being savvy, see "A Guide to Better Food Habits," *CN* 51, no. 7 (July 1955): 543.

109 Elizabeth Chant Robertson, *Nutrition for Today* (Toronto: McClelland & Stewart, 1951), 158–61, 178–9.

110 Doris L. Noble, "An Experiment in Nutrition Education," *CJPH* 43, no. 10 (October 1952): 431–2.

111 J.E. Monagle, "Nutrition and Health – A Critical Evaluation," *CJPH* 56, no. 11 (November 1965): 489.
112 Editorial, "Want in the Midst of Plenty," *CMAJ* 93, no. 11 (11 September 1965): 612. See also Sidney Katz, "Your Health and the Almighty Pill: Part One," *Maclean's* 75, no. 24 (1 December 1962): 60; David Lewis Stein, "A Doctor's Diagnosis of Nearly Everyone: Too Greedy," *Maclean's* 74, no. 1 (20 May 1961): 69; M. Elizabeth Campbell, "Vitamin D – Too Much or Too Little," *NSMB* 45, no. 8 (1966): 201–2, 212; "If a Little Bit Is Good, Isn't More Better?" *CMAJ* 93, no. 17 (23 October 1965): 938.
113 "Controversies in Medicine Fanned during Association Scientific Meeting," *CMAJ* 113, no. 1 (12 July 1975): 64.
114 For Hill, see "CMA Council on Community Health Reviews, Nutrition, Tropical Diseases, Abortion, Occupational Medicine, Seat Belts," *CMAJ* 113, no. 9 (8 November 1975): 889. For le Riche, see David Woods, "Nutritional for All: Medical Interest Seems to Be Awakening," *CMAJ* 116, no. 5 (5 March 1977): 533.
115 Irmin Stephen, "Limited on Two Fronts," *CD* 42, no. 3 (March 1976): 5.
116 For pharmacists, see "Health Happenings," *CN* 73, no. 6 (June 1977): 45. For nurses and dietitians, see Gertrude Lapointe, "A Nutrition Course for Nurses," *CN* 71, no. 1 (January 1975): 30–1.
117 Edward L. Cohen and Irma B. Cohen, "Report of a Survey of Full Diet Adult Menus in Urban Hospitals," *CJPH* 68, no. 1 (January/February 1977): 29. For problems in hospitals, see Lyse Genest and Marthe Hébert, "L'évaluation nutritionnelle," *UMC* 109, no. 4 (avril 1980): 522. For reply, see the letter from the Nutrition Committee of the Canadian Public Health Association, *CJPH* 68, no. 3 (May/June 1977): 253.
118 Eunice Misskey, "Teaching Teachers Nutrition," *CC* 6 (October 1976): 32; see also Heather MacDonald, "Organizational and Promotional Ideas for a Successful School Nutrition Program," *CAHPER* 47, no. 4 (March/April 1981): 11–14. For books available in stores, see Rita Christopher, "Eating Right," *Maclean's* 92, no. 48 (26 November 1979): 49.
119 Christopher, "Eating Right," 58; Jean Farmer, "Modern Meals: Marvel or Menace?" *CC* 2–3 (1972–73): 23; Bonnie Cornell, "Dietetic Dilemma," *Chatelaine* 49, no. 10 (October 1976): 25.
120 Pat Ramsey, "Health Food: Sense or Nonsense?" *Chatelaine* 44, no. 1 (January 1971): 36, 58–60. See also Christopher, "Eating Right," 50, 56.
121 Jacques Lorrain and Roger Gagnon, "Sélection préconceptionnelle du sexe," *UMC* 104, no. 5 (mai 1975): 803.
122 "Food Insufficiency Related to Overweight Children," results from the Canadian Community Health Survey, *INMD Newsletter* (Canada: Institute

of Nutrition, Metabolism and Diabetes, June 2007), 3. For the United States situation and its concern with the hunger of some of its citizens, see Levenstein, *Paradox of Plenty*, 148, 157.
123 Bill Jeffrey, "Canada's Food Guide vs https://www.choosemyplate.gov/," Centre for Science in the Public Interest, accessed 18 November 2014, https://www.cspinet.org/canada/pdf/canadasfoodguide-vs-usfoodplate.pdf

Chapter 2

1 "Obesity the Biggest Challenge in 1980s, Health Forum Told," *CMAJ* 123, no. 10 (22 November 1980): 1036.
2 "Review of *Obesity* by F.W. Christie (Toronto: Macmillan, 1937)," *CMAJ* 38, no. 61 (June 1938): 628; See also review of Marcel Labbe, *Maigreur et Obésité*, in *UMC* 62, no. 2 (février 1933): 176; review of Gilbert-Dreyfus, *Hygiène et régimes des obèses*, in *UMC* 63, no. 11 (novembre 1934): 1249–50; review of Maurice Perrin et Paul Mathieu, *L'obésité*, in *UMC* 52, no. 7 (juillet 1923): 324–5; "Review of *Nutrition and Diet in Health and Disease* by James S. McLester," in *CLP* 70, no. 3 (March 1928): 110.
3 "Séances du Comité des études médicales des étudiants en médecine d'l'Univercité [sic] de Montréal," *UMC* 52, no. 5 (mai 1923): 217; Edward H. Mason, "The Treatment of Obesity," *CMAJ* 14, no. 11 (November 1924): 1052; "On the Importance of Body Weight," *CMAJ* 16, no. 1 (January 1926): 64. For mention of papers on obesity, see "The Fifty-Fifth Annual Meeting of the Ontario Medical Association," *Ontario Medical Association Bulletin* 2, no. 1 (February 1935): 3–5.
4 Reprint from *The Lancet*, "Do You Carry Too Much Fat," in *Maclean's* 11, no. 10 (15 May 1927): 27. For obesity as unjustifiable, see "How About a Law for Fat People?" *Saturday Night* 39, no. 45 (27 September 1924): 1. For mental sluggishness, see James W. Barton, "Getting Rid of the Winter Surplus," *Maclean's* 38, no. 6 (15 March 1925): 20. For padding, etc., see Leonard Williams, "Claims Fat Is Dangerous Foe," *Maclean's* 40, no. 1 (1 January 1927): 24. Joke from "Maybe Adam Laughed at These," *Maclean's* 36, no. 13 (1 July 1923): 60.
5 *The Worker* was published by the Communist Party of Canada. For phrases, see Anne Frances Toews, "'Flesh, Bone, and Blood': Working-Class Bodies and the Canadian Communist Press, 1922–1956," in *Contesting Bodies and Nation in Canadian History*, ed. Patrizia Gentile and Jane Nicholas (Toronto: University of Toronto Press, 2013), 336–7.

6 Nellie Lyle Pattinson, "A Spring Tonic in Every Meal," *The Chatelaine* 1, no. 1 (March 1928): 42; Stella E. Pines, "Preparing for the Great Adventure," *The Chatelaine* 1, no. 8 (October 1928): 56; Grant Fleming, "Calories and Vitamins," *Maclean's* 44, no. 21 (1 November 1931): 34; *The Chatelaine* 1, no. 3 (May 1928): 44, advertisement for Tillson's Bran; H. Napier Moore, "In the Editor's Confidence," *Maclean's* 48, no. 15 (1 August 1935): 2.

7 Editorial, "Two Forgotten Aspects of Nutrition," *CPHJ* 36, no. 9 (September 1945): 374; E.W. McHenry, Ruth Crawford, and Lillian Barber, "The Heights and Weights of a Canadian Group," *CJPH* 38, no. 9 (September 1947): 437; E.W. McHenry, "Food in Canada: A Discussion of Canadian Nutritional Conditions," *Health* 16, no. 1 (January/February 1948): 22; René Blain, "La nutrition est un problème d'hygiène publique," *UMC* 73, no. 7 (juillet 1944): 799.

8 "Recent Accessions: A Classified List of Selected Books and Serials *Acquired by* the Library, Faculty of Medicine, the University of Manitoba, *January 1st, 1940 to November 1st 1941*," *ManMR* 21, no. 12 (December 1941): 231–4; J.-B. Boulanger, "Review of C.N. Armstrong, 'Considérations d'actualité sur le traitement des obèses,'" *UMC* 78, no. 11 (novembre 1949): 1345. J.C. Hossack, "Great Men," *ManMR* 28, no. 7 (July 1948): 379–80. *CD* 11, no. 6 (June 1945): 93, advertisement for Hook-Type Cuff; *OMR* 11, no. 1 (February 1944): 44, advertisement for Detecto scale.

9 "Cours de perfectionnement à Sainte-Justine," *UMC* 87, no. 12 (décembre 1958): 1579–80. For epidemic, see Peter H. Nash, "Health...and the Businessman," *Health* 24, no. 5 (September/October 1956): 10. For comments about obesity, see L.B. Pett and G.F. Ogilvie, "The Canadian Weight-Height Survey," *Human Biology* 28 (1956): 177. For frequency of obesity, see Rosario Robillard, "Preludin Treatment of Obesity in Diabetes Mellitus: Preliminary Report," *CMAJ* 76, no. 11 (11 June 1957): 938. For scourge, see Sidney Katz, "Are We Eating Too Much?" *Maclean's* 68, no. 12 (11 June 1955): 15, 98.

10 For blood pressure equipment, see *CD* 11, no. 6 (June 1945): 93, advertisement for Hook-Type Cuff. For abnormality, misfit, and obnoxious, see Peter H. Nash, "Health...and the Businessman," *Health* 24, no. 5 (September/October 1956): 10; *ManMR* 36, no. 6 (June 1956): 396, advertisement for Ambar; S. Vaisrub, "Editorial: Pleasure," *ManMR* 39, no. 3 (March 1959): 195. For McHenry, see Katz, "Are We Eating Too Much?" 15.

11 For women aging, see Adele White, "Age Old Signs," *Chatelaine* 19, no. 8 (August 1946): 47. For pity, see Blanche Bishop, "Things That Worry Me," *CN* 51, no. 9 (September 1955): 708.

12 For eight articles, see *CJPH* 58, no. 11 (November 1967): 479–507. For Maurice Verdy, see "Obésité: mortalité et morbidité," *CJPH* 58, no. 11 (November 1967): 494. For the OMA, see Helen Christie, "Obesity Is a Major Topic of Papers in Annual Scientific Meeting of OMA," *CMAJ* 108, no. 12 (23 June 1973): 1547. Interestingly, when a survey of practitioners was done in Ontario and Nova Scotia, the percentage of doctors' practices devoted to obesity (not specified as endocrine) was minimal: 0.5 per cent in Ontario and 1.1 per cent in Nova Scotia. See Kenneth F. Clute, *The General Practitioner: A Study of Medical Education and Practice in Ontario and Nova Scotia* (Toronto: University of Toronto Press, 1963), 248.
13 "How to Grow Slim without Trying: 2 Wafers, 1 Highball," *Maclean's* 75, no. 6 (24 March 1962): 65.
14 For epidemic, see Errol B. Marliss, "Protein Diets for Obesity: Metabolic Clinical Aspects" (Symposium on Obesity), *CMAJ* 119, no. 12 (23 December 1978): 1413. For endemic proportions, see Anne B. Kenshole, "Weight and Diabetes," *CFP* 18, no. 2 (February 1972): 41. For Lalonde, see Réjean Grenier, "L'hypokinétisme: la maladie du siècle," *UMC* 103, no. 3 (mars 1974): 487. In 1976, the estimate of 40 per cent obesity in young adults was bandied about. Adrienne Pitt, "Lunchtime at School," *CC* 6 (October 1976): 29. For 50 per cent overweight, see Susan Ross, "Nutrtition Assessment," *BCMJ* 16, no. 10 (October 1974): 296; and "Dr. Morrison's Worry List," *Harrowsmith* 3 (1978/79): 59.
15 For age, muscular, and race/ethnicity, see Guylaine Charbonneau-Roberts, Helga Saudny-Unterberger, Harriet V. Kuhnlein, and Grace M. Egeland, "Body Mass Index May Overestimate the Prevalence of Overweight and Obesity among the Inuit," *International Journal of Circumpolar Health* 64, no. 2 (2005): 164. For ethnicity, see World Health Organization, "Global Data Base on Body Mass Index: BMI Classification," 17 November 2006, accessed 25 November 2011, http://www.assessmentpsychology.com/icbmi.htm. For muscle mass, see also Michael L. Power and Jay Schulkin, *The Evolution of Obesity* (Baltimore, MD: John Hopkins University Press, 2009), 26.
16 For use of self-reports and measured reports, see G.M. Torrance, M.D. Hooper, and B.A. Reeder, "Trends in Overweight and Obesity among Adults in Canada (1970–1992)," *International Journal of Obesity* 26 (2002): 798; Margo Shields, Sarah Connor Gorber, Ian Janssen, and Mark S. Tremblay, "Bias in Self-Reported Estimates of Obesity in Canadian Health Surveys: An Update on Corrections for Adults," *Health Reports* 22, no. 3 (September 2011): 35.

17 For using waist circumference, see Sarah D. McDonald, "Commentary: Management and Prevention of Obesity in Adults and Children," *CMAJ* 176, no. 8 (10 April 2007): 1109–10; "Waistline Size New 'Vital Sign' for Doctors," *The Record*, 10 April 2007, A3. For neck, see [*McClatchy-Tribune*] "Fat Neck? You May Be Obese," *The Record*, 9 July 2010, C5. For an article describing the acceptance of the BMI, see Franklin White, "The Epidemiology of Weight – Implications for Atlantic Canada," *NSMB* 68, no. 1 (1989): 15–17.
18 I made this point in my book *Giving Birth in Canada 1900–1950* (Toronto: University of Toronto, 2002), 25. While I was looking at birth, I suspect it is somewhat the same for obesity.
19 William G. Rothstein, *Public Health and the Risk Factor: A History of an Uneven Medical Revolution* (Rochester, NY: University of Rochester Press, 2003), 153.
20 See "Measuring Up: Height-Weight Standards and Diagnosis," chapter 2 in *Childhood Obesity in America* by Laura Dawes (Cambridge, MA: Harvard University Press, 2014), 41–58.
21 An early scale appeared in *Eaton's Catalogue*, Spring/Summer 1932, 196.
22 R.L. Alsaker, "It's Always Wrong to Be Fat," *Maclean's* 35, no. 1 (1 June 1922): 40, reprint. For another equation, see Joan Flower, "Interesting Reasons Why You Are Thin," *Maclean's* 37, no. 9 (1 May 1924): 74.
23 *Chatelaine* 11, no. 5 (May 1938): 22, advertisement for Metropolitan Life Insurance Co. For heart and lung problems, see Leonard Williams, "Claims Fat Is Dangerous Foe," *Maclean's* 40, 1 (January 1, 1927): 24, reprint.
24 For the need to measure body build and chest circumference, see "On the Importance of Body Weight," 64. For bones and muscles, see E.F. Cathcart, "Standards on Food and Nutrition," *CMAJ* 41, no. 4 (October 1939): 397. For races, see Walter R. Campbell, "Obesity and Its Treatment," *CMAJ* 34, no. 1 (January 1936): 42.
25 F.W. Tidmarsh, "Malnutrition," *CMAJ* 13, no. 6 (June 1923): 426; "On the Importance of Body Weight," 66 (20 per cent); Campbell, "Obesity and Its Treatment," 42 (25 per cent plus).
26 MAB, "Getting Back to Normal after Summer," *The Chatelaine* 3, no. 9 (September 1930): 33; Annabelle Lee, "Your Beauty Problem," *Chatelaine* 6, no. 10 (October 1933): 68.
27 Amanda M. Czerniawski, "From Average to Ideal: The Evolution of the Height and Weight Table in the United States, 1836–1943," *Social Science History* 31, no. 2 (Summer 2007): 284. See also Josephine Lowman, "Tubby Hubby Diet: Obesity Top Killer, Watch Your Weight," *Globe and Mail*, 1 October 1953, 10 (for age twenty-five).

28 Harold N. Segall, "How to Be an Executive and Live," *Health* 26, no. 1 (January/February 1958): 28. See also F.S. Brien, "Obesity – Treatment," *OMR* 20, no. 4 (April 1953): 225 (for age in the thirties); Czerniawski, "From Average to Ideal," 288.
29 For the finding that the 1959 average for men was up five pounds but for women was five pounds lighter, see "Don't Diet, Get New Table: Maybe You're Underweight!" *Financial Post*, 7 November 1959, 35. For life experiences, see B.L. Frank, "De l'importance d'une alimentation appropriée dans la grossesse et la lactation, dans la croissance et le développement des enfants, et dans les états débilitants et la sénilité," *UMC* 83, no. 3 (mars 1954): 297.
30 Pett and Ogilvie, "The Canadian Weight-Height Survey," 187. For the need for a Canadian measurement, see E. Gordon Young, "An Appraisal of Canadian Nutriture," *Canadian Bulletin on Nutrition* 3, no. 1 (July 1953): 20; L.B. Pett, "A National Weight-Health Survey," *CJPH* 43, no. 11 (November 1952): 487. For details of the surveys from 1950, see Michael Gard, "Hearing Noises and Noticing Silence: Towards a Critical Engagement with Canadian Body Weight Statistics," in *Obesity in Canada: Critical Perspectives*, ed. Jenny Ellison, Deborah McPhail, and Wendy Mitchinson (Toronto: University of Toronto Press, 2016), 31–55.
31 Lionel M. Lindsay, "The Overweight Child," *CMAJ* 44, no. 5 (May 1941): 504.
32 W.W. Bauer, "Battle of the Bulges," *Maclean's* 59, no. 16 (15 August 1946): 9.
33 L.B. Pett and G.F. Ogilvie, "The Report on Canadian Average Weights, Heights, and Skinfolds," *Bulletin of Nutrition* 5, no. 1 (September 1957): 44.
34 Lionel Bradley Pett, "A Canadian Table of Average Weights for Height, Age and Sex," *American Journal of Public Health* 45, no. 7 (July 1955): 862. For an analysis of Pett's view of statistics, see Gard, "Hearing Noises and Noticing Silence," 35–7. For agreement on the problem of weight charts for children, see Helen Evans Reid, "Is Your Child Underweight?" *CHJ* 53, no. 4 (August 1956): 70
35 For the mathematical equation, see Iva L. Armstrong and Barbara McLaren, "'We Are What We Eat': Proper Choice of Food Can Make the Differences between Robust Health and a Mediocre Existence," *Health* 30, no. 5 (October 1962): 14. For ponderal index, see D.J. Ghent, "Want to Know When You'll Die?" *Maclean's* 79, no. 6 (19 March 1966): 3; for more on the ponderal index, see Dawes, *Childhood Obesity in America*, 52. For McLaren, see Ann Austen, "Diet Clubs Share Their Weight Losing Secrets," *Chatelaine* 42, no. 2 (February 1969): 66.
36 H.D. Oliver, "Obesity," *MSJ* 21 (September 1965): 217, 221. For other tests, see John R. Beaton, "Energy Balance and Obesity," *CJPH* 58, no. 11

(November 1967): 479; Patrick Vinay et al., "Obésité: revue générale," *UMC* 98, no. 5 (mai 1969): 781. R.G. Stennett and D.M. Cram, "Cross-Sectional, Percentile Height and Weight Norms for a Representative Sample of Urban, School-Aged Ontario Children," *CJPH* 60, no. 12 (December 1969): 465.

37 Daniel Cappon, *Eating, Loving and Dying: A Psychology of Appetites* (Toronto: University of Toronto Press, 1973), 53.

38 For 30 per cent, 12 per cent, and 5 to 15 pounds, see "Can You Say 'No' to Second Helping?" *Financial Post*, 27 July 1963, 28; extracts from a General Foods booklet in "What to Know about Weight Control," *Health* 39, no. 2 (Summer 1973): 14–15. John R. Brown and Roy J. Shephard, "Some Measurements of Fitness in Older Female Employees of a Toronto Department Store," *CMAJ* 97, no. 20 (11 November 1967): 1209, 1211.

39 Charlotte M. Young, "Body Composition and Body Weight: Criteria of Overnutrition," *CMAJ* 93, no. 17 (23 October 1965): 902; James A. Collyer, "The Unhappy Fat Woman," *CFP* 19, no. 5 (May 1973): 93.

40 Denis Craddock, *Obesity and Its Management*, 3rd ed. (Edinburgh, London and New York: Churchill Livingstone, 1978), 1. For staying the same weight, see Robert Musel, "L'obésité peut avoir des causes physiologiques," *UMC* 99, no. 9 (septembre 1970): 1722.

41 For Dr Sackett, see David Woods, "Two Epidemiologists Discuss Myths and Realities of Health Maintenance," *CMAJ* 109, no. 11 (1 December 1973): 1151.

42 Anthony W. Myers and David L. Yeung, "Obesity in Infants: Significance, Aetiology, and Prevention," *CJPH* 70, no. 2 (March/April 1979): 113.

43 R.W. Shepherd, "Diets Be Damned: Eat, Drink and Be Merry for Your Body Knows Best," *Maclean's* 83, no. 12 (December 1970): 66.

44 William Osler, *The Principles and Practice of Medicine* (New York: D. Appleton and Co., 1893), 1019; William Osler, *The Principles and Practice of Medicine*, 8th ed. (New York: D. Appleton and Co., 1912), 451; Thomas McCrae, ed., *The Principles and Practice of Medicine*, 10th ed. (New York: D. Appleton and Co., 1925), 445, and Henry A. Christian, ed., *The Principles and Practice of Medicine*, 16th ed. (New York: D. Appleton-Century Co., 1947), 604. For comments on more women being obese, see Aimé-Paul Heineck, "Excision massive de graisse sous-cutanée abdominale," *UMC* 54, no. 3 (mars 1925): 154.

45 W.F. Christie, *Ideal Weight: A Practical Handbook for Patients* (London: William Heinemann Ltd., 1938), 13; W.F. Christie, *Obesity: A Practical Handbook for Physicians* (London: Willam Heinemann Ltd., 1937), 59–61; Charles K.P. Henry, "'Queens and Sweets'" *CN* 35, no. 12 (December 1939): 687.

46 See Wendy Mitchinson, *Body Failure: Medical Views of Women, 1900–1950* (Toronto: University of Toronto Press, 2013), 58–60.
47 For rates, see N. Obney, "Obesity and Health," *Health* (September/October 1948): 7. For other percentages, see Lloyd Percival, "Our Flabby Muscles Are a National Disgrace," *Maclean's* 66, no. 8 (15 April 1953): 71 (39 per cent overweight); H.T. McAlpine, "Obesity," *OMR* 20, no. 2 (February 1953): 89 (28 per cent overweight); Brien, "Obesity – Treatment," 225 (25–30 per cent overweight); J.A.F. Stevenson, "Trends in Nutrition," *CSMJ* 12 (April 1956): 354 (20 per cent obese over age thirty). For the 1953 survey, see James A.F. Stevenson "[Review of] 'The Report on Canadian Average Weights, Heights, and Skinfolds' by L.B. Pett and G.F. Oglivie, *Canadian Bulletin on Nutrition* 5, no. 1 (1957), Nutrition Division, Dept of Nat. Health and Welfare," *CSMJ* 14 (November 1958): 751. For emphases on middle age, see "Shakespeare Wrong on Diet," *CD* 21, no. 6 (June 1955): 63; Editorial, "Two Forgotten Aspects of Nutrition," 374; Edward J. Stieglitz, "Geriatric Nutrition," *CN* 48, no. 9 (September 1952): 705–6. For age and sex, see Lucien Dubreuil, "L'obésité," *UMC* 81, no. 6 (juin 1952): 708. For age and obesity, see René Rolland, "La Société médicale de Montréal," *UMC* 84, no. 6 (juin 1955): 717. For executives, see F.M. Jones, "Health Hazards of Executives," *OMR* 16, no. 4 (August 1949): 90–5.
48 For psychology and physiology, see D.E. Rodger, J. Grant McFetridge, and Eileen Price, "The Management of Obesity," *CMAJ* 63, no. 3 (September 1950): 268. For estrogen, see Antonio Martel, "Prelundin (Phenmetrazine) in the Treatment of Obesity," *CMAJ* 76, no. 2 (15 January 1957): 120.
49 "Aging – A Project Report," *CN* 58, no. 7 (July 1962): 617.
50 For a damning assessment of the government, see Walter J. Vanast, "'Hastening the Day of Extinction': Canada, Québec, and the Medical Care of Ungava's Inuit, 1867–1967," *Études/Inuit/Studies* 15, no. 2 (1991): 55–84. See also Deborah McPhail, "'The White Man's Burden'? Obesity and Colonialism in the Developing North," chapter 4 in *Contours of the Nation: Making Obesity and Imagining Canada, 1945 1970* (Toronto: University of Toronto Press, 2017), 101–33, for more details on Indigenous people in Canada.
51 Verdy, "Obésité: mortalité et morbidité," 494.
52 For regions, see "48% of Canadians Are Too Fat," *Weekend Magazine* 28, no. 40 (7 October 1978): 3. For immigrants, see Mollie Gillen, "Is It True Some People Are Naturally Fat?" *Chatelaine* 44, no. 9 (September 1971): 101; and Cappon, *Eating, Loving and Dying*, 86.
53 For women, see Betty Thomas, "Interviewing the Patient about Diets," *CN* 56, no. 11 (November 1960): 967. For the north, see McPhail, "Canada

Weighs In," 335; Young, "Body Composition and Body Weight," 904–5. See also the advertisement in *CMAJ* 95, no. 12 (17 September 1966): 17. On the difference between women and men, see Vinay et al., "Obésité," 796; E.W. McHenry, "Canadian Women Are Too Fat," *Chatelaine* 33, no. 6 (June 1960): 25, 44. For women in the studies, see Doris L. Hirsch and W.I. Morse, "Emotional and Metabolic Factors in Obesity," *CPHJ* 51, no. 11 (November 1960): 450, 453. For men not admitting to being fat, see A. Cornacchia, "A Layman's View of Group Therapy in Weight Control," *CJPH* 58, no. 11 (November 1967): 507.

54 Gard, "Hearing Noises and Noticing Silence," 41–2.

55 For class, see A. Demirjian, *Anthropometry Report, Height, Weight and Body Dimensions: A Report from Nutrition Canada* (Ottawa: Minister of National Health and Welfare, 1980), 36. On young women, see A.W. Myers and Danièle Kroetsch, "The Influence of Family Income on Food Consumption Patterns and Nutrient Intake in Canada," *CJPH* 69, no. 3 (May/June 1978): 208. For older women, see Patricia D. Wolczuk, "Nutrition BC," *BCMJ* 17, no. 3 (March 1975): 81. For Indigenous and Inuit youth, see Krista Walters, "'A National Priority': Nutrition Canada's Survey and the Discipining of Aboriginal Bodies, 1964–1975," in *Edible Histories, Cultural Politics: Towards a Canadian Food History*, ed. Franca Iacovetta, Valerie J. Korinek, and Marlene Epp (Toronto: University of Toronto Press, 2012), 433–51. For the 1978 survey, see "48% of Canadians Are Too Fat," 3.

56 Most fat in our bodies is white fat, which is where energy is stored. White fat also produces hormones, one specifically, adiponetin, which "makes the liver and muscles sensitive to the hormone insulin." If a person is too fat, the production of adiponetin declines. Brown fat is found more in infants/children than in adults, and it keeps them warm. Brown fat is also found more in lean people, and some scientists think brown fat can burn white fat. According to some studies, women have more brown fat than men, and theirs is more active than the brown fat in men. Visceral fat is found around organs and is linked to serious health problems. Subcutaneous fat is found under the skin and is less problematic, especially when on the thighs and buttocks. Abdominal fat is both visceral and subcutaneous; the amount of abdominal fat is more significant than its type, because abdominal fat is unhealthy. In recent reports, it has been suggested that abdominal fat might even increase your urge to eat. See Kathleen Doheny, "The Truth about Fat: Everthing You Need to Know about Fat, Including an Explanation of Which Is Worse – Belly Fat or Thigh Fat," *WebMD*, 13 July 2009, accessed 6 March 2014, https://www.webmd.com/diet/features/the-truth-about-fat#1. For more on fat, see

Jennie Macdiarmid (1998) and Neville Rigby (rev. version, 2002), "The Global Challenge of Obesity and the International Obesity Task Force," International Union of Nutritional Sciences, accessed 22 November 2007, http://www.iuns.org/resources/the-global-challenge-of-obesity-and-the-international-obesity-task-force/; Amina Zafar, "Belly Fat Dangers Go Beyond Weight Scale," *CBC News*, 16 May 2012, accessed 4 September 2012, http://www.cbc.ca/news/health/belly-fat-dangers-go-beyond-weight-scale-1.1283980; Reuters Staff, "Why Those Fat Thighs May Help You Live Longer," *Reuters*, 12 January 2010, accessed 13 January 2010, https://www.reuters.com/article/us-fat-hips/why-those-fat-thighs-may-help-you-live-longer-idUSTRE60B4H920100112; Philip A. Wood, *How Fat Works* (Cambridge, MA: Harvard University Press, 2006), 13–14; Walter Gratzer, *Terrors of the Table: The Curious History of Nutrition* (Oxford: Oxford University Press, 2005), 224–5.

57 For food fats, see Wood, *How Fat Works*, 29. For the necessity for fat, see Paul Campos, *The Obesity Myth: Why America's Obsession with Weight Is Hazardous to Your Health* (New York: Gotham Books, 2004), 73.

58 Hillel Schwartz, *Never Satisfied: A Cultural History of Diets, Fantasies and Fat* (London: Collier Macmillan Publishers, 1986), 9, 58, 133, 147. Fat has more calories in weight than protein or carbohydrates, so it was assumed that reducing calories by eating less fat was the way to lose weight.

59 Mason, "The Treatment of Obesity," 1052. The perception of obesity "types" hasn't changed much over time. Even in 1950, there was a sense that endocrine obesity and "constitutional anomaly" obesity were two different types of obesity. One article even suggested that the former was an American way of understanding obesity, whereas European researchers tended to emphasize the latter. See Rodger, McFetridge, and Price, "The Management of Obesity," 265. But such a division was significantly out of date. Articles during the 1940s and later had been very clear that endocrine causes for obesity essentially reflected a minority of cases. For other early articles on obesity, see J.R. Pepin, "L'obésité est-elle réductible?" *UMC* 58, no. 5 (mai 1929): 261–2; Jean LeSage, "Review of *Embonpoint et Obésité*," *UMC* 61, no. 2 (février 1932): 436–7; Christie, *Obesity*, 34, 61; E.M. Watson, "Some Present-Day Views on Diet: Concluded," *CN* 26, no. 7 (July 1930): 368.

60 Christie, *Obesity*, 3–5 for quote and 19, 18, 34. For the importance of fat as fuel, see also Christie, *Ideal Weight*, 9. For the history of fat measurements, see Dawes, *Childhood Obesity in America*, 60–1, 65–6.

61 For fat needed to utilize other food, see John O'Neill, "Scientists Now Turn to Theory: Fat Person's Undernourished," *Saturday Night* (3 May 1949): n.p.

62 J.T. Phair and N.R. Speirs, *Good Health* (Toronto: Ginn and Company, 1945), 253. For active and inert fat, see Schwartz, *Never Satisfied*, 5. For cholesterol, see Henri Pichette, "Cholestérol et cataracte," *UMC* 75, no. 6 (juin 1946): 647–53. For the creation of cholesterol as a risk factor, see Jeremy A. Greene, *Prescribing by Numbers: Drugs and the Definition of Disease* (Baltimore, MD: Johns Hopkins University Press, 2007), chapter 5, 151–88.

63 Hilde Bruch, *The Importance of Overweight* (New York: W.W. Norton & Co., 1957), 148, 150; Elizabeth Chant Robertson, *Nutrition for Today* (Toronto: McClelland & Stewart, 1951), 158–61.

64 Alan Phillips, "Is This Your Heart's Worst Enemy?" *Maclean's* 68, no. 25 (10 December 1955): 23; L.B. Pett and Elaine Collett, "Low-Fat Meals to Help Your Husband's Heart," *Chatelaine* 30, no. 8 (August 1957): 15; Alick Little, "Letter, to Which the Heading 'Disagreement on Fats' Has Been Added," *Chatelaine* 30, no. 11 (November 1957): 3; E.W. McHenry, "Nutrition and Coronary Heart Disease," *OMR* 25, no. 8 (August 1958): 732–3, 774; Rothstein, *Public Health and the Risk Factor*, 284–5.

65 Todd Michael Olszewski, "Cholesterol: A Scientific, Medical, and Social History, 1908–1962" (PhD diss., Yale University, 2008), 103, 105.

66 "Diet and Heart Disease," *CMAJ* 88, no. 10 (9 March 1963): 33–4. On cholesterol, see also C.M. Harlow, "High Fish Diet, Obesity and Blood Cholesterol," *NSMB* 40, no. 11 (1961): 329–37.

67 J.M.R. Beveridge, "Your Diet and Your Heart," *Health* 28, no. 3 (June 1960): 20. For debate on the link between diet and heart problems, see Roy J. Shephard, "Exercise and Physical Fitness," *OMR* 35, no. 2 (February 1968): 81. Shephard dismissed low cholesterol diets for so-called "high-risk groups." See Nina Teicholz, *The Big Fat Surprise: Why Butter and Cheese Belong in a Healthy Diet* (Toronto: Simon & Schuster Canada, 2015), for a critique that suggests dieting by eliminating fat is not beneficial.

68 For Choloxin (dextrothyroxin), see *UMC* 97, no. 7 (juillet 1968): 13, advertisement.

69 Associated Press, "Sugar Industry Paid Scientists for Favourable Research, Documents Reveal," 13 September 2016, accessed 13 September 2016, http://www.cbc.ca/news/health/sugar-harvard-conspiracy-1.3759582.

70 For diet high in fat, see Ernest L. Wynder, "To Help People Live Younger and Longer," *Health* 38, no. 1 (Spring 1972): 28–30; "Are You Really Well Fed," *Health* 38, no. 3 (Fall 1972): 29; Canadian Fisheries Services, "How Seafoods Help Roll Away Pounds," *Health* 39, no. 3 (Autumn 1973): 17; "Le mal des pay développés: la suralimentation," *UMC* 101, no. 4 (avril 1972): 752. For saturated fat, see "What to Know about Weight Control,"

Health 39, no. 2 (Summer 1973): 21; Monique D. Gélinas, "L'alimentation de l'homme d'affaires," *Commerce* 75 (November 1973): 108–12. For gender, see "One Man's War on Cholesterol," *Financial Post Magazine*, June–July 1971, 18. The role fat played in providing estrogen long after menstruation had stopped was beginning to be understood. See "Fat and Fancy (letter)," *CFP* 21, no. 3 (March 1975): 139.

71 Health and Welfare Canada, reprint, "What Should You Eat for a Healthy Heart?" *Health* 44, no. 1 (Spring 1978): 11. For trials, see "Diet Therapy Pointers for Young Athletes," *CFP* 23, no. 5 (May 1977): 128; Health and Welfare Canada, "What Should You Eat?," 11. For Quebec, see Barbara Santich, *What the Doctors Ordered: 150 Years of Dietary Advice in Australia* (Victoria, AU: Hyland House, 1995), 186. For an article on fat and cholesterol that reflects the complexity, see Shirley R. MacIntosh, "Dietary Fat and Cholesterol," *NSMB* 58, no. 3 (1979): 84–5, 106.

72 *Health* 31, no. 2 (April 1963): 32, cartoon.

73 Young, "Body Composition and Body Weight," 907.

74 For fat cells, see S.S.B. Gilder, "The Fat Child," *CMAJ* 107, no. 11 (9 December 1972): 1068; Linda Oglov, "Canadian Dietetic Association Delegates at Annual Meeting Study Relationship of Diet to Exercise," *CMAJ* 117, no. 3 (6 August 1977): 289–90; L.C. Petrich, "Review of *The Psychology of Obesity: Dynamics and Treatment* by Norman Kiell," *CD* 41, no. 4 (April 1975): 81; "Problem of Obesity Said Frustrating to Doctor and Patient," *CMAJ* 112, no. 3 (8 February 1975): 350. For juvenile-onset obesity, see Bill Gladstone, "Beautiful Loser: His Story," *Chatelaine* 51, no. 7 (July 1978): 110; "Early Weaners More Obese?" *Chatelaine* 51, no. 11 (November 1978): 24. For fat cells not disappearing, see Peter Hahn, "Nutrition in Pregnancy and Early Infancy," *BCMJ* 15, no. 9 (October 1973): 260. For adults forming fat cells, see A. Angel, "Pathophysiological Changes in Obesity," *CMAJ* 119, no. 12 (23 December 1978): 1402.

75 Jean Himms-Hager, "Obesity May Be Due to a Malfunction of Brown Fat," *CMAJ* 121, no. 10 (17 November 1979): 1361–4. The italics are mine.

76 June Engel, "10 Worst Eating Habits," *Chatelaine* 53, no. 12 (December 1980): 36.

77 Sander L. Gilman, *Fat Boys: A Slim Book* (Lincoln, NB: University of Nebraska Press, 2004), 41, 84.

78 World Health Organization, "Controlling the Global Obesity Epidemic," accessed 28 October 2016, http://www.who.int/nutrition/topics/obesity/en/.

79 For correlations, see Rothstein, *Public Health and the Risk Factor*, 227. On risk, see Gabe Mythen and Sandra Walklate, eds., *Beyond the Risk Society:*

Critical Reflections on Risk and Human Security (Beckshire, UK: Open University Press, 2006). Kathleen Woodward, in her book *Statistical Panic: Cultural Politics and Poetics of the Emotions* (Durham, NC: Duke University Press, 2009), looks at how statistics have led to emotions and the fear of risk. See chapter 7, "Statistical Panics," 195–218.

80 Rothstein, *Public Health and the Risk Factor*, 3, 231. For more critical thinking on epidemiology, see Darlene McNaughton, "From the Womb to the Tomb: Obesity and Maternal Responsibility," *Critical Public Health* 21, no. 2 (June 2011): 181. On risk and epidemiology, see also Lisa McDermott, "A Critical Interrogation of Contemporary Discourses of Physical (In) Activity amongst Canadian Children: Back to the Future," *Journal of Canadian Studies* 42, no. 2 (Spring 2008): 23–4. For an early discussion, see P.C. Gordon, "Epidemiological Principles and Problems in Clinical Research Based on Hospitalized Patients," *NSMB* 46, no. 7 (1967): 141–4.

81 Nancy Krieger, "Epidemiology and the Web of Causation: Has Anyone Seen the Spider?" *Social Science and Medicine* 39, no. 7 (1994): 887–903. For more on epidemiology, see John Evans et al., *Education, Disordered Eating and Obesity Discourse: Fat Fabrications* (London: Routledge, 2008), 14.

82 Hans Krueger et al., *The Health Impact of Smoking and Obesity and What to Do About It* (Toronto: University of Toronto Press, 2007), 19.

83 Peter T. Katzmarzyk and Christopher I. Ardern, "Overweight and Obesity Mortality Trends in Canada, 1985–2000," *CJPH* 95, no. 1 (January–February 2004): 16; National Institutes of Health, National Heart, Lung and Blood Institute, and North American Association for the Study of Obesity, *The Practical Guide: Identification, Evaluation and Treatment of Overweight and Obesity in Adults*, NIH Publication no. 00-4084 (Washington, DC: National Institutes of Health, 2000), 18, accessed 15 June 2007, https://www.nhlbi.nih.gov/files/docs/guidelines/prctgd_c.pdf.

84 C.E. Adair, G. McVey, J. deGroot, et al., *Obesity and Eating Disorders: Seeking Common Ground to Promote Health*. A National Meeting of Researchers, Practitioners, and Policy Makers, Calgary, AB, November 2007, Final Discussion Document (n.p.: 2008), 5, https://www.ocoped.ca/PDF/Obesity_eating_disorders_discussion_document_2008.pdf; CBC TV, "While You Were Sleeping," *The Nature of Things*, season 2015–2016, episode 16, 10 March 2016, http://www.cbc.ca/player/play/2685061991, looked at sleeping and eating, and highlighted a study that showed people who sleep for nine hours eat "normally," while those who only get five hours of sleep eat more.

85 For fertility, see Tara Parker-Pope, "Can a 'Fertility Diet' Get You Pregnant," *New York Times*, 18 December 2007, accessed 20 December 2007,

http://www.nytimes.com/2007/12/18/health/nutrition/18well.html. For effect on the brain, see Olivia Judson, "Brain Damage," *New York Times*, 20 April 2010, accessed 26 April 2010, https://opinionator.blogs.nytimes.com/2010/04/20/brain-damage/. For mortality rates, see Katzmarzyk and Ardern, "Overweight and Obesity Mortality Trends in Canada," 16, 18. For shortening life expectancy, see D. Haslam, "Obesity: A Medical History," *Obesity Reviews* 8, supp. 1 (2007): 36. The generational argument was based on a researcher's offhand comment. Dawes, in *Childhood Obesity in America*, 212, still maintains that "generations of Y and Z may be the first generations in recent history to have a shorter life then their parents." For pregnancy health, see Tara Leanne Black, "Understanding Excessive Parental Weight Gain among First Nations Women" (MA thesis, University of Alberta, 2004), 1.

86 Bruce Ross, "Fat or Fiction: Weighing the 'Obesity Epidemic,'" chapter 5 in *The Obesity Epidemic: Science, Morality and Ideology* by Michael Gard and Jan Wright (London and New York: Routledge, Taylor & Francis Group, 2005), 98.

87 Heather M. Orpana et al., "BMI and Mortality: Results from a National Longitudinal Study of Canadian Adults," *Obesity* 18, no. 1 (2010): 214–18. The study, however, warned that people should not extrapolate from the findings about mortality to morbidity in overweight people, that is, the threshold for certain morbidity problems could be lower than that of mortality. Dr Bailey has seen more morbid obesity in her practice.

88 Osler, *The Principles and Practice of Medicine* (1893), 642, 665; Osler, *The Principles and Practice of Medicine* (1912), 451, 789, 843; McCrae, *The Principles and Practice of Medicine* (1925), 446, 445. In the eighteenth century, German physicians saw gluttony as a cause of haemorrhoids. Christopher E. Forth, *Masculinity in the Modern Weight: Gender, Civilization and the Body* (New York and Basingstoke, U.K.: Palgrave Macmillan, 2008), 81; see 101–3 for the nineteenth century in America.

89 For associated problems, see "On the Importance of Body Weight," 64–5. For kidneys, see May R. Mayers, "Normal Weight and Working Efficiency," *CMAJ* 19, no. 3 (September 1928): 374. For liver, see *The Lancet* reprint, "Do You Carry Too Much Fat?" *Maclean's* 11, no. 10 (15 May 1927): 27. For circulatory problems and dyspepsia, see "The Menace of Obesity," *CMAJ* 16, no. 11 (November 1926): 1373–4. For cancer, see "Protein in Food Favors Cancer," *Maclean's* 37, 4 (15 February 1924): 45. For surgical risk, see "On the Importance of Body Weight," 65. For all organs, see Williams, "Claims Fat Is Dangerous Foe," 24.

90 Mason, "The Treatment of Obesity," 1052. Being able to get pregnant was still a sign of weight loss success in 1946. See Leonora Hawirko and P.H. Sprague, "Treatment of Obesity by Appetite-Depressing Drugs," *CMAJ* 54, no. 1 (January 1946): 267.
91 "How About a Law for Fat People?" *Saturday Night* 39, no. 45 (27 September 1924): 1.
92 "On the Importance of Body Weight," 66.
93 "Overweight and Longevity," *CMAJ* 23, no. 2 (August 1930): 259.
94 For diseases, see L.H. Newburgh, "Normal Nutrition," *CMAJ* 40, no. 5 (May 1939): 491. For ill health, etc., see Sir Edward Mellanby, "Proper Feeding and Good Health," *CMAJ* 40, no. 6 (June 1939): 599. For sore feet, shortage of breath, and diverticulosis of colon, see Christie, *Obesity*, 51. For gallstones, see Henry, "'Queens and Sweets,'" 688. For back, etc., see George H. Ryan, "Some Back Injuries and Causes of Low Back Pain with Demonstration of Methods of Treatment," *MMAR* 18, no. 8 (August 1938): 145.
95 Christie, *Obesity*, 70.
96 E.W. McHenry, "Nutrition in a Public Health Program," *CN* 43, no. 3 (March 1947): 180; Hugo R. Rony, *Obesity and Leanness* (Philadelphia: Lea & Febiger, 1940), 224–5.
97 *CD* 15, no. 4 (April 1949): 56, advertisement for Iodobesin.
98 George S. Young, "How to Grow Old Successfully," *Health* 15, no. 3 (May/June 1947): 8; see also "Note," *Health* 16, no. 3 (May/June 1958): 31.
99 For decline of sex, see Sidney Katz, "Those Middle-Age Blues," *Maclean's* 62, no. 20 (15 October 1949): 36; Joan Phillips, "Watch Your Husband's Waistline," *CHJ* 45, no. 4 (August 1948): 42, 44. For executives, see Jones, "Health Hazards of Executives," 90, 92. For concern about men and their health, see also Metropolitan Life Insurance advertisement in *CHJ* 45, no. 6 (October 1948): 48.
100 For working class, see McPhail, "Canada Weighs In," 238, 241. For women, see Nash, "Health...and the Businessman," 11.
101 "Diabetes," *CN* 49, no. 7 (July 1953): 364.
102 John Gibson, "The Manic-Depressive Psychosis," *CN* 55, no. 10 (October 1959): 928; see also *CMAJ* 69, no. 4 (October 1953): 468, advertisement for Methedrine; *CMAJ* 74, no. 4 (15 February 1956): 333, advertisement for Dexedrine.
103 Rosario Robillard, "La pathogénie du diabète sucré," *UMC* 88, no. 19 (octobre 1959): 1193; Editorial, "Obesity and Heart Disease," *CMAJ* 71, no. 5 (November 1954): 501. For a modern analysis of diabetes and obesity, see Darlene McNaughton and Cynthia Smith, "Diabesity, or the 'Twin

Epidemics': Reflection on the Iatrogenic Consequences of Stigmatizing Lifestyle to Reduce the Incidence of Diabetes Mellitus in Canada," in Ellison, McPhail, and Mitchinson, *Obesity in Canada*, 122–47.

104 Young, "Body Composition and Body Weight," 901. For mortality rates, see "Mortality Trends in Relation to Blood Pressure and Build," *CMAJ* 82, no. 20 (14 May 1960): 1033. On mortality, see J.E. Monagle, "Nutrition and Health – A Critical Evaluation," *CJPH* 56, no. 11 (November 1965): 490; and Barbara A. McLaren, "Nutritional Control of Overweight," *CJPH* 58, no. 11 (November 1967): 483.

105 For hypertension, see *CMAJ* 82, no. 23 (4 June 1960): 38, advertisement for New Tenuate; Sister Marguerite Frances, "Hypertensive Heart Disease," *CN* 59, no. 5 (May 1963): 443. For atherosclerosis, see A. Lemaire et al., "Les bases biochimiques du régime dans l'athérosclérose," *UMC* 97, no. 5 (mai 1968): 565. For high blood pressure, see Elizabeth Chant Robertson, "What to Eat to Be Healthy," *Health* 29, no. 4 (August 1961): 26. For depression, see *CMAJ* 87, no. 8 (25 August 1962): 16, advertisement for Desbutal Gradumet. For diabetes, see "Le docteur Rosario Robillard traite du diabète et obésité," *UMC* 93, no. 4 (avril 1964): 482. For coronary heart, kidney, liver, and gallbladder problems, see Monagle, "Nutrition and Health," 490. For work injury, see Austin Henschel, "Obesity as an Occupational Hazard," *CJPH* 58, no. 11 (November 1967): 491. For pregnancy, see D.M. Sinclair, "Obesity as a Public Health Problem," *CJPH* 58, no. 11 (November 1967): 520. For psychological problems, see Monagle, "Nutrition and Health," 490. For infertility, see Vinay et al., "Obésité," 795. For accidents, see Rosario Robillard, "La sécurité routière et les maladies de la nutrition," *UMC* 89, no. 1 (janvier 1960): 71. For breathing, see Charles Lepine, "Review of 'Anomalies des échanges gazeux du poumon dans l'obésité,'" *UMC* 90, no. 3 (mars 1961): 303. For strokes, see Canada, Department of National Health and Welfare, Nutrition Division, *Healthful Eating* (Ottawa: Department of National Health and Welfare, 1963), 43.

106 For diabetes, see Georgina Faludi, Gordon Bendersky, and Philip Gerber, "Functional Hypoglycemia, The Link between Obesity and Diabetes," *CFP* 14, no. 2 (February 1968): 18. For diabetes leading to obesity, see also Maurice Verdy, "Traitement des obésités," *UMC* 96, no. 5 (mai 1967): 578. For more than two linkages, see Dr Jean Mayer, "Quotations from: Nutrition, Exercise and Cardiovascular Disease," *CFP* 14, no. 2 (February 1968): 19.

107 "Long, Hot Days of Summer Are Hazard to Industry's Fat Men," *Financial Post*, 5 August 1967, 26. For the Medical Care Act, see Marilyn

Dunlop, "Health Policy," *Canadian Encyclopedia*, 3 April 2015, accessed 23 February 2017, http://www.thecanadianencyclopedia.ca/en/m/article/health-policy/.

108 S.S.B. Gilder, "Obesity and Smoking Habits," *CMAJ* 106, no. 8 (22 April 1972): 875. Another estimate maintained that smoking twenty cigarettes in a day was as hard on the body as being 100 pounds overweight. Diane Birch, "Control: Cigarettes & Calories," *CN* 71, no. 3 (March 1975): 33.

109 "Dr. Morrison's Worry List," 59.

110 Christie, "Obesity Is a Major Topic of Papers," 1547, 1549.

111 Sidney Katz, "How We Must Live Healthily and Enjoy It More," *CMAJ* 111, no. 12 (21 December 1974): 1370.

112 Cappon, *Eating, Loving and Dying*, 17, 51.

113 June Engel with Elizabeth Parr, "Obesity: The Losing Battle That Can Sometime Be Won," *Chatelaine* 53, no. 11 (November 1980): 174. Vranic is cited in this article.

114 "Stand Up and Be Tested," *CN* 70, no. 9 (September 1974): 28; Oglov, "Canadian Dietetic Association Delegates," 290; W. Gifford-Jones, "Shut Up and Pass the Baked Alaska," *Maclean's* 88, no. 6 (June 1975): 77–8. See also Brenda Rabkin, "Hypertension: Medical World under Pressure," *Maclean's* 91, no. 28 (20 November 1978): 59.

Chapter 3

1 Daniel Cappon, "Review Article, Obesity," *CMAJ* 79, no. 7 (1 October 1958): 569.

2 For querying the equation, see Canada, Health and Welfare Canada, *Promoting Healthy Weights: A Discussion Paper* (Ottawa: Minister of National Health and Welfare, 1988), 34; Arya M. Sharma, "Why the Energy Balance Equation Results in Flawed Approaches to Obesity Prevention and Management," Dr. Sharma's Obesity Notes, 26 February 2014, accessed 4 November 2016, http://www.drsharma.ca/why-the-energy-balance-equation-results-in-flawed-approaches-to-obesity-prevention-and-management. Dr Sharma argues that "body weight itself may very much determine energy intake and output (and not just the other way around)." He suggests we should "shift our focus to the physiological (and psychological) factors (often dependent on our body weight) that ultimately dictate how much we 'choose' to eat or expend in physical activity."

3 For food in Canada and identity, see Dorothy Duncan, *Canadians at Table: Food, Fellowship and Folklore: A Culinary History of Canada* (Toronto: Dundurn Press, 2006).

4 Harvey A. Levenstein, *Revolution at the Table: The Transformation of the American Diet* (Berkeley: University of California Press, 2003), 177.
5 "On the Importance of Body Weight," *CMAJ* 16, no. 1 (January 1926): 64. For types of food, see Bernard Fantus, "What We Eat and Why," *CLP* 64, no. 4 (April 1925): 183.
6 Walter Campbell, "Obesity and Treatment," *CMAJ* 34, no. 1 (January 1936): 41. On Campbell, see Kerry Segrave, *Obesity in America, 1850–1939: A History of Social Attitudes and Treatment* (Jefferson, NC: McFarland & Co., 2008), 124.
7 Annabelle Lee, "Can You Live Up to Your Spring Hat?" *Chatelaine* 6, no. 4 (April 1933): 28.
8 E.W. McHenry, "Food in Canada: A Discussion of Canadian Nutritional Conditions," *Health* 16, no. 1 (January/February 1948): 15; *Maclean's* 62, no. 19 (1 October 1949): 34, advertisement for Westinghouse.
9 Henry A. Christian, ed., *The Principles and Practice of Medicine*, 16th ed. (New York: D. Appleton-Century Co., 1947), 602–4. For why people eat, see A. Keenberg, "Obesity and Its Treatment," *ManMR* 27, no. 5 (May 1947): 280.
10 *ManMR* 29, no. 7 (July 1949): 380, advertisement for Desoxyn; "Review of *Obesity and Leanness* by H.R. Rony," *CMAJ* 44, no. 5 (May 1941): 546; N.B.F., "Review of *Obesity and Leanness* by H.R. Rony," *CD* 6, no. 2 (February 1940): 46.
11 For anomaly, see D.E. Rodger, J. Grant McFetridge, and Eileen Price, "The Management of Obesity," *ManMR* 30, no. 5 (May 1950): 294; Cappon, "Review Article, Obesity," 572.
12 For more money, see Sidney Katz, "Are We Eating Too Much?" *Maclean's* 68, no. 12 (11 June 1955): 14. For a study of packaged food in the 1950s, see Laura Shapiro, *Something from the Oven: Reinventing Dinner in 1950s America* (New York: Penguin, 2004), 64, 79. For fast food, see Steve Penfold, *The Donut: A Canadian History* (Toronto: University of Toronto Press, 2008), 65, for Table 2.1 and a list of such chains in Canada 1953–1965.
13 For eating and drinking, see *Chatelaine* 32, no. 2 (February 1959): 3, advertisement for Metropolitan Life Insurance. For Quebec, see Lucien Dubreuil, "L'obésité," *UMC* 81, no. 6 (juin 1952): 707. For quote, see Jean Grignon, "L'obésité et la maigreur," *UMC* 81, no. 11 (novembre 1952): 1309.
14 L.B. Pett and Elaine Collett, "Low-Fat Meals to Help Your Husband's Heart," *Chatelaine* 30, no. 8 (August 1957): 15.
15 J.E. Parsons, "To a Wife," *Maclean's* 65, no. 19 (1 October 1952): 58, poem. For the tubby hubby, see Deborah McPhail, *Contours of the Nation: Making Obesity and Imagining Canada, 1945–1970* (Toronto: University of Toronto

Press, 2017), 53–5. See also Deborah McPhail, "What to Do with the 'Tubby Hubby'? 'Obesity,' the Crisis of Masculinity, and the Nuclear Family in Early Cold War Canada," *Antipode* 41, no. 5 (2009): 1021–2. Blaming the wife was also seen in 1930s Britain. Christopher E. Forth, *Masculinity in the Modern West: Gender, Civilization and the Body* (New York and Basingstoke, UK: Palgrave Macmillan, 2008), 186. For having health, see Harold S. Segall, "How to Be an Executive and Live," *Health* 26, no. 1 (January/February 1958): 11.

16 D.E. Rodger, J. Grant McFetridge, and Eileen Price, "The Management of Obesity," *CMAJ* 63, no. 3 (September 1950): 265–6. For the joy of eating, see Josephine Lowman, "Tubby Hubby Diet: Good Nutrition Provided in Weight-Cutting Menu," *Globe and Mail*, 30 September 1953, 10.

17 L. Bradley Pett, "Public Health, Ottawa Newsletter...Appetite Control and Obesity," *CMAJ* 76, no. 12 (15 June 1957): 1083. For blaming of wives and mothers, see also Deborah McPhail, "The 'Kitchen Demon' and the 'Tubby Hubby': Reproductive Labour and the Nuclear Family in Obesity Discourse," chapter 2 in *Contours of the Nation*, 55–74.

18 Paul Dumas, "Le traitement de l'obésité," *UMC* 87, no. 11 (novembre 1958): 1364.

19 "Salad Can Help You Look Better, Feel Better," *Health* 32, no. 3 (June 1964): 20.

20 For active eater and sedentary eater, see *CMAJ* 84, no. 9 (4 March 1961): 13, advertisement for Biphetamine. For night eaters, see *CMAJ* 90, no. 11 (14 March 1964): 15, advertisement for Prelutal. For compulsive eater, see *CD* 31, no. 7 (July 1965): 4, advertisement for Desbutal.

21 For fattening food, see Dr P. Jacquemart, *Échec à l'obésité et à la cellulite* (Paris: Librairie Maloine, 1961), 51; for a review of the preceding book, see *UMC* 91, no. 7 (juillet 1962): 806; see also *CMAJ* 86, no. 20 (19 May 1962): 5, advertisement for Limmits.

22 For carbohydrates being cheap, see Daniel Cappon, *Eating, Loving and Dying: A Psychology of Appetites* (Toronto: University of Toronto Press, 1973), 42. For refined carbohydrates, see Barbara Birchwood, "What's Wrong with Carbohydrates?" *CFP* 21, no. 4 (April 1975): 69–70. For Inuit, see O. Schaefer, "Pre- and Post-Natal Growth Acceleration and Increased Sugar Consumption in Canadian Eskimos," *CMAJ* 103, no. 10 (7 November 1970): 1059. For sugar and package labels, see D.J.R. Rowe, "Salt and Sugar in the Diet," *CMAJ* 119, no. 7 (7 October 1978): 790.

23 David Woods, "Two Epidemiologists Discuss Myths and Realities of Health Mainenance," *CMAJ* 109, no. 11 (1 December 1973): 1154. For Shephard, see Kaspars Dzeguze, "A Lean and Hungry Look," *Maclean's* 91, no. 15 (24 July 1978): 31.

24 For elderly, see "Aging – A Project Report," *CN* 58, no. 7 (July 1962): 617.
25 For fat cells, see Simeon Margolis and Dean H. Lockwood, "Obesity," in *The Principles and Practice of Medicine*, 18th ed., ed. A. McGehee Harvey et al. (New York: Appleton-Century Crofts, 1972), 919, 921. The fat cell theory remains significant to the 1980 edition. Arnold E. Andersen and Simeon Margolis, "Eating Disorders: Obesity and Anorexia Nervosa," in *The Principles and Practice of Medicine*, 20th ed., ed. A. McGehee Harvey et al. (New York: Appleton-Century Crofts, 1980), 825. A. Angel, "Pathophysiology of Obesity," *CMAJ* 110, no. 5 (2 March 1974): 548. For set-point, see C. Peter Herman and Janet Polivy, "Restrained Eating," in *Obesity*, ed. Albert J. Stundard (Philadelphia: W.B. Saunders, 1980), 210. For the overview, see J.E. Blundell and R.A. McArthur, *Annual Research Reviews: Obesity and Its Treatment*, vol. 1 (Montreal: Eden Press, 1979), 2.
26 Jana Evans Braziel and Kathleen LeBesco, "Introduction," in *Bodies Out of Bounds: Fatness and Transgression*, ed. Jana Evans Braziel and Kathleen LeBesco (Berkeley: University of California Press, 2001): 3. For the psychological "cause" of obesity, see Arya M. Sharma, "Is Obesity Part of the Mental Health Epidemic," *CONDUIT* 3, no. 2 (Summer 2009): 6; Robert D. Levitan and Caroline Davis, "Emotions and Eating Behaviour: Implications for the Current Obesity Epidemic," *University of Toronto Quarterly* 79, no. 2 (Spring 2010): 783–99.
27 For DSM-5, see Nora D. Volkow and Charles P. O'Brien, "Issues for DSM-V: Should Obesity Be Included as a Brain Disorder?" *American Journal of Psychiatry* 164 (May 2007): 708, accessed 29 October 2015, https://ajp.psychiatryonline.org/doi/full/10.1176/ajp.2007.164.5.708; Avner Offer, "Body Weight and Self-Control in the United States and Britain since the 1950s," *Social History of Medicine* 14, no. 1 (2001): 105.
28 For history of psychology, see Mona Gleason, *Normalizing the Ideal: Psychology, Schooling and the Family in Postwar Canada* (Toronto: University of Toronto Press 1999); Leonora Hawirko and P.H. Sprague, "Treatment of Obesity by Appetite-Depression Drugs," *CMAJ* 54, no. 1 (January 1946): 27. For dissatisfaction, see Hilde Bruch, *The Importance of Overweight* (New York: W.W. Norton & Co., 1957): 358. For insecurity, see News Briefs, "The Emotional Obese," *CD* 14, no. 3 (March 1948): 92. For defence, see Edward H. Rynearson and Clifford F. Gastineau, *Obesity*, American Lecture Series, no. 36, American Lectures in Endocrinology (Springfield, IL: Charles C. Thomas, 1949), 21, 29. For boredom, see Christian, *The Principles and Practice of Medicine* (1947), 603. For depression, see Rynearson and Gastineau, *Obesity*, 30. For the present, see Arya M. Sharma, "Benefits of (Excess) Weight Gain," Dr. Sharma's Obesity Notes,

2 September 2009, accessed 19 July 2010, http://www.drsharma.ca/benefits-of-excess-weight-gain.
29 Louis N. Sarbach, "Food Can Be a Drug," *Maclean's* 62, no. 1 (1 January 1949): 27.
30 Rynearson and Gastineau, *Obesity*, 29.
31 Bernard Laski, "The Overnourished and the Undernourished Child," *Health* 18, no. 4 (July/August 1950): 21; News Brief, "Shakespeare Wrong on Diet," *CD* 21, no. 6 (June 1955): 63; Peter H. Nash, "Health...and the Businessman," *Health* 24, no. 5 (September/October 1956): 10. For dislike of the psychological as a crutch, see E.W. McHenry, "Canadian Women Are Too Fat," *Chatelaine* 33, no. 6 (June 1960): 47.
32 For depression, see *CMAJ* 69, no. 4 (October 1953): 468, advertisement for Methdrine; for depresson leading to obesity, see also *CMAJ* 74, no. 4 (15 February 1956): 333, advertisement for Dexedrine. Cappon, "Review Article, Obesity," 568.
33 Rodger, McFetridge, and Price, "The Management of Obesity," 265, 268. For women and emotional obesity, see Josephine Lowman, "Why Grow Old? Tensions May Cause Overeating," *Globe and Mail*, 28 January 1956, 13. For postmenopause, see Antonio Martel, "Preludin (Phenmetrazine) in the Treatment of Obesity," *CMAJ* 76, no. 2 (15 January 1957): 120. Editorial, "Obesity and Anorexia," *CMAJ* 73, no. 5 (1 September 1955): 408.
34 Cappon, "Review Article, Obesity," 572. Hilde Bruch, *Eating Disorders: Obesity, Anorexia Nervosa, and the Person Within* (New York: Basic Books, 1973), 130. For fear, see Louis Palmer, "Causes of Obesity," *CN* 46, no. 8 (August 1950): 668.
35 Pett, "Public Health, Ottawa Newsletter," 1083.
36 For psychodietics, see Sidney Katz, "A Report on Eating," *Maclean's* 68, no. 12 (11 June 1955): 11; Dorothy Sangster, "The Tragedy of the Fat Child," *Maclean's* 72, no. 16 (1 August 1959): 35. For more on eating as an "emotional" problem, see "Eat and Grow Slim," *Chatelaine* 23, no. 9 (September 1950): 74–5. For Lowman, see McPhail, *Contours of the Nation*, 26, 53.
37 Editorial, "Treatment of Obesity," *CMAJ* 80, no. 8 (15 April 1959): 657; for others, see Grignon, "L'obésité et la maigreur," 1308–9.
38 Cappon, "Review Article, Obesity," 569.
39 Doris L. Hirsch and W.I. Morse, "Emotional and Metabolic Factors in Obesity," *CJPH* 51, no. 11 (November 1960): 451.
40 Hirsch and Morse, "Emotional and Metabolic Factors in Obesity," 450, 454–5. For emotional and mental health causation, see also *CMAJ* 87, no. 7 (18 August 1962): 33, advertisement for Eskatrol; "Review of *Les cellulites*

et obésités d'origine psychique de Marcel Rouet," *UMC* 92, no. 9 (septembre 1963): 1068; F.W. Hanley, "The Treatment of Obesity by Individual and Group Hypnosis," *CPAJ* 9, no. 4 (April 1967): 128.

41 F. Gerard Allison, "Modern Treatment of Obesity," *ManMR* 40, no. 7 (August–September 1960): 509. For ennui, see Linda Oglov, "Canadian Dietetic Association Delegates at the Annual Meeting Study Relationship of Diet to Exercise," *CMAJ* 117, no. 3 (6 August 1977): 290. D.R. Wilson, "Current Drug Therapy: Drugs for Obesity," *CMAJ* 91, no. 26 (26 December 1964): 1369.

42 Sheila Kieran, "What Diets Fail," *Chatelaine* 39, no. 12 (December 1966): 16.

43 Dorothy Sangster, "The Trouble with Middle-Aged Men," *Maclean's* 73, no. 12 (4 June 1960): 25.

44 S. Saint-Hilaire, "Emotions and Poor Food Habits," *CN* 61, no. 12 (December 1965): 964.

45 For psychological view of obesity as unbalanced, see Ethel Gillingham, "Who Says Anyone Can Lose Weight," *Chatelaine* 34, no. 6 (June 1961): 69. For Swedish study, see "Fat Women Less Anxious," *CN* 62, no. 10 (October 1966): 17. For American studies, see Gina Kolata, *Rethinking Thin: The New Science of Weight Loss – and the Myths and Realities of Dieting* (New York: Farrar, Straus and Giroux, 2007), 92, 94.

46 For this quote and more, see James Paupst, "A Whole Nation of Thin People, Wildly Signaling to Be Let Out," *Maclean's* 89, no. 17 (4 October 1976): 73–4.

47 For recognition of the psychological factor, see General Foods, "What to Know about Weight Control," *Health* 29, no. 2 (Summer 1972): 14; James C. Collyer, "Review of *Obesity and Its Management* by D. Craddock," *CFP* 19, no. 11 (November 1973): 153; Herman and Polivy, "Restrained Eating," 222; Kathleen McDonnell, "Obesity's Revamped Image," *Maclean's* 94, no. 34 (24 August 1981): 58; Barbara Edelstein, "How Teen Girls Can Fight against Fatness," *Toronto Star*, 4 August 1980, C1. For the case, see Rona Levitt, "Chronic Obesity in a Family," *CFP* 22, no. 7 (July 1976): 88.

48 For drugs, see Blundell and McArthur, *Annual Research Reviews*, 48–9. For depression as a cause and result of obesity, see James A. Collyer, "The Unhappy Fat Woman," *CFP* 19, no. 5 (May 1973): 93. For the two types, see Frank G. Sommers, "Psychophysiological Aspects in Treating Obesity," *CFP* 18, no. 2 (February 1972): 52. For image, see "Problem of Obesity Said Frustrating to Doctor and Patient," *CMAJ* 112, no. 3 (8 February 1975): 350. For Cappon, see Cappon, *Eating, Loving and Dying*, x. For a review of the book, see J.A. Collyer, "Review of *Eating, Loving and Dying* by D. Cappon," *CFP* 20, no. 3 (March 1924): 129.

49 For Cappon, see "What Kind of Eater Are You?" *CN* 68, no. 8 (August 1972): 44; Cappon, *Eating, Loving and Dying*, 22, 32, 58. For more on appestat, see Bert L. Fairbanks, "Exercise, Nutrition and Obesity," *Health* 44, no. 1 (Spring 1978): 9.
50 Susie Orbach, *Fat Is a Feminist Issue: The Anti-Diet Guide to Permanent Weight Loss* (New York: Berkley Books, 1979), 36. For the teacher, see McDonnell, "Obesity's Revamped Image," 58.
51 Kelly D. Brownell, *Food Fight: The Inside Story of the Food Industry, America's Obesity Crisis and What We Can Do About It* (New York, Chicago: McGraw-Hill Companies Inc., 2004), 27.
52 Claude Bouchard, "Is There a Biological Basis for the Obesity Epidemic?" in *Presentation and Poster Abstracts from the International Conference on Physical Activity and Obesity in Children* (Toronto: International Conference, 24–7 June, 2007), 14–16.
53 William Osler, *The Principles and Practice of Medicine* (New York: D. Appleton and Co., 1893), 1020; William Osler, *The Principles and Practice of Medicine*, 8th ed. (New York: D. Appleton and Co., 1912), 451; Thomas McCrae, ed., *The Principles and Practice of Medicine*, 10th ed. (New York: D. Appleton and Co., 1925), 445. For race and heredity, see "The Menace of Obesity," *CMAJ* 16, no. 11 (November 1926): 1373–4.
54 E.S. Mills, "Review of 'Studies of Relatively Normal Obese Individuals During and After Dietary Restrictions' by H.H. Fellows," *CMAJ* 24, no. 6 (June 1931): 875. The eugenic movement in Canada didn't see obesity as one of their issues. For the movement, see C. Elizabeth Koester, "An Evil Hitherto Unchecked: Eugenics and the 1917 Ontario Royal Commission on the Care and Control of the Mentally Defective and Feebleminded," *Canadian Bulletin of Medical History* 33, no. 1 (Spring 2016): 59–81; Angus McLaren, *Our Own Master Race: Eugenics in Canada, 1885–1945* (Toronto: Oxford University Press, 1988); Erica Dyck, *Facing Eugenics: Reproductions, Sterilization and the Politics of Choice* (Toronto: University of Toronto Press, 2013); and "History of Eugenics Revisited," *Canadian Bulletin of Medical History* 31, no. 1 (2014): 7–16, especially 7–12. For the early days of heredity, see Riko Bedford, "Heredity as Ideology: Ideas of the Woman's Christian Temperance Union of the United States and Ontario on Heredity and Social Reform, 1880–1910," *Canadian Bulletin of Medical History* 32, no. 1 (2015): 77–100.
55 E.S. Mills, "Review of 'Obesity Constitutional or Endocrine' by Solomon Silver and Julius Bauer," *CMAJ* 26, no. 3 (September 1931): 354–5. See also J.-E. Dubé, "Considérations générales sur la tension et l'hypertension artérielle," *UMC* 62, no. 11 (novembre 1933): 1123; J.R. Pepin, "L'obésité

est-elle réductible?" *UMC* 48, no. 5 (mai 1929): 262; W.F. Christie, *Obesity: A Practical Handbook for Physicians* (London: William Heinemann, 1937), 61; Christian, *The Principles and Practice of Medicine* (1947), 603. For looking at both nature and nurture, see Lennox G. Bell, "The Trials of Obesity," *ManMR* 20, no. 8 (August 1940): 143.

56 Adele Saunders, "How'd You Get That Way –?" *Chatelaine* 17, no. 5 (May 1944): 16.
57 "Review of *Obesity and Leanness* by H.R. Rony," *CMAJ* 44, no. 5 (May 1941): 546. For more on heredity, see Virginia Morris, "Meet the Man You Will Marry," *Chatelaine* 26, 7 (July 1953): 24.
58 Rynearson and Gastineau, *Obesity*, 40, 42.
59 For Bruch, see her book *The Importance of Overweight*, 88. For biological/social, see Jacquemart, *Échec à l'obésité et à la cellulite*, 10–11.
60 Cappon, "Review Article, Obesity," 570–1. For dismissing heredity, see J.R. Beaton, "Energy Balance and Obesity," *CJPH* 58, no. 11 (November 1967): 482. For family eating, see Nash, "Health…and the Businessman," 10; and Elizabeth Chant Robertson, "What to Eat to Be Healthy," *Health* 29, no. 4 (August 1961): 26. For the statistics, see Dubreuil, "L'obésité," 707.
61 For accepting heredity, see Katz, "Are We Eating Too Much?" 93; Byng Whitteker (as told to Robert Oslon), "I Like Being Fat…And Here Are My Reasons," *Maclean's* 70, no. 1 (26 October 1957): 68. Some spell Byng's last name as Whittaker. Florence James, "Letter," *Chatelaine* 33, no. 8 (August 1960): 112. Concerning the letter, see also Heather Molyneaux, "In Sickness and in Health: Representations of Women in Pharmaceutical Advertisements in the *Canadian Medical Association Journal*, 1950–1970" (PhD diss., University of New Brunswick, 2009), 189.
62 For family history, see "Problem of Obesity Said Frustrating to Doctor and Patient," 350. See also Susan C. Wooley and Orland W. Wooley, "Obesity and Women – 1. A Closer Look at the Facts," *Women's Studies International Quarterly* 2 (1979): 75. For 35 to 65 per cent variation in opinion on heredity as related to obesity, see M.K. Fajic et al., "Height-Weight Comparison of Canadian Schoolchildren," in *Physical Fitness Assessment: Principles, Practice and Application*, ed. Roy J. Shephard et al. (Springfield, IL, Charles C. Thomas Publisher, 1978), 73. *Chatelaine*, in an article on children, noted that if one parent was overweight, the odds were 40 per cent that the child would be overweight as well; the odds were 80 per cent if both parents were overweight. Naomi Mallovy, "Good Food Habits Last a Lifetime," *Chatelaine* 46, no. 6 (June 1973): 98.
63 Cappon, *Eating, Loving and Dying*, 4, 64.

64 For adopted children, see Pierre Biron, Jean-Guy Mongeau, and Denise Bertrand, "Letter to Editor," *CMAJ* 116, no. 2 (22 January 1977): 133. For an optimistic view, see Dr Winick in Oglov, "Canadian Dietetic Association Delegates," 289. For Inuit weight, see Fajic et al., "Height-Weight Comparison of Canadian Schoolchildren," 73.
65 C.H. Hollenberg, "Editorial: Human Obesity – a Survey and a Suggestion," *CMAJ* 119, no. 12 (23 December 1978): 1383. For genetic flaws, see Angel, "Pathophysiology of Obesity," 546. For being hardwired, see "Problem of Obesity Said Frustrating to Doctor and Patient," 350.
66 Mollie Gillen, "Is It True Some People Are Naturally Fat?" *Chatelaine* 44, no. 9 (September 1971): 44, 101.
67 James M. Rippe and Weight Watchers, *Weight Loss That Lasts: Break Through the 10 Big Diet Myths* (Hoboken, NJ: John Wiley & Sons, 2005), 127–8.
68 Harvey A. Levenstein, *Paradox of Plenty: A Social History of Eating in Modern America*, rev.ed. (Berkeley: University of California Press, 2003), 249–50; see also Philip A. Wood, *How Fat Works* (Cambridge, MA: Harvard University Press, 2006), 74, 172.
69 Walter Gratzer, *Terrors of the Table: The Curious History of Nutrition* (Oxford: Oxford University Press, 2005), 244; David A. Kessler, *The End of Overeating: Taking Control of the Insatiable North American Appetite* (Toronto: McClelland & Stewart, 2009), 8.
70 S.W. Keith et al., "Putative Contributors to the Secular Increase in Obesity: Exploring the Roads Less Traveled," *International Journal of Obesity* 30 (2006): 1584–94, accessed 21 March 2011, https://www.nature.com/articles/0803326.
71 Osler, *The Principles and Practice of Medicine* (1893), 1020; Osler, *The Principles and Practice of Medicine* (1912), 450–1. See Sander L. Gilman, *Fat Boys: A Slim Book* (Lincoln, NB: University of Nebraska Press, 2004), 5.
72 McCrae, *The Principles and Practice of Medicine* (1925), 445. For others, see Pepin, "L'obésité est-elle réductible?," 263; "Lose Fat as She Did," *The Chatelaine* 1, no. 6 (August 1928): 44, advertisement for Marmola–Prescription Tablets; *The Chatelaine* 2, no. 1 (January 1929): 38, advertisement for Marmola.
73 Edward Mason, "The Treatment of Obesity," *CMAJ* 14, no. 11 (November 1924): 1052.
74 J. Freigenbaum, "Review of *The Cause of Obesity* by L.H. Newburgh," *CMAJ* 26, no. 3 (March 1932): 368. For endocrine obesity, see E.M. Watson, "Some Present-Day Views on Diet: Concluded" *CN* 26, no. 7 (July 1930): 368; "Medical Library University of Manitoba: Current

Medical Literature," *MMAR* 18, no. 5 (May 1938): 101–2; Christie, *Obesity*, 18–19, 21.
75 For thyroid, see Campbell, "Obesity and Its Treatment," 41. For querying the connection, see P.M. MacDonnell, "Review of 'Blood Cholesterol and Hypometabolism: Suprarenal and Pituitary Deficiency, Obesity, and Miscellaneous Conditions' by Lewis M. Hurxthal," *CMAJ* 31, no. 3 (September 1934): 330.
76 Christie, *Obesity*, 11–12, 19–22, 24, 26; for women, see 29, 45; for men, see 46; for race, see 31.
77 Grant Fleming, "Calories and Vitamins," *Maclean's* 44, no. 21 (1 November 1931): 34.
78 See *Maclean's* 60, no. 6 (15 March 1947): 28, advertisement for Metropolitan Life Insurance Co.; Keenberg, "Obesity and Its Treatment," 280; Christian, *The Principles and Practice of Medicine* (1947), 602–3; Bell, "The Trials of Obesity," 143. For a discussion of the popularity of the endocrine theory, see Bruch, *The Importance of Overweight*, 6–8; Hugo R. Rony, *Obesity and Leanness* (Philadelphia: Lea & Febiger, 1940), 84. Rony also listed why endocrine problems and obesity might seem to be related, 90.
79 H.I. Cramer, "Physiological Considerations of the Etiology and Threatment of Obesity," *CMAJ* 55, no. 5 (November 1946): 505–6.
80 Rony, *Obesity and Leanness*, 107, 106; Rynearson and Gastineau, *Obesity*, 21, 35, on thyroid, 33, 92. For Iodobesin, see *CD* 10, no. 5 (May 1944): 45, advertisement; and *CD* 14, no. 3 (March 1948): 54, advertisement. For Clarkotabs, see *CD* 13, no. 4 (April 1947): 77, advertisement. For Probese, see *CD* 13, no. 4 (April 1947): 87, advertisement.
81 Dubreuil, "L'obésité," 707. For a similar division, see Fernand Joncas and Jean Bissonnette, "Obésité et diabète: évaluation clinique d'un nouvel anorexique: Préudine," *UMC* 86, no. 6 (juin 1957): 663. For a different way of dividing obesity, see Dumas, "Le traitement de l'obésité," 1363.
82 For menopause, see Martel, "Preludin (Phenmetrazine) in the Treatment of Obesity," 120. For puberty and after pregnancy, see Dubreuil, "L'obésité," 707; "Traitement de l'obésité," *UMC* 82, no. 12 (décembre 1953): 1438. For metabolism and women having more fat, see Elizabeth Chant Robertson, *Nutrition for Today* (Toronto: McClelland & Stewart, 1951), 178. For hypothalamus disorder, see Jean Mayer, "Effects of Obesity on Health: Physiologic Factors," *MMC* 13, no. 5 (May 1958): 194.
83 Chant Robertson, *Nutrition for Today*, 179.
84 See, for example, Paul-René Archambault, "[Review of] A. Blige and Mme M. Martin, 'Les obésités d'origine nerveuse,'" *UMC* 94, no. 2 (février 1965): 245; W. Schweisheimer, "Your Waistline Is Biggest Health

Hazard," *Executive* 7 (April 1965): 60; S.S.B. Gilder, "The Fat Child," *CMAJ* 107, no. 11 (9 December 1972): 1068; "Review of *Adolescent Nutrition and Growth*, edited by Felix P. Heald," *CMAJ* 102, no. 3 (28 February 1970): 433.
85 Angel, "Pathophysiology of Obesity," 546, 548.
86 For adrenal gland, see C.J. Pattee and R.R. Gilles, "Metabolic Studies in Obesity," *MSJ* 17 (July/August 1961): 525. For thyroid, see "Effect of Thyroid Hormone on Obesity," *CMAJ* 95, no. 4 (23 July 1966): 177; *CD* 27, no. 3 (March 1961): 23, advertisement for Probese; Jean Yack, "What's New in Dieting," *Chatelaine* 36, no. 4 (April 1963): 39. For hypothalamus, see L.-J. Poirer, A.-M. Mouren-Mathieu, and C.-L. Richer, "Obésité hypothlamique chez le singe," *UMC* 91, no. 1 (janvier 1962): 90; Archambault, "[Review of] A. Blige and Mme M. Martin, 'Les obésités d'origine nerveuse,'" 245; for hypothalamic injury, see Blundell and McArthur, *Annual Research Reviews*, 6. For hormones, see Maurice Verdy, "Traitement des obésités," *UMC* 96, no. 5 (mai 1967): 578; Beryl A. Chernick, "Blood Pressure and Body Weight Changes during Oral Contraceptive Treatment," *CMAJ* 99, no. 12 (28 September 1968): 593; Sir Ian G.W. Hill, "Must We Wear Out?" *CFP* 15, no. 11 (November 1969): 17; Barbara McLaren, "The Group Approach to Weight Loss," *Health* 39, no. 3 (Autumn 1973): 18; Barbara Edelstein, "On a Diet? Still Fat? You Must be a Woman," *Globe and Mail*, 7 September 1978, T1.
87 Margolis and Lockwood, "Obesity," 918–24.
88 For utilization of calories, see Margolis and Lockwood, "Obesity," 920. For metabolism, see Sheila Kieran, "A Frank Report on *Some* Diet Doctors," *Chatelaine* 46, no. 12 (December 1973): 68. For elderly, see Stan McFadden, "It's Easier to Stay Slim," *CHW* 17, no. 10 (January 1962): 4; Chant Robertson, "What to Eat to Be Healthy," 26.
89 Robbie Salter, "Origin of Obesity," *Health* 45, no. 1 (Spring 1979): 20.
90 A. Angel, "Pathophysiologic Changes in Obesity," *CMAJ* 119, no. 12 (23 December 1978): 1401.
91 Jean Himms-Hagen, "Obesity May Be Due to a Malfunctioning of Brown Fat," *CMAJ* 121, no. 10 (17 November 1979): 1361.
92 Ibid.
93 William L. Haskell, "Has There Been a Change in the Level of Sedentarism and the Pattern of Physical Activity of Children and Youth over Time?" in *Presentation and Poster Abstracts from the International Conference on Physical Activity and Obesity in Children* (Toronto: International Conference, 24–7 June, 2007), 9–10.

94 For exercise not helping weight loss, see Heather Sykes, *Queer Bodies: Sexualities, Genders, and Fatness in Physical Education* (New York: Peter Lang, 2011), 53. For obesity not being the result of a lack of activity, see Michael Gard, "Understanding Obesity by Understanding Desire," in *Critical Feminist Approaches to Eating Dis/orders*, ed. Helen Malson and Maree Burns (London: Routledge, 2009), 37. For the idea that being obese doesn't mean being sedentary, see Jeanne and Jennifer in Leanne Joanisse, "Reducing and Revisioning the Body: Women's Experiences of Weight Loss Surgery" (PhD diss., McMaster University, 2003), 135. For the meaning of activity, see Michael Gard and Jan Wright, *The Obesity Epidemic: Science, Morality and Ideology* (London and New York: Routledge, Taylor & Francis Group, 2005), 52, 57.

95 Osler, *The Principles and Practice of Medicine* (1893), 1020.

96 For age and exercise, see Maurice Boigny, "Effets physiologiques et l'exercise," *UMC* 50, no. 7 (juillet 1921): 287–95; Fleming, "Calories and Vitamins," 34; CMA, "What Should I Weigh?" *Maclean's* 43, no. 2 (15 January 1930): 44. For middle-aged people, see H.M. Harrison, "Good Habits – Good Health," *Health* 6, no. 3 (September 1938): 76.

97 Wendy Mitchinson, *Body Failure: Medical Views of Women, 1900–1950* (Toronto: University of Toronto, 2013), 29–32.

98 For winter, see James W. Barton, "Getting Rid of the Winter Surplus," *Maclean's* 38, no. 6 (15 March 1925): 20. For sedentary life, see "Vanity Box," *CHJ* 21, no. 4 (August 1924): 22.

99 *Eaton's Catalogue*, Spring/Summer 1920, 394; Annabelle Lee, "Work-A-day Beauty," *Chatelaine* 6, no. 11 (November 1933): 33; *Maclean's* 52, no. 7 (1 April 1939): 58, cartoon; *Maclean's* 60, no. 7 (1 April 1947): 48, cartoon.

100 For forty being the cut-off age, see *Maclean's* 54, no. 8 (15 April 1941): 24, advertisement for Metropolitan Insurance Co.; see also "Changing Emphasis," *CN* 45, no. 2 (February 1949): 124, for not doing overly strenuous exercise.

101 Lionel M. Lindsay, "The Overweight Child," *CMAJ* 44, no. 5 (May 1941): 506.

102 Rony, *Obesity and Leanness*, 80.

103 A. Corinne Trerice, "Slimming Can Be Healthy or Hazardous," *Health* 23, no. 3 (May/June 1955): 18. See also Grignon, "L'obésité et la maigreur," 1309; Grace A. Goldsmith, "Effects of Obesity on Health: Living Habits and Weight," *MMC* 13, no. 5 (May 1958): 189.

104 Lloyd Percival, "Can You Pass This Fitness Test?" *Chatelaine* 29, no. 2 (February 1956): 19. On women, see Christina McCall, "How to Be

338 Notes to pages 106–7

More Vital Than You Are," *Chatelaine* 32, no. 5 (May 1959): 58; Lloyd Percival, "Our Flabby Muscles Are a National Disgrace," *Maclean's* 66, no. 8 (15 April 1953): 71; Howard O'Hagan, "Why Have We Lost the Joy of Walking?" *Maclean's* 70, no. 10 (11 May 1957): 32. For business men, see "In Search of Physical Fitness," *Health* 26, no. 1 (January–February 1958): 12. See also McPhail, "What to Do with the 'Tubby Hubby'?," 1026. For older Canadians, see Morton Hunt, "Exercise is the Bunk – Relax," *Maclean's* 63, no. 8 (15 April 1950): 25. See also a survey of 51,555 Canadians by the Sports College, "Are Women the Fitter Sex?" *Health* 24, no. 2 (March/April 1956): 13.
105 Dubreuil, "L'obésité," 707.
106 McPhail, *Contours of the Nation*, 77–8.
107 About the obese not overeating, see "Did You Know ...," *CN* 73, no. 2 (February 1977): 10; Russ Kisby, "Exercise Is a 'Must,'" *Health* 34, no. 6 (December 1966): 17, 26. On fitness, see Roy J. Shephard, "Exercise and Physical Fitness," *OMR* 35, no. 2 (February 1968): 78. For the Inuit, see Andris Rode and Roy J. Shephard, "Growth and Fitness of Canadian Inuit: Secular Trends, 1970–1990," *American Journal of Human Biology* 6 (1994): 525. On physical fitness of the Inuit, see R.J. Shephard and A. Rode, *The Health Consequences of 'Modernization': Evidence from Circumpolar Peoples* (Cambridge: Cambridge University Press, 1996), chapter 5, 123–50.
108 CBC Radio, "Deliberating Man's Appearance in the Year 2000," *Sports College*, 9 December 1961, accessed 10 April 2007, http://www.cbc.ca/archives/entry/deliberating-mans-appearance-in-the-year-2000; CBC-TV, "Committing Armchair Suicide," *CBC Newsmagazine*, 16 July 1968, accessed 19 April 2007, http://www.cbc.ca/archives/entry/committing-armchair-suicide. For middle-age Canadians, see Chant Robertson, "What to Eat to Be Healthy," 26. For middle age beginning in the thirties, see Hugh A. Noble, "The Adult and 'Physical Fitness,'" *CAHPER* 27, no. 5 (June/July 1961): 31. For staying the same weight as a twenty-five-year-old, see Eileen Morris, "How Doctors Diet," *Chatelaine* 40, no. 10 (October 1967): 31. For exercise, see "Cycling for Fitness and Fun," *CN* 67, no. 9 (September 1971): 53. For fitness, see also J.V. Daniel, "Exercise Should Start at an Early Age," *Health* 42, no. 2 (Summer 1976): 13; E. Lee Macnamara, "Fitting Nursing into Fitness," *CN* 76, no. 4 (April 1980): 33; Judith Banning, "A Personal Commitment to Fitness Results in Healthier Clients," *CN* 76, no. 5 (May 1980): 40. Italics are mine.
109 E.W. Banister, S.R. Brown, H.R. Loewen, and H.C. Nordan, "The Royal Canadian Air Force 5BX Program: A Metabolic Evaluation," *MSJ* 23 (November 1967): 1237; John B. Armstrong, "Perspectives of Overweight

and Other Factors Related to Cardiovascular Disease," *CJPH* 58, no. 11 (November 1967): 498. See also Fairbanks, "Exercise, Nutrition and Obesity," 8; Elaine Collett, "Diet Facts," *Chatelaine* 45, no. 10 (October 1972): 77.

110 For walking, see Wes McVicar, "Here's How to Exercise If You Are Over Forty," *Health* 29, no. 3 (June 1961); 53. For golf, see Allison, "Modern Treatment of Obesity," 509.

111 Bert L. Fairbanks, "Exercise, Nutrition and Obesity," *CAHPER* 43, no. 3 (January/February 1977): 15. For LeRiche, see Woods, "Two Epidemiologists Discuss Myths," 1146.

112 Donnalu Wigmore, "20-Minutes-a-Day Fitness Program for Women," *Chatelaine* 44, no. 2 (February 1971): 72.

113 Campbell, "Obesity and Its Treatment," 41.

114 S.S.B. Gilder, "The London Letter," *CMAJ* 100, no. 23 (21 June 1969): 1110. For a more modern list of causes, see Christine L. Wells, "Exercise and Weight Control – What You Should Know," *CAHPER* 38, no. 3 (January/February 1972): 23.

115 For list of factors, see Dumas, "Le traitement de l'obésité," 1364; D.L. Keegan, "The Doctor's and the Patient's Problems in Treating Obesity," *CFP* 23, no. 8 (August 1977): 77. For a current list, see Jeannine Stein, "How to Fight Obesity: New Drugs, Chewing Gum among New Ways to Help Shed Weight Conference Learns," *The Record* [Kitchener], 2 November 2007, D1; Sheena Starky, *The Obesity Epidemic in Canada*, PRB 05–11E (Ottawa: Library of Parliament, 2005), 7, accessed 19 February 2007, https://lop.parl.ca/content/lop/ResearchPublications/prb0511-e.htm; Canadian Institutes of Health Research, *Obesity Research in Canada: Backgrounder* (Ottawa: Canadian Institutes of Health Research, 2004), 1, accessed 19 February 2007, http://www.cihr-irsc.gc.ca/e/20406.html (no longer online). For the quandary, see Andersen and Margolis, "Eating Disorders," 824.

116 For multifactorial, see Christie, *Obesity*, 57; Blundell and McArthur, *Annual Research Reviews*, 1, 58; National Institutes of Health, National Heart, Lung and Blood Institute, and North American Association for the Study of Obesity, *The Practical Guide: Identification, Evaluation and Treatment of Overweight and Obesity in Adults*, NIH Publication no. 00-4084 (Washington, DC: National Institutes of Health, 2000), accessed 15 June 2007, https://www.nhlbi.nih.gov/files/docs/guidelines/prctgd_c.pdf; Wood, *How Fat Works*, 9; John Kalbfleisch, "Fat Accompli," *Weekend Magazine*, 21 August 1976, 3. For no real cause, see Wooley and Wooley, "Obesity and Women – 1," 69.

Chapter 4

1 *CD* 21, no. 6 (June 1955): 98, cartoon. In December 1982 a similar anecdote was placed in the Large as Life newsletter, *The Bolster*. Jenny Ellison, "Let Me Hear Your Body Talk: Aerobics for Fat Women Only, 1981–1985," in *Gender, Health, and Popular Culture Historical Perspectives*, ed. Cheryl Krasnick Warsh (Waterloo, ON: Wilfred Laurier University Press, 2011), 205. The quotation in the title is from Barbara A. Davis and Daniel A.R. Roncari, "Behavourial Treatment of Obesity," *CMAJ* 119, no. 12 (23 December 1978): 1423.

2 William H. Dietz, "The Causes of the Obesity Epidemic in Children" in *Presentation and Poster Abstracts from the International Conference on Physical Activity and Obesity in Children* (Toronto: International Conference, 24–7 June, 2007), 7.

3 Rockefeller University, "Obesity and Metabolism: Why Weight Loss Is Difficult to Sustain," 14 October 2014, accessed 14 October 2014, http://centennial.rucares.org/index/php?page=Weight_Loss. See also Michael I. Goran, "Energy Metabolism and Obesity," *Medical Clinics of North America* 84, no. 2 (March 2000): 347–62, accessed 14 October 2014, https://www.ncbi.nlm.nih.gov/pubmed/10793646; Claude Bouchard, "Is There a Biological Basis for the Obesity Epidemic?" in *Presentation and Poster Abstracts from the International Conference on Physical Activity and Obesity in Children* (Toronto: International Conference, 24–7 June, 2007), 14–16.

4 For the "global epidemic," see Kate Lunau, "Don't Just Sit There," *Maclean's* 126, no. 1 (14 January 2013): 56. For the 2011 report and for Dr Sharma, see Sharon Kirkey, "Obesity Report Panned by Critics as Misleading, Simplistic," *PostMedia News*, 20 June 2011, accessed 9 August 2011, http://www.canada.com/health/obesity+report+panned+critics+misleading+simplistic/4976590/story.html. Others suggest that it doesn't take much activity to hold obesity at bay; see Jesse Singal, "Going from Extremely Lazy to Pretty Lazy Could be Lifesaving," *New York Magazine*, 14 January 2015, accessed 24 January 2015, http://nymag.com/scienceofus/2015/01/sorta-lazy-is-much-healthier-than-extremely-lazy.html.

5 William Osler, *The Principles and Practice of Medicine* (New York: D. Appleton and Co., 1893), 1020; William Osler, *The Principles and Practice of Medicine*, 8th ed. (New York: D. Appleton and Co., 1912), 451.

6 "The Physical Education of Girls," *CMAJ* 12, no. 11 (November 1922): 816. For age, see Maurice Boigny, "Effets physiologiques et l'exercice," *UMC* 59, no. 7 (juillet 1921): 287; and George S. Young, "The Relations between

Periodic Health Examinations and Improper Living Habits," *OMR* 2, no. 2 (March 1935): 43.
7 For the obese, see W. Ford Connell, "Review of 'On the Control of Obesity' by A.H. Douthwaite," *CMAJ* 31, no. 6 (December 1934): 688. For exercise for the dieter, see R. Tait McKenzie, *Exercise in Education and Medicine*, 3rd ed. (Philadelphia and London: W.B. Saunders Co., 1923), 533, 540, 543.
8 W.F. Christie, *Ideal Weight: A Practical Handbook for Patients* (London: William Heinemann Ltd., 1938), 103. For increasing appetite, see CMA, "What Should I Weigh?" *Maclean's* 43, no. 2 (15 January 1930): 44; and R. L. Alsaker, "It's Always Wrong to Be Fat," *Maclean's* 35, no. 11 (1 June 1922): 40, reprint. For firming, see Grant Fleming, "Calories and Vitamins," *Maclean's* 44, no. 21 (1 November 1931): 34.
9 For not using up energy, see D.E. Rodger, J. Grant McFetridge, and Eileen Price, "The Management of Obesity," *ManMR* 30, no. 5 (May 1950): 295; F.S. Brien, "Obesity – Treatment," *OMR* 20, no. 4 (April 1953): 227; Elizabeth Chant Robertson, *Nutrition for Today* (Toronto: McClelland & Stewart, 1951), 184. For increasing appetite, see Edward H. Rynearson and Clifford F. Gastineau, *Obesity*, American Lecture Series, no. 36, American Lectures in Endocrinology (Springfield, IL: Charles C. Thomas, 1949), 104; W.H. Sebrell Jr, "Effects of Obesity on Health: Metabolic Facts and Fallacies," *MMC* 13, no. 5 (May 1958): 190; Paul Dumas, "Le traitement de l'obésité," *UMC* 87, no. 11 (novembre 1958): 1367. For health problems, see Hugo R. Rony, *Obesity and Leanness* (Philadelphia: Lea & Febiger, 1940), 266. For older people, see "Review of *You Don't Have to Exercise! Rest Begins at Forty* by Peter J. Steincrohm," *CD* 9, no. 1 (January 1943): 44; Jean Grignon, "L'obésité et la maigreur," *UMC* 81, no. 11 (novembre 1952): 1310.
10 Rodger, McFetridge, and Price, "The Management of Obesity," 266. Quote from "In the Waiting Room," *CD* 6, no. 10 (October 1940): 70. For humour about patients rejecting exercise, see *CD* 6, no. 5 (May 1940): 22.
11 Morton Hunt, "Exercise is the Bunk – Relax," *Maclean's* 63, no. 8 (15 April 1950): 24, 41; Sidney Katz, "Are We Eating Too Much?" *Maclean's* 68, no. 12 (11 June 1955): 14; Josephine Lowman, "Tubby Hubby Diet: Don't Count on Exercise to Reduce," *Globe and Mail*, 21 March 1952, 15; Josephine Lowman, "Why Grow Old? Hubby Hollow Chested? He May Need Exercise," *Globe and Mail*, 8 July 1952, 11.
12 For 5BX and 10BX, see chapter 3 of this volume. For ParticipACTION, see Peggy Edwards, "No Country Mouse: Thirty Years of Effective Marketing and Health Communications," *CJPH* 95, suppl. 2 (May/June 2004): S6–S13; Victoria Lamb Drover, "ParticipACTION, Healthism and the Crafting of a Social Memory (1971–1999)," *Journal of the Canadian Historical*

Association, n.s., 25, no. 1 (2014): 277–306. For emphasis on fitness in the 1970s, see CBC-TV, "Mandatory Fitness in Manitoba," *What's New*, 25 May 1978, accessed 9 February 2016, http://www.cbc.ca/archives/entry/mandatory-fitness-in-manitoba; "Your Move," *CN* 73, no. 6 (June 1977): 42; E. Lee Macnamara, "Fitting Nursing into Fitness," *CN* 76, no. 4 (April 1980): 33–5; John Robertson, "You Know the 60-year-old Swede Who's Fitter Than a 30-Year-Old Canadian? To Hell with Him," *Maclean's* 90, no. 12 (13 June 1977): 70. For Marc Lalonde, see "Introduction," in *Obesity in Canada: Critical Perspectives*, ed. Jenny Ellison, Deborah McPhail, and Wendy Mitchinson (Toronto: University of Toronto Press, 2016), 7.

13 For Slim Jym, see *Chatelaine* 43, no. 1 (January 1970): 62, advertisement. For spas, see Eveleen Dollery, "Body-Job," *Chatelaine* 42, no. 6 (June 1969): 38.

14 For support for exercise leading to weight loss, see Bonnie Cornell, "Chatelaine's FAB Diet," *Chatelaine* 48, no. 1 (January 1975): 46; Peter Elson, "Chatelaine's Fitness Plan for Women," *Chatelaine* 49, no. 1 (January 1976): 1–2. For being overweight and fit, see Ethel Gillingham, "Who Says Anyone Can Lose Weight?" *Chatelaine* 34, no. 6 (June 1961): 69.

15 Wilfred Leith, "Experiences with the Pennington Diet and the Royal Victoria Hospital, Montreal," *CMAJ* 84, no. 25 (24 June 1961): 1411; "Fit! Fat! Fad!" *Health* 32, no. 5 (October 1964): 22, advertisement for Sun Life; *Maclean's* 76, no. 22 (16 November 1963): 6, advertisement for Metropolitan Life Insurance Co.; L. Lee Coyne, "'A Positive Attitude to Health': The Role of Physical Education," *ManMR* 46, no. 4 (April 1966): 246; Davis and Roncari, "Behavioural Treatment of Obesity," 1423; *Health* 38, no. 4 (Winter 1972/1973): 29, advertisement for PreSate; "Cycling for Fitness and Fun," *CN* 67, 9 (September 1971): 53; André Boyer, "Le troisième congrès international de l'obésité," *UMC* 109, no. 11 (novembre 1980): 1667; Walter Kempner et al., "Losing Weight Need Not Be Unpleasant," *MMC* 31, no. 9 (October 1976): 942; M. Kindl and Peggy Brown, "Effective Treatment of Obesity in the Community," *CFP* 23, no. 6 (June 1977): 79. For support of exercise as a weight-loss method, see John A. Carmichael, "Psychological Methods of Obesity Reduction in Adolescent Girls" (PhD diss., University of Victoria, 1975), 29.

16 D.R. Wilson, "Current Drug Therapy: Drugs for Obesity," *CMAJ* 91, no. 26 (26 December 1964): 1369; J.B. Firstbrook, "What Physical Fitness Can Do for You," *Health* 31, no. 3 (June 1963): 17; Sandy Keir, "Keynote Address 2," *CJPH* 67, suppl. 2 (September/October 1976): 27–30. Bert L. Fairbanks, "Exercise, Nutrition and Obesity," *Health* 44, no. 1 (Spring 1978): 25. For supporters of exercises, see Jean Mayer, "Overweight and Exercise," *Health* 42, no. 2 (Summer 1976): 8.

17 For massage and hydrotherapy, see Edward H. Mason, "The Treatment of Obesity," *CMAJ* 14, no. 11 (November 1924): 1052. See also J.R. Pepin, "L'obésité est-elle réductible?" *UMC* 58, no. 5 (mai 1929): 266. For electricity, see Thomas McCrae, ed., *The Principles and Practice of Medicine*, 9th ed. (New York: D. Appleton and Co., 1920), 442.

18 For Renulife Violet Ray, see *Maclean's* 33, no. 3 (15 February 1920): 72, advertisement. For soap, see *The Chatelaine* 2, no. 1 (January 1929): 44, advertisement for Osmos. For the belt, see *Maclean's* 39, no. 6 (15 March 1926): 46, advertisement. It is unclear whether tightening the belt was reducing weight. For the roller, see *The Chatelaine* 1, no. 9 (November 1928): 52, advertisement. For the corset, see *Maclean's* 50, no. 19 (1 October 1937): 52, advertisement for Beasley Reducing Corset.

19 Gordon Sinclair, "I'm Reducing," *Maclean's* 58, no. 1 (1 January 1945): 43. For the steam bath, see *Eaton's Catalogue*, Spring/Summer 1959, 279. For the Relax-A-Cisor, see *Chatelaine* 32, no. 1 (January 1959): 52, advertisement. For purchasing exercise machines, see Barbara Moon, "Can You Loaf Your Way to a Better Figure?" *Maclean's* 72, no. 3 (1 January 1959): 16. For salons, see *Chatelaine* 32, no. 7 (July 1959): 77, advertisement for Stauffer Salon.

20 *CN* 45, no. 5 (May 1949): 328, advertisement for Spencer Supports; *CD* 14, no. 10 (October 1948): 26, advertisement for Camp Support; *CMAJ* 76, no. 1 (1 January 1957): 56, advertisement for Camp Support.

21 For Exercycle, see *Health* 28, no. 4 (August 1960): 4, advertisement. For shapers, see Eveleen Dollery, "Keep in Trim the Beauty-Spa Way," *Chatelaine* 38, no. 9 (September 1965): 136. For belt massage, see *Eaton's Catalogue*, Spring/Summer 1968, 333.

22 *Maclean's* 81, no. 11 (November 1968): 62, advertisement for i-sometric-isotonic. For "exercise" in no time, see *Maclean's* 91, no. 5 (6 March 1978): 45, advertisement for Synometrics.

23 For staplepuncture, see Bonnie Cornell "Diet by Ear," *Chatelaine* 48, no. 4 (April 1970): 10.

24 *CD* 46, no. 1 (January 1980): 18, cartoon; Robertson, "You Know the 60-Year-Old Swede," 70; Drover, "ParticipACTION," 289. For cold environment, see W.J. O'Hara, C. Allen, and R.J. Shepard, "Treatment of Obesity by Exercise in the Cold," *CMAJ* 117, no. 3 (8 October 1977): 786. For Friedman, see John Hofsess, "How to Survive Middle Age," *Maclean's* 86, no. 10 (October 1973): 37.

25 Keith Walden, "The Road to Fat City: An Interpretation of the Development of Weight Consciousness in Western Society," *Historical Reflections/Réflexions historiques* 12, no. 3 (1985): 341.

26 For stages, see Lee F. Monaghan, *Men and the War on Obesity: A Sociological Study* (London: Routledge, 2008), 76, 80–1. For Sharma, see Arya M. Sharma, "Why Diet and Exercise Is Not a Treatment for Obesity," Dr. Sharma's Obesity Notes, 20 June 2011, accessed 9 August 2011, http://www.drsharma.ca/obesity-why-diet-and-exercise-is-not-a-treatment-for-obesity.

27 Hillel Schwartz, *Never Satisfied: A Cultural History of Diets, Fantasies and Fat* (London: Collier Macmillan Publishers, 1986), 17–18, 21, 37. For the meaning of diet, see Peter N. Stearns, *Fat History: Bodies and Beauty in the Modern West*, rev. ed. (New York: New York University Press, 2002), 6. For men, see Katharina Vester, "Regime Change: Gender, Class, and the Invention of Dieting in Post-Bellum America," *Journal of Social History* 44, no. 1 (Fall 2010): 46. For women, see Kerry Segrave, *Obesity in America, 1850–1939: A History of Social Attitudes and Treatment* (Jefferson, NC: McFarland & Co., 2008), chapter 4, 48–70.

28 Osler, *The Principles and Practice of Medicine* (1893), 1020. For today, see Kris Gunnars, "23 Studies on Low-Carb and Low-Fat Diets – Time to Retire the Fad," *Healthline*, 22 June 2017, accessed 12 September 2017, https://www.healthline.com/nutrition/23-studies-on-low-carb-and-low-fat-diets/. Studies found that low-carb diets result in more weight loss.

29 "The Menace of Obesity," *CMAJ* 16, no. 1 (January 1926): 1373–4.

30 Mason, "The Treatment of Obesity," 1052–3.

31 Thomas McCrae, ed., *The Principles and Practice of Medicine*, 10th ed. (New York: D. Appleton and Co., 1925), 445–6. For 1924 legislation, see L.I. Pugsley, "The Administration and Development of Federal Statutes on Foods and Drugs in Canada," *MSJ* 23, no. 3 (March 1967): 410. On saccharin, see Carolyn de la Peña, *Empty Pleasures: The Story of Artificial Sweeteners from Saccharin to Splenda* (Chapel Hill, NC: University of North Carolina Press, 2010). For the uselessness of saccharin, see James M. Rippe and Weight Watchers, *Weight Loss That Lasts: Break Through the 10 Big Diet Myths* (Hoboken, NJ: John Wiley & Sons, 2005), 108.

32 Lulu Hunt Peters, "If You Are Obese, Shrink Your Stomach," *CN* 19, no. 5 (May 1923): 287.

33 For bad and good diets, see "Overweight and Longevity," *CMAJ* 23, no. 2 (August 1930): 160; Walter R. Campbell, "Obesity and Its Treatment," *CMAJ* 34, no. 1 (January 1936): 42–4, 48.

34 For a good diet, see Hugh Grant Rowell, "Eating," *Maclean's* 48, no. 4 (15 February 1935): 50. For the warnings, see CMA, "What Should I Weigh?" 44. For the popularity of fasting, see Marcella, "Slimness by Way of the

Kitchen," *CM* (February 1930): 22. For extremes, see Fleming, "Calories and Vitamins," 34.

35 For food to avoid, see Lennox G. Bell, "The Trials of Obesity," *ManMR* 20, no. 8 (August 1940): 144; A. Keenberg, "Obesity and Its Treatment," *ManMR* 27, no. 5 (May 1947): 280. For the uselessness of cutting down carbohydrates, see Rippe and Weight Watchers, *Weight Loss That Lasts*, 111.

36 H.I. Cramer, "Physiological Considerations of the Etiology and Treatment of Obesity," *CMAJ* 55, no. 5 (November 1946): 507–8. For a more positive view of the 400- to 600-calorie diet, see Rony, *Obesity and Leanness*, 244. For support of hospitalization, see Editorial, "Overnutrition," *CMAJ* 49, no. 1 (July 1943): 53.

37 For calories, see W.W. Bauer, "The Bread You Eat," *CN* 54, no. 2 (February 1958): 152; Brien, "Obesity – Treatment," 227; "Weight Reduction," *MMC* 10, no. 7 (July 1955): 120. For fat, see Reta Wright, "Cream on Your Diet," *CHJ* 50, no. 7 (November 1953): 6. Wright was referencing her doctor when disparaging fat in food.

38 For the 1956 survey and other options, see Barbara A. McLaren, "Nutritional Control of Overweight," *CJPH* 58, no. 11 (November 1967): 484–5. For more on studies, see Rodger, McFetridge, and Price, "The Management of Obesity," 265–9.

39 Sinclair, "I'm Reducing," 40, 43; James Bannerman, "They Used to Call Me Fatty," *Maclean's* 62, no. 4 (15 February 1949): 22, 30–2. Bannerman was a pseudonym for John Charles Kirkpatrick McNaught, accessed 7 June 2017, http://archives.mcmaster.ca/index.php/james-bannerman-fonds. For men in the United States, see Jesse Berrett, "Feeding the Organization Men: Diet and Masculinity in Postwar America," *Journal of Social History* 30, no. 4 (Summer 1997): 805–25.

40 For cutting back calories, see Canada, Department of National Health and Welfare, Nutrition Division, "A Study in Frustration: The Diagnosis and Treatment of Obesity, Part II," *Canadian Nutrition Notes* 19, no. 9 (1963): 100. For more small meals, see S.S.B. Gilder, "The London Letter: Frequent Meals and Obesity," *CMAJ* 94, no. 25 (18 June 1966): 1321.

41 Dean H. Lockwood and Simeon Margolis, "Obesity," in *The Principles and Practice of Medicine*, 19th ed., ed. A. McGehee Harvey et al. (New York: Appleton-Century Crofts, 1976), 1030.

42 For restricted diet vs fasting, see Charles G. Roland, "Editorial: Some Recent Studies of Obesity," *CFP* 14, no. 2 (February 1968): 4. For fasting, see A. Rapoport et al., "Some Studies in Starvation," *CMAJ* 90, no. 7 (15 February 1964): 485.

43 Leith, "Experiences with the Pennington Diet," 1411. For percentages on dieting, see F. Gerard Allison, "Modern Treatment of Obesity," *ManMR* 40, no. 7 (August–September 1960): 511.
44 For "long-range" plan, see Wilson, "Current Drug Therapy," 1369. For "lifelong problem," see Kenneth G. Rothwell, "A Review of the Overweight Problem," *CFP* 14, no. 2 (February 1968): 13, 14. For addiction, see Patrick Vinay et al., "Obésité: revue générale," *UMC* 98, no. 5 (mai 1969): 796.
45 Iva L. Armstrong and Barbara McLaren, "'We Are What We Eat': Proper Choice of Food Can Make the Difference," *Health* 30, no. 5 (October 1962): 14.
46 D.R., "Pour prévenir l'obésité: information et education précoce," *CMAJ* 120, no. 7 (7 April 1979): 873.
47 Auréa Cormier, "Group versus Individual Dietary Instruction in the Treatment of Obesity," *CJPH* 63, no. 4 (July/August 1972): 327, 331. For mechanism, see *CMAJ* 102, no. 2 (31 January 1970): 118–19, advertisement for Vimicon.
48 Fairbanks, "Exercise, Nutrition and Obesity," 25.
49 Virginia Lea, "Eating Off Weight," *CM* 72, no. 4 (October 1929): 42; Virginia Lea, "Join the Slimmers," *CM* 73 (May 1930): 21. For more on the 18-day diet, see "Eighteen-Day Diet for Reducing Is Spreading and Has Hit Sycamore," *True Republican*, 21 August 1929, Illinois Digital Newspaper Collection, accessed 18 July 2015, http://idnc.library.illinois.edu/; "'18 Day Reducing Diet' Disowned by Mayo Clinic," *Chicago Tribune*, 10 July 1929, 34, accessed 18 July 2015, http://chicagotribune.newspapers.com/.
50 Marcella, "Slimness by Way of the Kitchen," 22.
51 "Topics of Current Interest," *CMAJ* 32, no. 4 (April 1935): 451, reprint from *JAMA* (2 February 1935). For more on William Howard Hay, see Walter Gratzer, *Terrors of the Table: The Curious History of Nutrition* (Oxford: Oxford University Press, 2005), 198.
52 *CD* 7, no. 11 (November 1941): 78, humour anecdote. For "racketeers," see Bell, "The Trials of Obesity," 144. See also L.B. Pett, "Food Fads and Fancies," *CHW* 2, no. 5 (February 1947): 5. For the milk days, see Henry A. Christian, ed., *The Principles and Practice of Medicine*, 16th ed. (New York: D. Appleton-Century Co., 1947), 606.
53 A. Corinne Trerice, "Slimming Can Be Healthy or Hazardous," *Health* 23, no. 3 (May/June 1955): 18. For superstition, etc., see A. Corinne Trerice, "Food Fads at Face Value," *Health* 23, no. 5 (September/October 1955): 14–15.
54 Library and Archives Canada, Department of Health, RG 29, Nutrition Division, 1921–1971, vol. 934, file 386, 5–4, part 1, Nutrition Services,

Foods, Request for Special Dietary Foods, August 1956–63, Letter from Mrs B., 2 July 1959.
55 Katz, "Are We Eating Too Much?," 14, 93, 95.
56 E.W. McHenry, "Canadian Women Are Too Fat," *Chatelaine* 33, no. 6 (June 1960): 50; Lawrence Galton, "A New Look at Reducing Diets," *Chatelaine* 33, no. 11 (November 1960): 13.
57 For snack diet, see "Shape Up '68: *Chatelaine*'s New Snack Diet," *Chatelaine* 41, no. 1 (January 1968): 29. For the thinking woman's diet, see Rebecca Hawke, "The Thinking Woman's Diet," *Chatelaine* 42, no. 11 (November 1969): 46–7, 109–10. For the *Diet Cook Book*, see *Chatelaine* 42, no. 12 (December 1969): 67, advertisement. For the Queen's diet, see Dennis Eisenberg, "How the Queen Diets," *Chatelaine* 44, no. 3 (March 1971): 28–9, 61–2. For many others, see Margaret A. Wood, "The Slob Diet & Exercise Program: Or, How I Lost 30 Pounds in Just 1,001 Days," *Chatelaine* 50, no. 7 (July 1977): 22, 78–9; Cornell, "Chatelaine's FAB Diet," 44–6, 60; Ellen Roseman, "Alternatives: The Wages of Fat," *Weekend Magazine* 26 (17 April 1976): 23; Margaret Allan, "The British Quick Milk Diet," *Chatelaine* 48, no. 11 (November 1975): 28–9, 128–30; Zalman Amit and E. Ann Sutherland, "Stay Slim for Good," *Chatelaine* 49, no. 7 (July 1976): 24, 28, 74–6.
58 Eric Hutton, "The One Weight-Control System That Works Every Time," *Maclean's* 74, no. 14 (15 July 1961): 8; Bob Blackburn, "Eat, Drink...and Feel Smug," *Maclean's* 79, no. 5 (5 March 1966): 22; Sidney Katz, "Drab-Food and No-Food Diets," *Maclean's* 81, no. 12 (December 1968): 80.
59 For Pennington's diet, see Leith, "Experiences with the Pennington Diet," 1412.
60 Barbara Croft, "LP (Liquid Program) Diet," *Chatelaine* 39, no. 2 (February 1966): 17–19. For letters, see "Readers Report on Losing Weight with Liquids," *Chatelaine* 39, no. 5 (May 1966): 108.
61 Greg Critser, *Fat Land: How Americans Became the Fattest People in the World* (Boston, New York: Mariner Books, 2004), 49–50.
62 Roseman, "Alternatives: The Wages of Fat," 23. For quackery, see Jelia C. Witschi and Frederick J. Stare, "Nutrition Quackery: 'Bigger Fraud in the Health Field,'" *Health* 40, no. 1 (Spring 1974): 25.
63 *CN* 20, no. 2 (February 1924): 122, advertisement for Nujol dressing. For Bovril, see *Maclean's* 42, no. 22 (15 November 1929): 87, advertisement. For Tillson's bran, see *The Chatelaine* 1, no. 3 (May 1928): 44, advertisement. For salts, see *Maclean's* 45, no. 12 (15 June 1932): 56, advertisement. For more on salts, see Carvell MacIntosh, "Quackery in Medicine," *DMJ* 3, no. 3 (November 1938): 31. For Standard Brands, see *Chatelaine* 10, no. 2

(February 1937): 29, advertisement. For gender in Standard Brands, see *CHJ* 34, no. 7 (November 1937): 29, advertisement.
64 *Chatelaine* 30, no. 4 (April 1957): 96, advertisement for Vita-Thin.
65 Ian Mosby, "'Food Will Win the War': The Politics and Culture of Food and Nutrition during the Second World War" (PhD diss., York University, 2011), 266.
66 For diet foods, see *CMAJ* 77, no. 7 (15 July 1957): 176, advertisement for Kraft skim milk cheese; *Chatelaine* 32, no. 10 (October 1959): 124, advertisement for E.D. Smith low-calorie spreads. For D-Zerta ads, see *CD* 22, no. 8 (August 1956): 26; *CD* 23, no. 7 (July 1957): 32. For cyclamate sodium, see *Health* 27, no. 1 (January/February 1959): 24; *Chatelaine* 31, no. 1 (January 1958): 27; *MMC* 13, no. 12 (December 1958): 118; *CHJ* 54, no. 8 (December 1957): 53. For Sucaryl, see "Sugar Substitute," *CN* 46, no. 10 (October 1950): 836–7; "New Product, Sucaryl Sodium," *ManMR* 30, no. 8 (October 1950): 570.
67 L.S. White, "Weight Watchers Brighten Meals with Special Diets," *Health* 27, no. 1 (January/February 1959): 12. For medical support of Sucaryl, see Brien, "Obesity – Treatment," 227. On sweeteners, see Thomas Land, "See 'No Risk' in Food Sweeteners," *Financial Post*, 21 May 1966, 23, and Canada's investigation of them. For legislation, see John Rosseel, "What Would You Do?" *Financial Post*, 9 May 1970, 6. See also de la Peña, *Empty Pleasures*; Bee Wilson, *Swindled: The Dark History of Food Fraud, from Poisoned Candy to Counterfeit Coffee* (Princeton, NJ: Princeton University Press, 2008), 242–7.
68 For cyclamate, see Calorie Control Council, "Cyclamate," accessed 3 February 2016, https://caloriecontrol.org/cyclamate/. Cyclamates were also "acquitted" in the United States. Deal Edell, *Eat, Drink and Be Merry: Doctor Tells You Why the Health Experts Are Wrong* (New York: Quill, 2000), 25.
69 For those who shouldn't diet, see Mason, "The Treatment of Obesity," 1052–3; Campbell, "Obesity and Its Treatment," 42; A.E. Fowler, "Diets," *CN* 29, no. 4 (April 1933): 179–80; Cramer, "Physiological Considerations," 507–8. For a more positive view of the 400- 600-calorie diet, see Rony, *Obesity and Leanness*, 244. For support of hospitalization, see Editorial, "Overnutrition," 53.
70 W. Ford Connell, "Adiposity and Atherosclerosis," *CMAJ* 70, no. 3 (March 1954): 252. Henry W. Brosin, "Psychiatric Aspects of Obesity," *MMC* 10, no. 2 (February 1955): 106. For diets for different people, see "Review of *The Special Diet Cook Book*," *CN* 49, no. 3 (March 1953): 205.
71 L. Bradley Pett, "Public Health, Ottawa Newsletter...Appetite and Obesity," *CMAJ* 76, no. 12 (15 June 1957): 1083. See also Chant Robertson, *Nutrition for Today*, 185.

72 For Stillman, see Irwin Stillman and Samm Sinclair Baker, *The Doctor's Quick Weight Loss Diet* (New York and Tokyo: Ishi Press, 2011 [first published 1967]). For quote, see Carole Spitzack, *Confessing Excess: Women and the Politics of Body Redemption* (Albany, NY: State University of New York Press, 1990), 22. Carol Cooper remembers the popularity of Stillman's diet.
73 "Those Liquid Diets," *Health* 43, no. 4 (Winter 1977/1978): 26; see also "High Mortality Linked with Liquid Protein Diets," *CFP* 24, no. 8 (August 1978): 743. For forty deaths, see CP, "Liquid Protein Diet Fad Losing Popularity since Link with 40 Deaths Cited," *Globe and Mail*, 15 February 1979, T5.
74 Kaspars Dzeguze, "A Lean and Hungry Look," *Maclean's* 91, no. 15 (24 July 1978): 28–38.
75 For reducing as a "fetish," see R.W. Shepherd, "Diets Be Damned: Eat, Drink and Be Merry for Your Body Knows Best," *Maclean's* 83, no. 12 (December 1970): 66. For irritability, etc., see David M. Garner et al., "Cultural Expectations of Thinness in Women," *Psychological Reports* 47, no. 2 (1980): 490. For charlatans, see "Most Diabetics Can Be Handled by Diet: MD," *CFP* 22, no. 12 (December 1976): 25. For crash diets, see J. Edgar Monagle, "Malnutrition Can Lead to Accidents," *Health* 43, no. 4 (Winter 1977/1978): 14–15.
76 For Hollenberg, see "Problems of Obesity Said Frustrating to Doctor and Patient," *CMAJ* 112, no. 3 (8 February 1975): 350. For a list of reasons for its futility, see D.L. Keegan, "The Doctor's and the Patient's Problems in Treating Obesity," *CFP* 23, no. 8 (August 1977): 76. For Winick, see Linda Oglov, "Canadian Dietetic Association Delegates at Annual Meeting Study Relationship of Diet to Exercise," *CMAJ* 117, no. 3 (6 August 1977): 290.
77 Errol B. Marliss, "Protein Diets for Obesity: Metabolic and Clinical Aspects," *CMAJ* 119, no. 12 (23 December 1978): 1413.
78 National Institutes of Health, National Heart, Lung and Blood Institute, and North American Association for the Study of Obesity, *The Practical Guide: Identification, Evaluation and Treatment of Overweight and Obesity in Adults*, NIH Publication no. 00-4084 (Washington, DC: National Institutes of Health, 2000), 3, accessed 15 June 2007, https://www.nhlbi.nih.gov/files/docs/guidelines/prctgd_c.pdf.
79 Campbell, "Obesity and Its Treatment," 43, 44, 48; Keenberg, "Obesity and Its Treatment," 281.
80 On psychiatry, see Leona Crabb, "Minor Tranquilizing Drugs and the Medicalization of Everyday Life in English-Speaking Canada, 1945–1962" (PhD diss., Carleton University, 1997), 56; G.H. Stevenson, "Report on the Formation of the Canadian Psychiatric Association," *CMAJ* 65 (December

1951): 592–4. In 1951, the CPA had only 185 active members. See Isabel Dickson, "The Canadian Psychiatric Association, 1951–1958," *CJP* 25, no. 1 (February 1980): 89; see also Quentin Rae-Grant, *Psychiatry in Canada: 50 Years (1951 to 2001)* (Ottawa: Canadian Psychiatric Association, 2001).

81 Daniel Cappon, "Review Article, Obesity," *CMAJ* 79, no. 7 (1 October 1958): 573. For psychotherapy, see Rodger, McFetridge, and Price, "The Management of Obesity," 266; Brosin, "Psychiatric Aspects of Obesity," 106; Brien, "Obesity – Treatment," 227. For support of psychotherapy and the emotional origin of obesity, see Grignon, "L'obésité et la maigreur," 1310.

82 Pett, "Public Health, Ottawa Newsletter," 1083. For charts and tests, see Brosin, "Psychiatric Aspects of Obesity," 106. For group therapy, see "The Handicaps of Overweight," *CN* 48, no. 11 (November 1952): 932. For conditioning and the Faculty Food Services, see McLaren, "Nutritional Control of Overweight," 483. For psychiatry/psychology in the United States, see Berrett, "Feeding the Organization Men," 817.

83 Leith, "Experiences with the Pennington Diet," 1411; Doris L. Hirsch and W.I. Morse, "Emotional and Metabolic Factors in Obesity," *CJPH* 51, no. 1 (November 1960): 455; Vinay et al., "Obésité," 795.

84 For Biphetamine (Resin Complexes of d- and dl-Amphetamine) see *CMAJ* 94, no.21 (2 May 1966): 28, advertisement. For Ionamin (Phentermine Resin), see *CMAJ* 93, no. 18 (30 October 1965): 17, advertisement. For others in the *CMAJ*, see 87, no. 8 (25 August 1962): 16, advertisement for Desbutal Gradmet; 94, no. 4 (22 January 1966): 22, advertisement for Eskatrol Spansule; 94, no. 15 (9 April 1966): 14, advertisement for Ionamin; 94, no. 16 (16 April 1966): 23, advertisement for Biphetamine-T.

85 For the optimistic view, see S.S.B. Gilder, "Health Education about Obesity," *CMAJ* 95, no. 2 (9 July 1966): 81. For agreement on psychological/psychiatric issues causing obesity, see "Review of *The Thin Book of a Formerly Fat Psychiatrist* by Theodore Isaac Rubin," *CD* 32, no. 6 (June 1966): 73. See also Wilson, "Current Drug Therapy," 1369; Vinay et al., "Obésité," 789.

86 Kenneth Clute, *The General Practitioner: A Study of Medical Education and Practice in Ontario and Nova Scotia* (Toronto: University of Toronto Press, 1963), 307, 353.

87 For electroshock, see "Shocked Out of Fat," *Chatelaine* 39, no. 9 (September 1966): 17; see also Barbara Frum, "They Learn to 'Cure' Themselves with Shock," *Maclean's* 79, no. 22 (19 November 1966): 24–5, 44–5. For hypnosis, see F.W. Hanley, "The Treatment of Obesity by Individual and Group Hypnosis," *CJP* 12 (1967): 549–51; for hypnosis in the 1970s, see

Steven Crainford, "Role of Hypnosis in Medical Practice," *OMR* 45, no. 11 (November 1978): 523.
88 Daniel Cappon, *Eating, Loving and Dying: A Psychology of Appetites* (Toronto: University of Toronto Press, 1973), 99; Daniel Cappon, "Deliver Us from the Evil of Fat," *Maclean's* 86, no. 7 (July 1973): 32–3, 44.
89 For Breitman, see Oglov, "Canadian Dietetic Association Delegates," 290. For a discussion of psychiatric treatment, see Louise A. Demers-Desrosiers, "Considérations psychiatriques sur l'obésité et l'anorexie," *UMC* 107, no. 6 (juin 1978): 575–6, 578–9, 582.
90 For counselling, see P.M. Crockford and P.A. Salmon, "Hormones and Obesity: Changes in Insulin and Growth Hormone Secretion," *CMAJ* 103, no. 2 (18 July 1970): 147. For daily trips, see Helen Christie, "Obesity Is a Major Topic of Papers at Annual Scientific Meeting of OMA," *CMAJ* 108, no. 12 (23 June 1973): 1549. For the optimists, see S.S.B. Gilder, "Mental Changes in Fasting Patients," *CMAJ* 105, no. 5 (4 September 1971): 460.
91 For behaviour therapy, see Sidney Katz, "Advance Report on Behavior Therapy: A New, Simpler, Faster Way to Treat Mental Trouble," *Maclean's* 76, no. 14 (27 July 1963): 14, 40–2. For tricks, see Eveleen Dollery, "3 Dazzling Diet Successes," *Chatelaine* 36, no. 4 (April 1963): 40–5. See also Eveleen Dollery, "Three Diet Winners Discover New Beauty," *Chatelaine* 37, no. 4 (April 1964): 30–5. For addiction treatment and Bell, see Jim Hartford, "Now Gluttons Can Take the Pledge, Too," *Maclean's* 79, no. 6 (19 March 1966): 4. For group therapy, see Ann Austen, "Diet Clubs Share Their Weight Losing Secrets," *Chatelaine* 42, no. 2 (February 1969): 67.
92 For twenty types of behaviour modification, see John Raeburn and Joan Soler, "Behavior Therapy Approach to Psychiatric Disorder," *CN* 67, no. 10 (October 1971): 36; Davis and Roncari, "Behavourial Treatment of Obesity," 1423, 1425.
93 For support of behaviour modification, see Léo Boyer, André Boyer, et Pierre Biron, "Contrôle global de l'obésité: résultats chez 1225 patients après 5 ans," *UMC* 106, no. 6 (juin 1977): 887; "Treatment of Obese Can Prove Disastrous," *BCMJ* 15, no. 2 (February 1973): 48-C; Anthony W. Myers and David L. Yeung, "Obesity in Infants: Significance, Aetiology, and Prevention," *CJPH* 70, no. 2 (March/April 1979):117. For Mrs G., see Madeleine Levason, "The New 'Behaviorist' Diet," *Chatelaine* 45, no. 9 (September 1972): 66, 108–11.
94 Robert Pool, *Fat: Fighting the Obesity Epidemic* (New York: Oxford University Press, 2001), 218.
95 Betty Thomas, "Interviewing the Patient about Diets," *CN* 56, no. 11 (November 1960): 987; *Maclean's* 74, no. 17 (26 August 1961): 24, cartoon.

96 For TOPS, OA, and Weight Watchers, see Sarah Henry, "A Consumer's Guide to Diet Clubs in Canada: Battling Obesity with Moral Support and Guidance," *CMAJ* 119, no. 12 (23 December 1978): 1434. For TOPS, see David Lewis Stein, "How Some Fat Women Shame Pounds Off Each Other," *Maclean's* 74, no. 8 (22 April 1961): 91; Kae McColl, "TOPS... to Take Off Pounds," *CHJ* 54, no. 7 (November 1957): 24–5, 41–2. For tricks, see McColl, "TOPS," 41. For membership, see A. Cornacchia, "A Layman's View of Group Therapy in Weight Control," *CJPH* 58, no. 11 (November 1967): 505.

97 Beverley A. Burgess, "You Don't Have to Be Fat," CMAJ 107, no. 3 (5 August 1972): 193. For medical support of these organizations, see Anne B. Kenshole, "Weight and Diabetes," CFP 18, no. 2 (February 1972): 43; Ruth Sky, "Watching Your Weight – and Other People's – in Group Therapy," CFP 18, no. 2 (February 1972): 48.

98 For smaller groups, see Henry, "A Consumer's Guide to Diet Clubs in Canada," 1434. In Montreal, see D.R., "Pour les obèses: cesser de manger avec compulsion," *CMAJ* 120, no. 3 (3 February 1979): 369. For evaluation of clinics, see D.R., "Pour prévenir l'obésité," 873.

99 For TOPS and men, see Cornacchia, "A Layman's View of Group Therapy in Weight Control," 507; Julia Elwell, "How Harvey Tipped the Scales to Success," *Montreal Gazette*, 16 February 1980, 45.

100 Roslyn Nudell, "Fat Teen-Agers Suffering," *Winnipeg Free Press*, 11 June 1980, 29.

101 "Weight Watchers Introduce Canadian Family Meal Plan," *Health* 38, no. 3 (Fall 1972): 12–13. On Weight Watchers, see W. Gifford-Jones, "Shut Up and Pass the Baked Alaska," *Maclean's* 88, no. 6 (June 1975): 78. For the history of Weight Watchers in the United States, see Joyce Hendley, "Weight Watchers at Forty: A Celebration," *Gastronomica* 3, no. 1 (February 2003): 16–21.

102 For Stuart, see *Health* 44, no. 3 (Autumn 1978): back cover, advertisement. For references to the "behavioral modification," see *Health* 45, no. 1 (Spring 1979): inside back cover, advertisement. On Stuart's program, see Richard B. Stuart and Barbara Davis, *Slim Chance in a Fat World: Behavioral Control of Obesity* (Champaign, IL: Research Press Company, 1972), 25, 27; and Richard B. Stuart, *Act Thin, Stay Thin: New Ways to Lose Weight and Keep It Off* (New York: W.W. Norton & Company, 1978). Stuart wrote the latter book while working as a psychological director for Weight Watchers.

103 For the Personal Exercise Plan, see *Health* 45, no. 2 (Summer 1979): inside back cover, advertisement.

104 For Counterweight, see *Health* 39, no. 2 (Summer 1973): 2, advertisement. For the menu, see Bonnie Cornell, "Weight Watchers *New* Diet," *Chatelaine* 50, no. 2 (February 1977): 48. For newer menus, see *Health* 46, no. 4 (Winter 1980/1981): back cover, advertisement. For the national association, see "Weight Watchers Introduce Canadian Family Meal Plan," 13.

105 For self-acceptance, see "Obesity in Children Equally Intractable," *CMAJ* 112, no. 3 (8 February 1975): 350. For psychological support, see "Controversies in Medicine Fanned during Association Scientific Meeting," *CMAJ* 113, no. 1 (12 July 1975): 64.

106 For being positive about weight organizations, see Sky, "Watching Your Weight," 49; Saskatchewan, Legislative Assembly Debates (Hansard), 19th Legislature, 2nd Session (3 April 1980): 1449, accessed 6 October 2015, http://docs.legassembly.sk.ca/legdocs/Legislative%20Assembly/Hansard/19L2S/800403Debates.pdf.

107 David M. Garner, "Perceptual/Conceptual Disturbances in Anorexia Nervosa and Obesity" (PhD diss., York University, 1975), 2. The success estimate for behavioural modification was 15 per cent. For identity after losing weight, see Eda LeShan, "Reflections on a New Image," *Globe and Mail*, 1 January 1980, 1.

Chapter 5

1 CMA Committee on Pharmacy, "Report of the Committee on Pharmacy," *CMAJ* 85, no. 10 (2 September 1961): 559. The quote in the chapter title is from Sheila Kieran, "A Frank Report on *Some* Diet Doctors," *Chatelaine* 46, no. 12 (December, 1973): 71.

2 Jeremy A. Greene and Scott H. Podolsky, "Keeping Modern in Medicine: Pharmaceutical Promotion and Physician Education in Postwar America," *Bulletin of the History of Medicine* 83, no. 2 (Summer 2007): 376; Andrea Tone, *The Age of Anxiety: A History of America's Turbulent Affair with Tranquilizers* (New York: Basic Books, 2009); Richard DeGrandpre, *The Cult of Pharmacology: How America Became the World's Most Troubled Drug Culture* (Durham, NC: Duke University Press, 2006); David T. Courtwright, *Forces of Habits: Drugs and the Making of the Modern World* (Cambridge, MA: Harvard University Press, 2001). In Canada, studies are not numerous, but there are several excellent primary sources: Joel Lexchin, *The Real Pushers: A Critical Analysis of the Canadian Drug Industry* (Vancouver, BC: New Star Books, 1984); Myron J. Gordon and David J. Fowler, *The Drug Industry: A Case Study of the Effects of Foreign Control on the Canadian Economy*

(Ottawa: Canadian Institute for Economic Policy, 1981); Royal Commission on Health Services, *Provision, Distribution, and Cost of Drugs in Canada* (Ottawa: Queen's Printer, 1965).

3 For the United States and throughout the world, see Alicia Mundy, *Dispensing with the Truth: The Victims, the Drug Companies, and the Dramatic Story behind the Battle over Fen-Phen* (New York: St Martin's Press, 2001).

4 For physicians, pharmaceuticals, and gender, see Wendy Mitchinson, "Educating Doctors about Obesity: The Gendered Use of Pharmaceutical Advertisements," in *Bodily Subjects: Essays on Gender and Health, 1800–2000*, ed. Tracy Penny Light, Barbara Brookes, and Wendy Mitchinson (Montreal and Kingston: McGill-Queen's University Press, 2014), 268–302.

5 For the close relationship between medicine and pharmaceutical companies, see "Doctor-Pharma Industry Ties Examined in 'Embarrassing' Report," *CBC News*, 8 January 2016, accessed 9 January 2016, http://www.cbc.ca/news/canada/british-columbia/doctor-pharma-industry-ties-report-1.3394539.

6 For sales, see Barbara Millar, "The Pharmaceutical Industry's Influence on the Role of the Medical Profession" (MA thesis, University of Manitoba, 1986), 129. For profits, see Joel Lexchin, *Canadian Drug Prices and Expenditures: Some Statistical Observations and Policy Implications* (Ottawa: Canadian Centre for Policy Alternatives, 2007), 6. For more on drugs, see Joel Lexchin, *Drug Safety and Health Canada: Going, Going...Gone?* (Ottawa: Canadian Centre for Policy Alternatives, 2009), 3, accessed 3 February 2016, http://www.policyalternatives.ca/sites/default/files/uploads/publications/National_Office_Pubs/2009/Drug_Safety_and_Health_Canada.pdf.

7 Millar, "The Pharmaceutical Industry's Influence," 21, 94, 100 (quote).

8 Jeremy A. Greene and David Herzberg, "Hidden in Plain Sight: Marketing Prescription Drugs to Consumers in the Twentieth Century," *American Journal of Public Health* 100, no. 5 (May 2010): 794. For the history of US and Canadian legislation on patent medicine from 1870 to the 1960s, see R.G. Guest, "The Development of Patent Medicine Legislation," *Applied Therpeutics* 8, no. 9 (September 1966): 786–9. For the United States, see Nancy Tomes, "The Great American Medicine Show Revisited," *Bulletin of the History of Medicine* 79, no. 4 (Winter 2005): 627–63.

9 Jeremy A. Greene, "The Afterlife of the Prescription: The Sciences of Therapeutic Surveillance," in *Prescribed: Writing, Filling, Using, and Abusing the Prescription in Modern America*, ed. Jeremy A. Greene and Elizabeth Siegel Watkins (Baltimore, MD: Johns Hopkins University Press, 2012), 234.

10 For 1906 to 1962, see Jeremy A. Greene and Elizabeth Siegel Watkins, "Time Line of Federal Regulations and Rulings Related to the Prescription," in Greene and Watkins, *Prescribed*, 257–8. For more on the 1938 law, see Dominque A. Tobbell, *Pills, Power, and Policy: The Struggle for Drug Reform in Cold War America and Its Consequences* (Berkeley: University of California Press, 2012), 16. For the 1951 legislation, see DeGrandpre, *The Cult of Pharmacology*, 147. For 1962 and the FDA, see John E. Calfee, "Public Policy Issues in Direct-to-Consumer Advertising of Prescription Drugs," *Journal of Public Policy & Marketing* 21, no. 2 (Fall 2002): 174; and Dominique A. Tobbell, "Allied Against Reform: Pharmaceutical Industry – Academic Physician Relations in the United States, 1945–1970," *Bulletin of the History of Medicine* 82, no. 4 (Winter 2008), 890, accessed 24 December 2012, http://muse.jhu.edu/article/255756.
11 Calfee, "Public Policy Issues in Direct-to-Consumer Advertising of Prescription Drugs," 174.
12 Jeremy A. Greene, "Pharmaceutical Marketing Research and the Prescribing Physician," *Annals of Internal Medicine* 146, no. 19 (2007): 742, accessed 24 December 2012, http://annals.org/aim/fullarticle/734723/pharmaceutical-marketing-research-prescribing-physician; Tobbell, *Pills, Power, and Policy*, 69.
13 Greene and Podolsky, "Keeping Modern in Medicine," 340–1.
14 See Greene and Herzberg, "Hidden in Plain Sight," 799; Greene and Podolsky, "Keeping Modern in Medicine," 331–77; Scott H. Podolsky and Jeremy A. Greene, "A Historical Perspective of Pharmaceutical Promotion and Physician Education," *JAMA* 300, no. 7 (2008): 831.
15 Tobbell, "Allied Against Reform," 910. Dominique A. Tobbell, "'Who's Winning the Human Race?' Cold War as Pharmaceutical Political Strategy," *Journal of the History of Medicine and Allied Sciences* 64, no. 4 (October 2009): 429–73.
16 See D.R. Kennedy, "One Hundred Years of Pharmacy Legislation," in *One Hundred Years of Pharmacy in Canada, 1867–1967: Centennial Symposium, Canadian Academy of the History of Pharmacy, Toronto, Canada, 15 August 1967*, ed. E.W. Stieb (Toronto: Canadian Academy of the History of Pharmacy, 1969), 28. For some regulation of drugs in 1908 and 1911, see Catherine Carstairs, *Jailed for Possession: Illegal Drug Use, Regulation, and Power in Canada, 1920–1961* (Toronto: University of Toronto Press, 2006), 6.
17 Gary Gnirss, "A History of Food Law in Canada," *Food in Canada*, May 2008, 38, accessed 5 December 2015, http://www.bizlink.com/foodfiles/PDFs/may2008/38.pdf. For adulteration of food and drug legislation, and for patent medicine, see L.I. Pugsley, "The Administration and

Development of Federal Statutes on Food and Drugs in Canada," *MSJ* 23, no. 3 (March 1967): 387–449, especially 395–6, 401–2, and 408–9. For drugs, see Guest, "The Development of Patent Medicine Legislation," 787–8.

18 For 1934 to 1939 amendments and for the 1941 change, see Kennedy, "One Hundred Years of Pharmacy Legislation," 15–16, 30. For 1939 legislation, see Leona Crabb, "Minor Tranquilizing Drugs and the Medicalization of Everyday Life in English-Speaking Canada, 1945–1962" (PhD diss., Carleton University, 1997), 142. See also Carstairs, *Jailed for Possession*, 61–2. For a history of amphetamine, see Nicolas Rasmussen, *On Speed: The Many Lives of Amphetamine* (New York: New York University Press, 2008). For the way in which amphetamines work, see Courtwright, *Forces of Habits*, 78.

19 For the Drug Advisory Committee, see Crabb, "Minor Tranquilizing Drugs," 188. For 1951 to the 1970s, see Joel Lexchin, "Drug Makers and Drug Regulators: Too Close for Comfort. A Study of the Canadian Situation," *Social Science & Medicine* 31, no. 11 (1990): 1257–9. For thalidomide, see Denyse Baillargeron et Susanne Commend, "Un médicament 'monstrueux': débats publics et couverture médiatique de la tragédie de la thalidomide au Canada, 1961–1963," *Canadian Bulletin of Medical History* 33, no. 1 (Spring 2016): 131–53.

20 Joel Lexchin, "Canadian Marketing Codes: How Well Are They Controlling Pharmaceutical Promotion," *International Journal of Health Services* 24, no. 2 (1994): 92–3. Barbara Millar's thesis gives the date of PAAB's creation as 1976; see Millar, "The Pharmaceutical Industry's Influence," 182.

21 For advertising, see Scott H. Podolsky, Jeremy A. Greene, and David S. Jones, "The Evolving Roles of the Medical Journal," *New England Journal of Medicine* 366, no. 16 (19 April 2012): 1457. For more on the *CMAJ* and the role played by advertisements in its financing, subscription, and readership, see Heather Molyneaux, "In Sickness and in Health" (PhD diss., University of New Brunswick, 2009), 17–18, 23–6; Lexchin, *The Real Pushers*; "Announcement," *OMR* 2, no. 1 (February 1935): 2. For more on the power that the pharmaceutical companies had over the medical profession, see Millar, "The Pharmaceutical Industry's Influence." To connect to the public, see Greene and Herzberg, "Hidden in Plain Sight," 798.

22 Hillel Schwartz, *Never Satisfied: A Cultural History of Diets, Fantasies and Fat* (London: Collier Macmillan Publishers, 1986), 98, 113.

23 *The Chatelaine* 1, no. 2 (April 1928): 72, advertisement for Marmola. For endocrine obesity, see *The Chatelaine* 1, no. 2 (April 1928): 72, advertisement for Marmola. For other Marmola ads, see *The Chatelaine* 1,

no. 7 (September 1928): 48; *The Chatelaine* 2, no. 1 (January 1929): 38; *The Chatelaine* 1, no. 1 (March 1928): 60; *Maclean's* 40, no. 7 (1 April 1927): 95.

24 For Iodesin, see *CMAJ* 20, no. 6 (May 1929): xv, advertisement. In the 1930s, the same drug appears to be called "Iodobesin," made with the same ingredients and by the same company. *CD* 3, no. 3 (March 1937): 47, advertisement; *CD* 5, no. 11 (November 1939): 3, advertisement. For more on ovarian extract, see J.R. Pepin, "L'obésité est-elle réductible?" *UMC* 58, no. 5 (mai 1929): 264. For use of thyroid extract, see "The Menace of Obesity," *CMAJ* 16, no. 11 (November 1926): 1373–4; William Osler, *The Principles and Practice of Medicine*, 8th ed. (New York: D. Appleton and Co., 1912), 452; Thomas McCrae, ed., *The Principles and Practice of Medicine*, 10th ed. (New York: D. Appleton and Co., 1925), 446; "La maigreur esthétique," *UMC* 53, no. 4 (avril 1924): 200.

25 Edward H. Mason, "The Treatment of Obesity," *CMAJ* 14, no. 11 (November 1924): 1052; and R. Tait McKenzie, *Exercise in Education and Medicine*, 3rd ed. (Philadelphia and London: W.B. Saunders Co., 1923), 542.

26 G. Harvey Agnew, "What a Nurse Should Know about Basal Metabolism," *CN* 20, no. 3 (March 1924): 157. For concern that the extracts were uncontrolled, see Mason, "The Treatment of Obesity," 1056.

27 For opponents of thyroid extract, see P.M. MacDonnell, "Review of 'Blood Cholesterol and Hypometabolism: Suprarenal and Pituitary Deficiency, Obesity, and Miscellaneous Conditions' by L.M. Hurxthal," *CMAJ* 31, no. 3 (September 1934): 330; W. Ford Connell, "Review of 'On the Control of Obesity' by A.H. Douthwaite," *CMAJ* 31, no. 6 (December 1934): 688. For supporters, see Henry A. Christian, ed., *The Principles and Practice of Medicine*, 13th ed. (New York: D. Appleton-Century Co., 1938), 545; Walter Campbell, "Obesity and Its Treatment," *CMAJ* 34, no. 1 (January 1936): 47. For thyroid extract use, see also Campbell's 1936 article, 41. For approving thyroid extract, see the review by L.-Henri Gariépy of Samuel Simkins's "Le dinitrophénol et l'extrait thyroïdien dans le traitement de l'obésité" in *UMC* 66, no. 12 (décembre 1937): 1251–2.

28 For thyroid extract prescription, see Pierre Berton, "Nightmare Pills," *Maclean's* 61, no. 9 (1 May 1948): 61. For Clarkotabs, see *CD* 13, no. 4 (April 1947): 77, advertisement. For Probese A, B, or C, see *CD* 13, no. 4 (April 1947): 87, advertisement. L. Bradley Pett, "Public Health, Ottawa Newsletter...Appetite Control and Obesity," *CMAJ* 76, no. 12 (15 June 1957): 1083. For other literature against thyroid preparations, see "Review of *Obesity: Its Cause, Classification and Care* by Robert E. Hodges," *CMAJ* 78, no. 2 (15 January 1958): 160; Bernard Laski, "The Overnourished and the Undernourished Child," *Health* 18, no. 4 (July/August 1950): 21.

29 *CMAJ* 65, no. 2 (August 1951): 173, advertisement for Dexedrine. Dexedrine is no longer approved for treatment of obesity.
30 Schwartz, *Never Satisfied*, 189. For its use in the United States, see Christian, *The Principles and Practice of Medicine* (1938), 545. For a history of amphetamine use as an antidepressant, see Nicolas Rasmussen, "Making the First Anti-Depressant: Amphetamine in American Medicine," *Journal of the History of Medicine and Allied Sciences* 61, no. 3 (July 2006): 289; Rasmussen, *On Speed*, 117.
31 For amphetamine, see Rasmussen, *On Speed*, 55, 82. For American physicians worrying, see Susan Yager, *The Hundred Year Diet: America's Voracious Appetite for Losing Weight* (New York: Rodale Inc., 2010), 50. For British Columbia, see Rasmussen, *On Speed*, 99–100.
32 Leonora Hawirko and P.H. Sprague, "Treatment of Obesity by Appetite-Depressing Drugs," *CMAJ* 54, no. 1 (January 1946): 26–9. For the use of Benzedrine for narcolepsy, see Rasmussen, "Making the First Anti-Depressant," 312. Hawirko and Sprague's support for d-amphetamine might have been influenced by the Council on Pharmacy and Chemistry of the American Medical Association, which in 1943 had criticized the use of Benzedrine for obesity treatment and had recently approved the use of amphetamine sulphate. Edward H. Rynearson and Clifford F. Gastineau, *Obesity*, American Lecture Series, no. 36, American Lectures in Endocrinology (Springfield, IL: Charles C. Thomas, 1949), 100. D-amphetamine (Dextroamphetamine) was often described simply as amphetamine. Amphetamine molecules are structured with right and left versions "known as 'optical isomers.'" Benzedrine was "an equal ... mixture of left- and right-handed amphetamines." When the two versions were separated, the right-handed dextro-amphetamine (or d-amphetamine) didn't give rise to the kinds of side effects as were seen with the left-handed version. Rasmussen, *On Speed*, 51. For information about salyrgan, see Carter Smith, "The Use of Salyrgan in One Patient, Over a Period of Three Years, for Recurring Ascites and Edema Associated with Cardic Failure," *JAMA* 102, no. 7 (17 February 1934): 532, doi:10.1001/jama.1934.62750070001009.
33 R. Gordon Bell, "A Noted Doctor Talks about Alcohol and Tranquilizers," *Maclean's* 71, no. 4 (15 February 1958): 38.
34 For Dexedrine advertisements, see *CMAJ* 77, no. 10 (15 November 1957): 99; *CD* 24, no. 5 (May 1958):18; *UMC* 84, no. 7 (juillet 1955): 52.
35 For various uses of Dexedrine, see *CMAJ* 86, no. 14 (12 April 1962): 34, advertisement for Dexedrine. For assurances, see *CMAJ* 86, no. 8 (24

February 1962): 23, advertisement for Dexedrine. For its fifteen years of use, see *CMAJ* 87, no. 22 (1 December 1962): 30, advertisement for Dexedrine.

36 Antonio Martel, "Preludin (Phenmetrazine) in the Treatment of Obesity," *CMAJ* 76, no. 2 (15 January 1957): 117–20. For other articles supporting Preludin, see P. Szenas and C.J. Attee, "Phenmetrazine – A New Anti-Appetite Drug," *CSMJ* 13 (March 1957): 195–9; W. Leith and J.C. Beck, "The Use of Phenmetrazine Hydrochloride (Preludin) in the Obese Diabetic," *CMAJ* 79, no. 11 (1 December 1958): 897.

37 For example, see *CMAJ* 80, no. 10 (1 May 1959): 75, advertisement for Preludin. For articles that approve of Preludin, see Rosario Robillard, "Preludin Treatment of Obesity in Diabetes Mellitus: Preminary Report," *CMAJ* 76, no. 11 (11 June 1957): 938–40; Fernand Joncas, "Obésité," *UMC* 86, no. 3 (mars 1957): 328; Rosario Robillard, "Étude préliminaire sur la Préludine au cours du traitement de l'obésité dans le diabète sucré," *UMC* 86, no. 6 (juin 1957): 652–6.

38 For Prelutal, see *CMAJ* 90, no. 11 (14 March 1964): 15, advertisement.

39 Lawrence Galton, "Now There's Relief for Obesity," *Chatelaine* 35, no. 7 (July 1962): 10. For more on HCG, see Laura Fraser, *Losing It: America's Obsession with Weight and the Industry That Feeds It* (New York: Penguin, 1997), 90.

40 Jean Yack, "What's New in Dieting?" *Chatelaine* 36, no. 4 (April 1963): 39.

41 "U.S. Food and Drug Administration Insists on Label Change for Hormone Used to Treat Obesity," *CFP* 21, no. 3 (March 1975): 27. For critique of HCG, see Maurice Verdy, "L'obésité: la maladie nutritionnelle la plus importante de notre société," *UMC* 109, no. 5 (mai 1980): 632; Léo Boyer et al., "Les régimes amaigrissants," *UMC* 108, no. 4 (avril 1979): 381.

42 For New Tenuate, see *CMAJ* 82, no. 23 (4 June 1960): 38, advertisement. For diabetes, see *CMAJ* 90, no. 5 (February 1964): 3, advertisement for DBI, DBI-TD brand of Phenformin HCl; for DBI and DBI-TD, see also *OMR* 31, no. 3 (March 1964): 242, advertisement.

43 For Bamadex, see *CMAJ* 83, no. 25 (17 December 1960): 1340, advertisement. On the history of meprobamate in Canada, see Crabb, "Minor Tranquilizing Drugs." For Eskatrol, see *CD* 35, no. 2 (February 1969): 76, advertisement. For Ambar #2 Extentabs, see *CD* 32, no. 11 (November 1966): 6, advertisement. For Probesil, see *MMC* 20, no. 3 (March 1965): 188, advertisement.

44 For concern about the use of thyroid extract, see Elinor F.E. Black, "The Uses and Abuses of Endocrine Therapy," *ManMR* 25, no. 11 (November 1945): 475. For support for thyroid extract use, see advertisements for

Iodobesin, *CD* 6, no. 10 (October 1940): 3; *CD* 9, no. 6 (June 1943): 42. For use in non-endocrine obesity, see Lionel M. Lindsay, "The Overweight Child," *CMAJ* 44, no. 5 (May 1941): 506.

45 H. le Riche, "A Study of Appetite Suppressants in a General Practice," *CMAJ* 82, no. 9 (27 February 1960): 467; see also W. Harding le Riche and G.E. van Belle, "A Long-Term Study on the Use of Appetite Suppressants," *CMAJ* 85, no. 12 (16 September 1961): 673–6.

46 Wilfred Leith, "Experiences with the Pennington Diet in the Management of Obesity," *CMAJ* 84, no. 25 (24 June 1961): 1411; D.R. Wilson, "Current Drug Therapy: Drugs for Obesity," *CMAJ* 91, no. 26 (26 December 1964): 1369.

47 W. Harding le Riche, "Study of Phendimentrazine Bitartrate as an Appetite Suppressant in Relation to Dosage, Weight Loss and Side Effects," *CMAJ* 87, no. 1 (7 July 1962): 29.

48 *CD* 22, no. 3 (March 1956): 73, advertisement for Probese.

49 *CMAJ* 89, no. 2 (13 July 1963): 33, advertisement for Dexedrine.

50 For an action image, see *CMAJ* 90, no. 12 (21 March 1964): 25, advertisement for Dexedrine.

51 *CMAJ* 96, no. 16 (22 April 1967): 28–9, advertisement for Biphetamine T. See also an advertisement for Dexamyl that stresses a multipronged solution to weight loss: *CMAJ* 98, no. 15 (13 April 1968): 11.

52 *CD* 31, no. 1 (January 1965): 13, advertisement for Pre-Sate.

53 Letter about Dexedrine and Dexamyl, *CMAJ* 103, no. 12 (5 December 1970): 1306, advertisement.

54 For a Ponderal advertisement, see *CMAJ* 107, no. 8 (1 October 1972): 728. The fine print for a Pondimin advertisement contained the following statement: "[For use] as a short-term (few weeks') adjunct in the medical management of exogenous obesity." But the main text and visual graphic emphasized its use for twelve weeks, not a "few weeks." See *CMAJ* 116, no. 5 (5 March 1977): 532–3, advertisement for Pondimin. For a Pre-sate advertisement, see *CD* 39, no. 9 (September 1973): 82–3.

55 J.E. Blundell and R.A. McArthur, *Annual Research Reviews: Obesity and Its Treatment*, vol. 1 (Montreal: Eden Press, 1979), 45.

56 *Chatelaine* 7, no. 1 (January 1934): 24, advertisement for Metropolitan Life Insurance Co.; John W.S. McCullough, "Too Fat? Too Thin?" *The Chatelaine* 4, no. 7 (July 1931): 15; Trenholme L. Fisher, "Some New Therapeutic Agents," *CN* 31, no. 3 (March 1935): 101.

57 "Dintrophenal in Obesity," *CMAJ* 33, no. 1 (July 1935): 209–10, reprint from *JAMA*; Gariépy, review of "Le dinitrophénol et l'extrait thyroïdien," 1251–2; Christian, *The Principles and Practice of Medicine* (1938), 545.

58 *CD* 6, no. 5 (May 1940): 22, cartoon showing a patient who wants pills to help lose weight and the doctor who wants him to exercise; Berton, "Nightmare Pills," 61; *Maclean's* 61, no. 10 (15 May 1948): 34, advertisement for Metropolitan Life Insurance Co.
59 "Many Pill 'Cures' Phony: Crackdown Coming," *Maclean's* 72, no. 1 (3 January 1959): 1.
60 *Chatelaine* 24, no. 5 (May 1951): 3, advertisement for Metropolitan Life Insurance Co.
61 Sidney Katz, "Are We Eating Too Much?" *Maclean's* 68, no. 12 (11 June 1955): 95; Lawrence Galton, "Pregnancy Weight," *Chatelaine* 31, no. 9 (September 1958): 8; Lawrence Galton, "Weight Control," *CHJ* 54, no. 7 (November 1957): 10. For Levenor, see Lawrence Galton, "New Aid for the Overweight," *CHJ* 54, no. 12 (April 1958): 12–13; see also Lawrence Galton, "Drugs for Reducing Weight," *Chatelaine* 32, no. 6 (June 1959): 9.
62 For criticism of amphetamine, see *CMAJ* 93, no. 24 (11 December 1965): 17–30, advertisement for Pre-Sate; *CMAJ* 87, no. 7 (18 August 1962): 33, advertisement for Abstin; *CMAJ* 94, no. 16 (16 April 1966): 30, advertisement for Desbutal Gradumet; *CMAJ* 97, no. 9 (26 August 1967): 21, advertisement for Ioanamin; and *UMC* 96, no. 8 (août 1967): 49, advertisement.
63 Stan McFadden, "It's Easier to Stay Slim," *CHW* 17, no. 10 (January 1962): 5. For psychosis, see "'Pep' Pill: The Schizophrenic Shadow," *Financial Post*, 16 April 1966, 37. For foreign countries, see CMA, "Non-Medical Use of Drugs with Particular Reference to Youth," *CMAJ* 101, no. 13 (27 December 1969): 72–88.
64 See, for example, an advertisement for DBI and DBI-TD (Phenformin hydrochloride), *CMAJ* 90, no. 5 (1 February 1964): 3.
65 *CMAJ* 90, no. 11 (14 March 1964): 15, advertisement for Prelutal.
66 Sidney Katz, "New Addictions: The Menace of the 'Harmless' Drugs," *Maclean's* 73, no. 20 (24 September 1960): 19.
67 For the CMA and Morrison, see "F.D.D. Watching for Abuse of Anorexiants," *CMAJ* 106, no. 1 (1 January 1972): 81. See also Basil Jackson, "Why Use of Mood-Modifying Drugs Worries the Doctors," *Financial Post*, 22 May 1971, 34.
68 D.A. Geekie, "Amphetamine Controls," *CMAJ* 106, no. 10 (20 May 1972): 1124A.
69 Lexchin, *The Real Pushers*, 182, 194.
70 For Pondimin, see *CMAJ* 105, no. 3 (7 August 1971): 302–3, advertisement; and *Ontario Medical Review* 39, no. 3 (March 1972): 182, advertisement. For a study in support of fenfluramine, see J.P. Sedgwick, "The Usefulness of

Fenfluramine in Treating Simple Obesity," *CFP* 18, no. 2 (February 1972): 3, 55–7. For criticism, see Anne B. Kenshole, "Weight and Diabetes," *CFP* 18, no. 2 (February 1972): 43; "Colloque international sur la fenfluramine tenu à Montréal du 19 au 21 janvier 1972," *UMC* 101, no. 5 (mai 1972): 954–62; from the same conference, see S. Garattini, "Différences et similitudes entre la fenfluramine et l'amphétamine," *UMC* 101, no. 5 (mai 1972): 954; and B.C. Sproule, "Traitement de l'obésité excessive avec des doses massives de fenfluramine," *UMC* 101, no. 5 (mai 1972): 956. For the scandal, see Mundy, *Dispensing with the Truth*.

71 Health Canada, "Cardiac Adverse Reactions in Patients Following the Use of FEN PHEN (a Combination of Fenfluramine and Phentermine)," Recalls and Safety Alerts (archived), 11 July 1997, accessed 30 July 2015, http://healthycanadians.gc.ca/recall-alert-rappel-avis/hc-sc/1997/14700a-eng.php.

72 Kieran, "A Frank Report on *Some* Diet Doctors," 50, 68–71. For a response to Kieran's article, see Pat Connelly, "Letter," *Chatelaine* 47, no. 3 (March 1974): 72.

73 This conclusion was based on looking at individual (and separate) ads for a drug, but not including subsequent repeats of the same ads. Based on that criteria, the advertisements in the 1950s showed 27 per cent women, 18 per cent men, 9 per cent both, and 45 per cent no people; in the 1960s, ads showed 42 per cent, 23 per cent, 6.5 per cent, and 28.5 per cent, respectively; and in the 1970s, 23.5 per cent, 17.6 per cent, 11.7 per cent, and 45 per cent, respectively. Note the increase of ads showing women in the 1960s and the decline in the 1970s.

74 *The Chatelaine* 1, no. 7 (September 1928): 48, advertisement for Marmola.

75 *CMAJ* 68, no. 1 (January 1953): 91, advertisement for Dexedrine. For a gendered analysis of tranquilizers and how they appealed to men, see David Herzberg, *Happy Pills in America: From Miltown to Prozac* (Baltimore, MD: Johns Hopkins University Press, 2009), 48. One of the tranquilizers (Dexamyl) was also used as a diet pill, 59. For more on Dexamyl, see David Healy, *The Creation of Psychopharmacology* (Cambridge, MA: Harvard University Press, 2002), 68–9.

76 *CMAJ* 69, no. 4 (October 1953): 463, advertisement for Dexedrine; for home setting, see also the Dexamyl (dextroamphetamine and amobarbital) advertisement in *CMAJ* 88, no. 7 (16 February 1963): 26.

77 Molyneaux, "In Sickness and in Health," 178.

78 For Biphetamine (having 2 isomers – molecules that have the same molecular formula as amphetamine but different chemical structures) and

Ionamin (phentermine, i.e., phenyl-tertiary-butalamine), see *CMAJ* 84, no. 9 (4 March 1961): 12, advertisement.
79 For Ionamin, see *CMAJ* 97, no. 9 (26 August 1967): 21, advertisement.
80 Molyneaux, "In Sickness and in Health," 168, found a similar dichotomy. For women, the need to lose weight was deemed trivial, whereas for men it was regarded as important for their health. For looking anxious, see *CMAJ* 68, no. 3 (March 1953): 311, advertisement for Dexamyl. For lacking something in their lives, see *CMAJ* 73, no. 10 (15 March 1955): 479, advertisement for Dexedrine. For clothes, see *CMAJ* 87, no. 8 (25 August 1962): 16, advertisement for Desbutal Gradumet.
81 Rasmussen, *On Speed*, 135.
82 *CD* 15, no. 12 (December 1949): 77, advertisement for Probese. For other nude drawings for Probese and Dexobese, see *CD* 17, no. 10 (October 1951): 20; *CD* 19, no. 3 (March 1953): 69; *CD* 21, no. 11 (November 1955): 79.
83 For the man being weighed, see *CMAJ* 89, no. 17 (26 October 1963): 26, advertisement for Ionamin. For the trampoline, see *CMAJ* 89, no. 6 (10 August 1963): 22, advertisement for Ionamin and Biphetamine.
84 For the bathing suit, see *CMAJ* 89, no. 6 (10 August 1963): 20, advertisement for Ionamin and Biphetamine. For the other advertisements, see *CMAJ* 89, no. 8 (24 August 1963): 28; and *CMAJ* 89, no. 10 (7 September 1963): 22.
85 *CMAJ* 73, no. 3 (1 February 1958): 225, advertisement for Dexedrine.
86 For Probese A, B, or C, see *CD* 13, no. 4 (April 1947): 87, advertisement; *CD* 13, no. 10 (October 1947): 73, advertisement; and *CD* 15, no. 12 (December 1949): 77, advertisement.
87 *CMAJ* 76, no. 10 (15 May 1957): 915, advertisement for Dexedrine. For more on ads assuring doctors of "protection *from* the patient," see Leona Crabb, "'Mother's Little Helper': Minor Tranquilizers and Women in the 1950s" (MA thesis, Concordia University, 1992), 77.
88 *CMAJ* 85, no. 20 (11 November 1961): 7, advertisement for Tenuate Dospan; *CMAJ* 93, no. 3 (17 July 1965): 19, advertisement for Probese.
89 Dexedrine advertisement, *CD* 14, no. 10 (October 1948): 109. For safety concerns about drugs in general, see Mark Nickerson and John P. Gemmell, "Doctors, Drugs and Drug Promotion," *CMAJ* 80 (1 April 1959): 521.
90 For a Dexedrine advertisement on use by pregnant women, see *CMAJ* 75, no. 7 (1 October 1956): 617. For diabetes and hypertension, see advertisements for Dexedrine in *CMAJ* 75, no. 7 (1 October 1956): 617; and *CMAJ* 73, no. 3 (1 February 1958): 225. For heart problems, see New Tenuate (diethylpropion) advertisement, *CMAJ* 82, no. 23 (4 June 1960):

38. See Didrex (benzphetamine) advertisement, *CMAJ* 86, no. 15 (14 April 1962): 18–19, for secondary problems that complicate any kind of weight loss.
91 *CMAJ* 63, no. 3 (March 1953): 311, advertisement for Dexamyl. For Dexamyl, see also *CN* 55, no. 4 (April 1959): 363, advertisement. For more on the history of Dexamyl, see DeGrandpre, *The Cult of Pharmacology*, 163; Rasmussen, *On Speed*, 126, 137.
92 Probese and Dexobese advertisement, *CD* 17, no. 2 (February 1951): 12; *CMAJ* 69, no. 4 (October 1953): 463, advertisement for Dexedrine.
93 For Adjudets, see advertisements in *CD* 18, no. 4 (April 1952): 26; *CN* 48, no. 2 (February 1952): 89; *MMC* 8, no. 2 (February 1953): 94. For Probese, see *CD* 23, no. 4 (April 1957): 13, advertisement. For Revicaps, see *MMC* 10, no. 3 (March 1955): 2, advertisement.
94 Kenneth Clute, *The General Practitioner: A Study of Medical Education and Practice in Ontario and Nova Scotia* (Toronto: University of Toronto Press, 1963), 351, 354.
95 Lexchin, *The Real Pushers*, 93–4.
96 On the two types of surgery, see Leanne Joanisse, "Reducing and Revisioning the Body: Women's Experiences of Weight Loss Surgery" (PhD diss., McMaster University, 2003), 254. Intestinal malabsorption is designed to "decrease the intestinal tract, thereby decreasing nutrient and calories absorption." Gastric restriction creates "a small gastric pouch and outlet to decrease food intake." For gastric banding, see Arya M. Sharma, "Obesity Mangement: Handguns Versus Slingshots?" Dr. Sharma's Obesity Notes, 7 December 2010, accessed 1 January 2011, http://www.drsharma.ca/obesity-management-handguns-versus-slingshots. For more on gastric band surgery, see C. Cobourn, "Outpatient Laparosceopic Adjustable Gastric Band Surgery – Results of 2000 Consecutive Cases in Canada," *Applied Physiology, Nutrition and Metabolism* 34, no. 2 (April 2009): 249. For criticism of gastric banding, see Paul Taylor, "Small Doses: Risks of Weight-loss Surgery," *Globe and Mail*, 25 March 2011, L4.
97 Canadian Institute for Health Information, *Bariatric Surgery in Canada* (Ottawa: Canadian Institute for Health Information, 2014), 13, accessed 13 January 2016, https://secure.cihi.ca/free_products/Bariatric_Surgery_in_Canada_EN.pdf.
98 Aimé-Paul Heineck, "Excision massive de graisse sous-cutanée abdominale," *UMC* 54, no. 3 (mars 1925): 153–68; J.H. Duncan, "A Case of Ovarian Fibroma," *CMAJ* 28, no. 6 (June 1933): 655; Campbell, "Obesity and Its Treatment," 47.

99 On surgery in the United States, see Lawrence Galton, "Operation for Obesity," *Chatelaine* 36, no. 4 (April 1963): 20; "Obesity Operation Proving Successful," *CN* 62, no. 4 (April 1966): 10. For referencing surgery, see Barbara A. McLaren, "Nutritional Control of Overweight," *CJPH* 58, no. 11 (November 1967): 485. For the first US surgery in 1954, see Jean-Phillipe Gendron, "Une première chirurgie de l'obésité: la longue controverse du court-circuit jéjuno-iléal (1954–1980)," *Scientia Canadensis* 33, no. 1 (2010): 39.
100 For cosmetic surgery, see Bonnie Buxton, "Cosmetic Surgery: The Instant Makeover," *Chatelaine* 41, no. 8 (August 1968): 34, 56.
101 Jeffrey Sobal, "The Medicalization and Demedicalization of Obesity," in *Eating Agendas: Food and Nutrition as Social Problems*, ed. Donna Maurer and Jeffery Sobal (New York: Aldine De Gruyter, 1995), 74.
102 Helen Christie, "Obesity Is a Major Topic of Papers at Annual Meeting of OMA," *CMAJ* 108, no. 12 (23 June 1973): 1549. Unclear is whether the 148 cases were Salmon's patients. For statistics on death, see Jenny Ellison, "Large as Life: Self-Acceptance and the Fat Body in Canada, 1977–2000" (PhD diss., York University, 2010), 161.
103 Dr Kate Bailey shared this information with me.
104 "Problem of Obesity Said Frustrating to Doctor and Patient," *CMAJ* 112, no. 3 (8 February 1975): 350. R.C. Bowen and L. Shepal, "Physical and Psychological Complications after Intestinal Bypass for Obesity," *CMAJ* 116, no. 5 (23 April 1977): 871. For mention of surgery, see M. Kindl and Peggy Brown, "The Team Approach: Effective Treatment of Obesity in the Community," *MMC* 31, no. 11 (November 1976): 1031; Carol Herbert, "Intestinal Bypass for Obesity: The Family Physician's Concern," *CFP* 21, no. 7 (July 1975): 56–9; Charles G. Roland, "Editorial: Some Recent Studies of Obesity," *CFP* 14, no. 2 (February 1968): 4; John A. Carmichael, "Psychological Methods of Obesity Reduction in Adolescent Girls" (PhD diss., University of Victoria, 1975), 31. For more symptoms, see Peter Corrodi et al., "Intestinal Flora after Bypass for Obesity," *MMC* 33, no. 6 (June 1978): 935; Allen H. Spanier et al., "Weight-Reducing Surgery May Cause Malnutrition," *MMC* 32, no. 5 (May 1977): 628.
105 Gendron, "Une première chirurgie de l'obésité," 58.
106 Arnold E. Andersen and Simeon Margolis, "Eating Disorders: Obesity and Anorexia Nervosa," in *The Principles and Practice of Medicine*, 20th ed., ed. A. McGehee Harvey et al. (New York: Appleton-Century Crofts, 1980), 831.
107 Verdy, "L'obésité," 632.
108 Paul Dumas, "Le traitement de l'obésité," *UMC* 97, no. 11 (novembre 1958): 1363; Louise A. Demers-Desrosiers, "Considérations psychiatriques

sur l'obésité et l'anorexie," *UMC* 107, no. 6 (juin 1978): 575–6, 578–9, 582. For obesity as insolvable, see Kindl and Brown, "The Team Approach," 39. For the present day, see Denise Mann, "New Genes Linked to Obesity, Belly Fat," *WebMD*, 11 October 2010, accessed 8 November 2010, https://www.webmd.com/diet/news/20101011/new-genes-linked-to-obesity-belly-fat#1.

109 *CFP* 18, no. 2 (February 1972): 48, cartoon. For global approach, see Suzanne Simard-Mavrikakis, "Le traitement de l'obésité," *CFP* 21, no. 4 (April 1975): 162; Kindl and Brown, "The Team Approach," 1034; Léo Boyer, André Boyer, et Pierre Biron, "Contrôle global de l'obésité: résultats chez 1225 patients après 5 ans," *UMC* 106, no. 6 (juin 1977): 887; Maurice Larocque et Robert Prescott, "Comparison de différentes approches de l'obésité," *UMC* 109, no. 6 (juin 1980): 947. For team work, see David C.W. Lau, "Call for Action: Preventing and Managing the Expansive and Expensive Obesity Epidemic," *CMAJ* 160, no. 4 (23 February 1999): 505; C.E. Adair, G. McVey, J. deGroot, et al., *Obesity and Eating Disorders: Seeking Common Ground to Promote Health*. A National Meeting of Researchers, Practitioners, and Policy Makers, November 2007, Calgary, AB, Final Discussion Document (n.p.: 2007), 5, 8–9, https://www.ocoped.ca/PDF/Obesity_eating_disorders_discussion_document_2008.pdf; Sarah D. McDonald, "Management and Prevention of Obesity in Adults and Children," *CMAJ* 176, no. 8 (19 April 2007): 1109; A.P. Brozic et al., "The Bariatric Medical Clinic at Hamilton Health Sciences: Starting from Scratch" *Applied Physiology, Nutrition and Metabolism* 34, no. 2 (April 2009): 273.

110 Susan Billard, "What Are Family Physicians' Attitudes and Practices Toward Managing Adult Obesity in Nova Scotia?" (MA thesis, Mount Saint Vincent University, 2000), 47, 52. For chronic disease, see National Institutes of Health, National Heart, Lung and Blood Institute, and North American Association for the Study of Obesity, *The Practical Guide: Identification, Evaluation and Treatment of Overweight and Obesity in Adults*, NIH Publication no. 00-4084 (Washington, DC: National Institutes of Health, 2000), 31, accessed 15 June 2007, https://www.nhlbi.nih.gov/files/docs/guidelines/prctgd_c.pdf. For transforming culture, see Leanne Joanisse and Anthony Synnott, "Fighting Back: Reactions and Resistance to the Stigma of Obesity," in *Interpreting Weight: The Social Management of Fatness and Thinness*, ed. Jeffery Sobal and Donna Maurer (New York: Aldine de Gruyter, 1999), 50; Michael Gard and Jan Wright, *The Obesity Epidemic: Science, Morality and Ideology* (London and New York: Routledge, Taylor & Francis Group, 2005), 190.

Chapter 6

1 Alan Brown, *The Normal Child: Its Care and Feeding* (Toronto: F.D. Goodchild Company Publishers, 1923), 107.
2 For the foetus in utero, see Greg Critser, *Fat Land: How Americans Became the Fattest People in the World* (Boston, New York: Mariner Books, 2004), 129–30; see also Z. Ferraro, D. Prud'homme, and K.B. Adamo, "Exploring Maternal Obesity and the Intrauterine Environment: Can Attenuation of Gestational Weight Gain through a Lifestyle Intervention Reverse the Programming of Pediatric Obesity?" *Applied Physiology, Nutrition and Metabolism* 34, no. 2 (April 2009): 277–8. For diabetic mothers, see Gary Taubes, *Good Calories, Bad Calories: Challenging the Conventional Wisdom on Diet, Weight Control, and Disease* (New York: Alfred A. Knopf, 2007), 402. For older mothers, see S.W. Keith et al., "Putative Contributors to the Secular Increase in Obesity: Exploring the Roads Less Traveled," *International Journal of Obesity* 30 (2006): 1585–94, accessed 21 March 2011, https://www.nature.com/articles/0803326. For PCBs, see Susan Yager, *The Hundred Year Diet: America's Voracious Appetite for Losing Weight* (New York: Rodale Inc., 2010), 206. For obese mothers, see Leanne Joanisse, "Reducing and Revisioning the Body: Women's Experiences of Weight Loss Surgery" (PhD diss., McMaster University, 2003), 252. For birth weights, see Timothy Lobstein, "What Are the Factors Contributing to the Obesity Epidemic among Children and Youth?" in *Presentation and Poster Abstracts from the International Conference on Physical Activity and Obesity in Children* (Toronto: International Conference, 24–7 June, 2007), 13. For native children and high birth weight, see Tara Leanne Black, "Understanding Excessive Parental Weight Gain among First Nations Women" (MA thesis, University of Alberta, 2004), 21. For sleeping, see Todd Neale, "Obesity: Mother, Baby Risk Factors Predict Child's Obesity," *MedPage Today*, 3 October 2011, accessed 10 October 2011, https://www.medpagetoday.com/meetingcoverage/obesity/28847; Brian Goldman, "The Cure for Childhood Obesity Parents Will Hate," White Coat, Black Art (CBC Radio blog), accessed 10 November 2015, http://www.cbc.ca/radio/whitecoat/blog/the-cure-for-childhood-obesity-parents-will-hate-1.3014981. For discussion of breast feeding, see Dorothy H. Broom and Jane Dixon, "Introduction" in *The Seven Deadly Sins of Obesity: How the Modern World Is Making Us Fat*, ed. Jane Dixon and Dorothy Broom (Sydney, AU: University of New South Wales, 2007), 6; Laurie Twells and Leigh Anne Newhook, "Can Exclusive Breastfeeding Reduce the Likelihood of Childhood Obesity in Some Regions of Canada?" *CJPH* 101, no. 1 (2010): 38.

3 For too much weight in pregnancy, see Stella Pines, "Preparing for the Great Adventure," *The Chatelaine* 1, no. 8 (October 1928): 56. For the Toronto study, see E.W. McHenry, "Nutrition in Toronto," *CPHJ* 30, no. 1 (January 1939): 6–7; Alan Brown and Elizabeth Chant Robertson, *The Normal Child* (Toronto: McClelland & Stewart, 1948), 2–6. For weight gain of 25 to 30 pounds in pregnancy, see Donatien Marion, "Examen prénatal," *UMC* 75, no. 11 (November 1946): 1378.
4 For various weight gains, see Marie-Nöel Chabamel, "L'alimentation chez la femme enceinte," *CN* 48, no. 5 (May 1952): 410; George H. Beaton, "Les besoins nutritifs durant la grossesse," *CN* 54, no. 3 (March 1958): 217; W.A. Cochrane, "Overnutrition in Prenatal and Neonatal Life: A Problem," *CMAJ* 93, no. 17 (23 October 1965); 893–9; Earl Damude, "Pregnancy Weight Gain," *Chatelaine* 42, no. 6 (June 1969): 12; Réal Martineau et Antoine Habre, "Grossesse et obésité," *UMC* 96, no. 10 (octobre 1967): 1243. For diabetes, see Elizabeth Laugharne and Felicity Duncan, "Gestational Diabetes – When Teaching Is Important," *CN* 69, no. 3 (March 1973): 34. For weight in the 1970s, see A. Cecilia Pope (letter), "Weight Gain Inaccurate?" *CN* 66, no. 10 (October 1970): 4; Clive Cocking, "Putting on Weight: Baby, It's Worth It," *Maclean's* 91, no. 26 (6 November 1978): 52; BC Dairy Association advertisement, *BCMJ* 19, no. 5 (May 1977): 175; Gilles Amyot, "Les soins prénataux," *UMC* 104, no. 10 (octobre 1975): 1515. For appetite suppressants and pregnancy, see advertisements in *Chatelaine* 31, no. 9 (September 1958): 8, Preludin (phenmetrazine); *MMC* 6, no. 7 (July 1951): 53, Dexedrine; *ManMR* 41, no. 2 (February 1961): 128, Eskatrol Spansule (dextroamphetamine and prochlorperazine – a dopamine and an antipsychotic). For use of phermetrazine, see Martineau et Habre, "Grossesse et obésité," 1247.
5 Executive Committee, Perinatal Programme of BC, "BC's New Prenatal Record," *BCMJ* 17, no. 5 (May 1975): 156; "What Kind of Eaters Are You?" *CN* 68, no. 8 (August 1972): 44.
6 Laura Dawes, *Childhood Obesity in America: Biography of an Epidemic* (Cambridge, MA: Harvard University Press, 2014), 130.
7 For the nineteenth century, see Sander L. Gilman, *Fat: A Cultural History of Obesity* (Cambridge: Polity Press, 2008), 62. For the twentieth century, see the section "Bigger Babies Are Better Babies," in *The One Best Way? Breastfeeding History, Politics and Policy in Canada*, by Tasnim Nathoo and Aleck Ostry (Waterloo, ON: Wilfrid University Press, 2009), 72–4.
8 For Donald Baldock, see *The Chatelaine* 2, no. 11 (November 1929): 45, advertisement for Red River Cereal. For Virol, see *CHJ* 26, no. 12 (April 1930): 109, advertisement.

9 For formula advertisements, see the following: for Horlick's Malted Milk, see *Maclean's* 33, no. 1 (January 1920): 70; for Borden Eagle Brand milk, see *Maclean's* 33, no. 21 (15 November 1920): 10; for LilyWhite Corn Syrup, see *Maclean's* 38, no. 5 (1 March 1925): 55; for Nestle's Milk Food, see *Maclean's* 38, no. 10 (15 May 1925): 38; for Glaxo, see *Maclean's* 34, no. 13, (July 1921): 63; for St Charles Milk, see *Chatelaine* 10, no. 9 (September 1937): 61. For milk ads and their appeal, see E. Melanie DuPuis, *Nature's Perfect Food: How Milk Became America's Drink* (New York: New York University Press, 2002), 120. For Carnation Milk, see *Chatelaine* 16, no. 9 (September 1943): 22, advertisement.
10 *CD* 20, no. 9 (September 1954): 20, advertisement for Heinz. For "precious" pounds, see *Chatelaine* 27, no. 1 (January 1954): 57, advertisement for Heinz. For fat being desirable, see *CMAJ* 82, no. 10 (5 March 1960): 56, advertisement for Farmer's Wife milk.
11 M.J. Carney, "Feeding of the New Born Infant," *NSMB* 8, no. 3 (1929): 151. For Chandler, see Aleck Samuel Ostry, *Nutrition Policy in Canada, 1870–1939* (Vancouver, BC: UBC Press, 2006), 36. For the VON clinic, see "From a Victorian Order Nurse," *CN* 16, no. 11 (November 1920): 671. For the weight scale, see A.B. Chandler, "Breast Feeding in Health Centres," *CN* 25, no. 11 (November 1929): 664.
12 Hilary B. Bourne, "Breast Feeding," *CN* 46, no. 12 (December 1950): 970; Bernard Laramée, "Quelques considérations sur l'allaitement maternel," *UMC* 86, no. 12 (décembre 1957): 1404, 1406; Anne (Gelineau) Sharkey, "Starting Baby Off," *CN* 48, no. 3 (March 1952): 189; Albert Royer, "L'état actuel de l'alimentation chez le nourrisson," *UMC* 85, no. 2 (février 1956): 157; Victor D. McLaughlin, "Prenatal Care," *CN* 57, no. 12 (December 1961): 1118; Albert Royer, "Problems in Infant Feeding," *CN* 58, no. 11 (November 1962): 991; Dorothy Metie Grant, "Breast Feeding May Be a Dying Art," *CN* 64, no. 8 (August 1968): 47; Derrick B. Jelliffe et E.F. Patrice Jelliffe, "Le lait maternel: imitable, mais inégalable," *UMC* 101, no. 10 (octobre 1972): 2198, 2203, 2206; Micheline Brault-Dubuc, "Nutrition du nourrison," *CFP* 24, no. 12 (December 1978): 1303; Catherine Armstrong, Patricia Latner, and Carol R. Sage, *Current Issues in Infant Feeding: A Guide for Professionals* (Toronto: Ontario Ministry of Health, 1977), 16–17; Beverly MacLellan, "Matthew My Son: Prepared Childbirth at the General," *CN* 72, no. 3 (March 1976): 39; Marie-Elizabeth Taggart, "A Practical Guide to Breast-Feeding," *CN* 72, no. 3 (March 1976): 26. For statistics on breast feeding and different rates in various regions, see Canadian Paediatric Society Nutrition Committee, "Infant Feeding: A Statement by the Canadian Paediatric Society Nutrition Committee," *CJPH* 70, no. 6 (November/December 1979): 376–7.

13 Brown, *The Normal Child* (1923), 134–6, 139–40, 154, 156, 158; Alton Goldbloom, *The Care of the Child* (Toronto: Longmans, Green and Co., 1928), 83–4; 150; Alton Goldbloom, "A Twenty-five Year Retrospect of Infant Feeding," *CN* 41, no. 4 (April 1945): 279, 284; Brown and Chant Robertson, *The Normal Child* (1948), 55–6, 58, 107–8, 119. For different schedules, see "Alimentation des enfants entre douze et quinze mois," *UMC* 74, no. 10 (octobre 1945): 1460–1; Marcel Langlois, "La nutrition chez le nourrisson et chez l'enfant d'âge préscolaire," *UMC* 76, no. 4 (avril 1947): 396.

14 For Swift Strained Meats, see *Maclean's* 57, no. 22 (15 November 1944): 55, advertisement. For bacon, see *Chatelaine* 17, no. 9 (September 1944): 46, advertisement for Swift bacon. For baby food as a business, see Sidney Katz, "A Report on Eating," *Maclean's* 68, no. 12 (11 June 1955): 13.

15 Goldbloom, *The Care of the Child* (1928), 73, 3 for quotes; Brown, *The Normal Child* (1923), 107; see also Alan Brown, "Keeping the Well Child Well," *Maclean's* 35, no. 19 (1 October 1922): 22–3, 43–4; Brown and Chant Robertson, *The Normal Child* (1948), 75. For the *Chatelaine* Baby Clinic, see John W.S. McCullough, "No. 5 Artificial Feeding," *Chatelaine* 6, no. 6 (June 1933): 62. For recognition of infant overfeeding, see Carney, "Feeding of the New Born Infant," 151; Gordon Wiswell, "Proprietary Foods in Infant Feeding," *NSMB* 13, no. 10 (1934): 483–5.

16 L.L. Kulczycki, "Some Observations on Infants' Feeding and Development in Swan Valley Area," *ManMR* 32, no. 9 (November 1952): 567. For mothers, see Bernard Laski, "The Overnourished and the Undernourished Child," *Health* 18, no. 4 (July/August 1950): 21. For recognition of obesity in infancy and blaming the mother, see Jean Grignon, "L'obésité et la maigreur," *UMC* 81, no. 11 (novembre 1952): 1308–9.

17 L. Bradley Pett, "Public Health Ottawa Newsletter...Appetite Control and Obesity," *CMAJ* 76, no. 12 (15 June 1957): 1083; for Pett's quote, see Janice Tyrwhitt, "Are Our Children Growing Up Too Fast?" *Maclean's* 71, no. 8 (12 April 1958): 66; W.A. Cochrane, "Nutritional Excess in Infancy and Childhood," *CMAJ* 81, no. 6 (15 September 1959): 454; Cochrane, "Overnutrition in Prenatal and Neonatal Life," 893–9. The weight of babies at three to four months comes from Cochrane's 1959 article.

18 For bottle feeding and measurement of obesity, see Royer, "Problems in Infant Feeding," 992. For Mil-ko, see *CN* 51, no. 8 (August 1955): 655, advertisement. For Heinz baby foods, see *CD* 27, no. 11 (November 1961): 50, advertisement.

19 For Hill, see "Obesity in Children Equally Intractable," *CMAJ* 112, no. 3 (8 February 1975): 350. For fat cells, see "Problem of Obesity Said

Frustrating to Doctor and Patient," *CMAJ* 112, no. 3 (8 February 1975): 350 (quote). For more on fat cells, see Linda Oglov, "Canadian Dietetic Association Delegates at Annual Meeting Study Relationship of Diet to Exercise," *CMAJ* 117, no. 3 (6 August 1977): 289–90. For Yeung, see "Health Professionals Learn More about Latest in Infant Nutrition," *CN* 75, no. 10 (November 1979): 12. Yeung was from H.J. Heinz Co., Toronto.

20 T. Hancock, "Letter to Editor re 'Breast-feeding,'" *CMAJ* 113, no. 5 (6 September 1975): 362. See also "Bottle-Feeding Linked with Early Doubling of Birthweight," *CFP* 21, no. 7 (July 1975): 19; Platon J. Collipp, "Obesity in Childhood," in *Obesity*, ed. Albert J. Stunkard (Philadelphia: W.B. Saunders, 1980), 407; A.W. Myres, "Obesity: Is It Preventable in Infancy and Childhood?" *CFP* 21, no. 4 (April 1975): 75.

21 Canadian Paediatric Society, Nutrition Committee, "Infant Feeding Practices Revisted," *CMAJ* 122, no. 9 (10 May 1980): 987; see also J. Elizabeth Miles, "Tip the Scales in Your Favour," *CC* (June 1975): 23. Miles suggested that there was little difference in obesity rates between breast and formula feeding due to the increase of early weaning from both.

22 For weaning at six weeks to two months, see Earl Damude, "Early Overweight," *Chatelaine* 44, no. 12 (December 1971): 8. For rates for the nation and also for native people, see Nathoo and Ostry, *The Best Way?*, 109. For age of weaning and double-feeding, see Myres, "Obesity," 75.

23 Anthony W. Myres and David L. Yeung, "Obesity in Infants: Significance, Aetiology and Prevention," *CJPH* 70, no. 2 (March/April 1979): 113, 115–16.

24 For after birth, see Canadian Paediatric Society, Nutrition Committee, "Infant Feeding," 383.

25 For infants of four to nine months, see Maurice Verdy, "L'obésité: la maladie nutritionnelle la plus importante de notre société," *UMC* 109, no. 5 (mai 1980): 632. For the problem of some milk, see Carol Raebiger Sage, "The Neglected Age in Nutrition Education: Facts for Change," *CN* 74, no. 1 (January 1978): 47. For low-fat food, see Stephen A. Haines, "Feeding for the Future to Improve Health," *Health* 46, no. 4 (Winter 1980/81): 26.

26 For obesity rates, see Karen C. Roberts, Margot Shields, Margaret de Groh, Alfred Azis, and Jo-Anne Gilbert, "Overweight and Obesity in Children and Adolescents: Results from the 2009 to 2011 Canadian Health Measures Survey," *Health Reports* 23, no. 3 (2012), Table 1, accessed 6 December 2012, https://www.statcan.gc.ca/pub/82-003-x/2012003/article/11706-eng.htm. For the poor, see Kim D. Raine, *Overweight and Obesity in Canada: A Population Health Perspective* (Ottawa: Canadian Institute for Health Information, 2004), 9, 33; S.A Phipps et al., "Poverty and the Extent of

Child Obesity in Canada, Norway and the United States," *Obesity Reviews* 7 (2006): 8. For multi-ethnic, see Raine, *Overweight and Obesity in Canada*, 9. For First Nations, see Noreen D. Willows, "Overweight in First Nations Children: Prevalence, Implications and Solutions," *Journal of Aboriginal Health* 2, no. 1 (March 2005): 76–86; for off the reserves, see "Girls in Canada 2005: A Report Prepared for the Canadian Women's Foundation" (n.p.: Canadian Women's Foundation, 2005), 31. For concern about children today, see "Child Obesity Charts Open Door to Treatment," *CBC News*, 30 March 2015, accessed 8 January 2016, http://www.cbc.ca/news/health/child-obesity-charts-open-door-to-treatment-1.3014832.

27 Laurie K. Twells and Leigh A. Newhook, "Obesity Prevalence Estimates in a Canadian Regional Population of Preschool Children Using Variant Growth References," *BMC Pediatrics* 11 (2011), accessed 6 April 2013, https://bmcpediatr.biomedcentral.com/articles/10.1186/1471-2431-11-21. For why the BMI is used and for other ways of measuring without using the BMI, see Geoff C.D. Ball and Linda J. McCargar, "Childhood Obesity in Canada: A Review of Prevalence Estimates and Risk Factors for Cardiovascular Diseases and Type 2 Diabetes," *Canadian Journal of Applied Psychology* 28, no. 1 (2003): 124; see also L. Twells and L. Newhook, "What Is the Most Reliable and Valid Index for the Classification of Childhood Obesity?" *Applied Physiology, Nutrition and Obesity* 34, no. 2 (April 2009): 263; Margot Shields, *Measured Obesity: Overweight Canadian Children and Adolescents*. Issue no. 1 of Nutrition: Findings from the Canadian Community Health Survey (Ottawa: Statistics Canada, 2005), 12, http://www.statcan.gc.ca/pub/82-620-m/2005001/pdf/4193660-eng.pdf. For the problem of BMI and age, etc., see Laura Lovett, "The Popeye Principle: Selling Child Health in the First Nutrition Crisis," *Journal of Health Politics, Policy and Law* 30, no. 5 (October 2005): 827. For an analysis of child statistics, see Michael Gard, "Hearing Noises and Noticing Silence: Towards a Critical Engagement with Canadian Body Weight Statistics," in *Obesity in Canada: Critical Perspectives*, ed. Jenny Ellison, Deborah McPhail, and Wendy Mitchinson (Toronto: University of Toronto Press, 2016), 43–4.

28 For diabetes in the United States, see Critser, *Fat*, 133–40. For diabetes in Indigenous children, see Raine, *Overweight and Obesity in Canada*, 13. For blood pressure, etc., see Mark Grenier, "The Increase of Childhood Obesity in a Limited Sample of Canadian Children between 1979 and 1998" (MA thesis, University of Ottawa, 1998), 9. For an example of the belief that the current generation may not live as long as their parents and other concerns, see "Curse of Generation XL," *The Record*, 28 March 2007, A1–2. This idea came from a conversation between a scientist and a reporter

about the possible future. For psychological problems, see Lobstein, "What Are the Factors?"; Raine, *Overweight and Obesity in Canada*, 14; C.E. Adair, G. McVey, J. deGroot, et al., *Obesity and Eating Disorders: Seeking Common Ground to Promote Health*. A National Meeting of Researchers, Practitioners, and Policy Makers, Calgary, AB, November 2007, Final Discussion Document (n.p.: 2008), 5, https://www.ocoped.ca/PDF/Obesity_eating_disorders_discussion_document_2008.pdf.

29 Moss Edward Norman, "Living in the Shadow of an 'Obesity Epidemic': The Discursive Construction of Boys and Their Bodies" (PhD diss., University of Toronto, 2009).

30 For challenging the health issue, see Kirsten Bell, Darlene McNaughton, and Amy Salmon, "Medicine, Morality and Mothering: Public Health Discourses on Foetal Alcohol Exposure, Smoking around Children and Childhood Overnutrition," *Critical Public Health* 19, no. 2 (June 2009): 158; Twells and Newhook, "Obesity Prevalence Estimates."

31 Bell, McNaughton, and Salmon, "Medicine, Morality and Mothers," 159.

32 According to Sander L. Gilman, concern about childhood obesity existed in the early part of the nineteenth century, not in terms of health but in terms of the morality of fat. Stearns in *Fat History* differentiated Americans from the French by their different parenting approaches. French parents worried about the health implications of being fat and so were careful about their children's eating habits. The French expected children to eat at mealtimes; if they didn't, they had to wait until the next meal. Americans seemed to worry about their children getting enough to eat and so were lenient in allowing them to eat on demand. Harvey A. Levenstein looked at the situation in the two countries slightly differently. Unlike in France, the consumption of food in the United States was more hurried and less involved, which could very well lead to a different consumption pattern learned at an early age. Gilman, *Fat*, 62; Peter N. Stearns, *Fat History: Bodies and Beauty in the Modern West*, rev. ed. (New York: New York University Press, 2002), 195–201; Harvey A. Levenstein, *Revolution at the Table: The Transformation of the American Diet* (Berkeley: University of California Press, 2003), 8.

33 Dawes, *Childhood Obesity in America*, 17. For Canada, see Elise Paradis, "'Obesity' as Process: The Medicalization of Fatness by Canadian Researchers, 1971–2010," in Ellison, McPhail, and Mitchinson, *Obesity in Canada*, 60.

34 Bird T. Baldwin, "The Use and Abuse of Weigth-Height-Age Tables as Indexes of Health Nutrition," *JAMA* 82, no. 1 (5 January 1924): 1. For the malnourished and the underweight, see G.A. Lamont, "The Pre-School

Child," *CN* 25, no. 12 (December 1929): 709–14. For several early US weight-height standards, see Dawes, *Child Obesity in America*, chapter 1, "Quantifying Children's Size," 21–40.

35 Querying charts and health, see H. Jean Leeson, E.W. McHenry, and W. Mosley, "The Value of the Wetzel Grid in the Examination of School Children, " *CJPH* 38, no. 10 (October 1947): 494; L.B. Pett and R.W. Hanley, "A Nutrition Survey on a Nova Scotia Island," *CMAJ* 59, no. 3 (September 1948): 232.

36 Stanley Garn, "The Applicability of North American Growth Standards in Developing Countries," *CMAJ* 93, no. 17 (23 October 1965): 918.

37 William Osler, *The Principles and Practice of Medicine* (New York: D. Appleton and Company, 1893), 1019; William Osler, *The Principles and Practice of Medicine*, 8th ed. (New York: D. Appleton and Company, 1912), 451; Brown, *The Normal Child* (1923), 139–40, 145–6. For a danger point of 20 per cent overweight, see K.E. Dowler, "Co-Relating Health Education in a City Secondary School," *CN* 25, no. 10 (October 1929): 624; Goldbloom, *The Care of the Child* (1928), 5–6; Brown, *The Normal Child* (1923), 59.

38 Lionel M. Lindsay, "The Overweight Child," *CMAJ* 44, no. 5 (May 1941): 504–6; Elizabeth Chant Robertson, "My Child Is Too Fat," *Chatelaine* 21, no. 1 (February 1948): 10. On doctors and a clinical exam, see Lindsay, "The Overweight Child," 504. For problems of the charts, see Leeson, McHenry, and Mosley, "The Value of the Wetzel Grid," 494. For children growing more quickly, see Cochrane, "Nutritional Excess in Infancy and Childhood," 454. The Wetzel Grid was more popular in America; see Dawes, *Child Obesity in America*, 52–4.

39 Laski, "The Overnourished and the Undernourished Child," 21; W.R. Feasby, "Review of *The Importance of Overweight* by Hilde Bruch," *OMR* 24, no. 7 (July 1957): 526. For excesses, see Cochrane, "Nutritional Excess in Infancy and Childhood," 454. On youth obesity in a medical program, see "Cours de perfectionnement à Sainte-Justine," *UMC* 87, no. 12 (décembre 1958): 1579–80. For "Miss C. Diet Book," see *Chatelaine* 39, no. 3 (March 1966): 79, advertisement. For magazine articles, see Catherine Hoare Mahoney, "Teen Talk about Food," *Health* 28, no. 4 (August 1960): 32, 40–2; Jane Becker, "Medicine Discovers the Teen-agers," *Maclean's* 74, no. 24 (2 December 1961): 26. For Bruch and how she saw mothers in the United States over time, see Dawes, *Childhood Obesity in America*, 116–22.

40 For 20 per cent over average, see S.S.B. Gilder, "The Fat Child," *CMAJ* 107, no. 11 (9 December 1972): 1068. For calipers, see Miroslava Kindl and Peggy Brown, "A Programme to Treat Childhood Obesity," *MMC* 33, no. 5 (May 1978): 662.

41 For 80 per cent probability, see Reva T. Frankle, "When Is a Child a Good Eater?" *Health* 44, no. 1 (Spring 1978): 13. For 2 to 15 per cent prevalence, see A. Angel, "Pathophysiology of Obesity," *CMAJ* 110, no. 5 (2 March 1974): 540. For Canada's rates, see Don Bailey, "Physical Activity Vital for All Children," *Health* 45, no. 2 (Summer 1979): 11.
42 Patricia D. Wolczuk, "Nutrition BC," *BCMJ* 17, no. 3 (March 1975): 79.
43 For malnourishment, see H. Medovy, "The Malnourished Child," *CN* 27, no. 3 (March 1931): 117. For fatigue, see G.A. Lamont, "Fatigue in Children," *CMAJ* 36 (January 1937): 48. As a handicap, see M. Frances Huchs, "Food and Health," *Chatelaine* 7, no. 5 (May 1934): 68; E.P. Cathcart, "Standards in Food and Nutrition," *CMAJ* 41, no. 4 (October 1939): 397.
44 Lindsay, "The Overweight Child," 504–6.
45 Elizabeth Chant Robertson, "The Tragedy of the Fat Child," *Chatelaine* 31, no. 1 (January 1958): 45–6; Grignon, "L'obésité et la maigreur," 1308.
46 Sam Landa, "The Adolescent and 'Physical Fitness,'" *CAHPER* 27, no. 5 (June/July 1961): 13. For future obesity, see Royer, "Problems in Infant Feeding," 992; D.M. Sinclair, "Editorial: Obesity as a Public Health Problem," *CJPH* 58, no. 11 (November 1967): 520. For anorexia, see R.F. Farquharson and H.H. Hyland, "Anorexia Nervosa: The Course of 15 Patients Treated from 20 to 30 Years Previously," *CMAJ* 94, no. 9 (26 February 1966): 411–19. For the future of the nation, see John R. Beaton, "Energy Balance and Obesity," *CJPH* 58, no. 11 (November 1967): 480.
47 For physical health, see Robbie Salter, "Origin of Obesity," *Health* 45, no. 1 (Spring 1979): 7. For hypertension, see "Hypertension: Pediatric Hypertension – Think about It," *CN* 75, no. 4 (April 1979): 32. For inferiority, see Salter's article in *Health* 45, no. 1 (Spring 1979): 7; and Daniel Cappon, *Eating, Loving and Dying: A Psychology of Appetites* (Toronto: University of Toronto Press, 1973), 55, 74. For fear of child obesity leading to adult obesity, see Kindl and Brown, "A Programme to Treat Childhood Obesity," 662; Myres and Yeung, "Obesity in Infants," 113.
48 Lexa Denne, "Nutrition," *PHJ* 19, no. 9 (September 1928): 443.
49 Lindsay, "The Overweight Child," 504, 506; France L. Ilg, "The Child's Idea of What and How to Eat," *CN* 45, no. 7 (July 1949): 514; Brown and Chant Robertson, *The Normal Child* (1948), 151; Alan Brown and Elizabeth Chant Robertson, *The Normal Child* (Toronto: Harlequin Books, 1958), 124. See also D.E. Rodger, J.Grant McFetridge, and Eileen Price, "The Management of Obesity," *CMAJ* 63, no. 3 (September 1950): 265–6.
50 For snacks, see *CMAJ* 93, no. 16 (16 October 1965): 45, advertisement for Preludin. For teens overeating, see Mahoney, "Teen Talk about Food," 32.

For eating contests, see Steve Penfold, *The Donut: A Canadian History* (Toronto: University of Toronto Press, 2008), 79.

51 Beaton, "Energy Balance and Obesity," 481–2; A.M. Bryans, "Childhood Obesity – Prelude to Adult Obesity," *CJPH* 58, no. 11 (November 1967): 488; J.E. Monagle, "Canada's Food Guide: A Route Map to Health," *Health* 30, no. 5 (October 1962): 28.

52 For fat cells, see L.C. Petrich, "Review of *The Psychology of Obesity: Dynamics and Treatment* by Norman Kiell," *CD* 41, no. 4 (April 1975): 81; A.W. Myres, "Summary: Obesity: Is it Preventable in Infancy and Childhood?" *CFP* 21, no. 4 (April 1975): 2; and the article itself, "Obesity," 74; Anne B. Kenshole, "Weight and Diabetes," *CFP* 18, no. 2 (February 1972): 41. For "juvenile-onset obesity," see Bill Gladstone, "Beautiful Loser: His Story," *Chatelaine* 51, no. 7 (July 1978): 110; "Early Weaners More Obese?" *Chatelaine* 51, no. 11 (November 1978): 24. For a different view of fat cells, see Richard Goldbloom, "Pediatrics: Obesity in Childhood," *CMAJ* 113, no. 2 (26 July 1975): 139.

53 For lunch programs, see J. Ellestad-Sayed, J.C. Haworth, and H. Medovy, "Nutrition Survey of School Children in Greater Winnipeg," *CMAJ* 116, no. 5 (5 March 1977): 490. For school vending machines and cafeterias, see Adelaide Daniels, "Study of Nutrition and Teenage Health," *Health* 40, no. 1 (Spring 1974): 20. For lack of nutritional education, see Naomi Mallovy, "Good Habits Last a Lifetime," *Chatelaine* 46, no. 6 (June 1973): 98.

54 F.M Clydesdale, "The Obese Child and the Role of Exercise," *Health* 41, no. 3 (Autumn 1975): 9, 25.

55 See Wendy Mitchinson, "Mother Blaming and Obesity: An Alternative Perspective," in Ellison, McPhail, and Mitchinson, *Obesity in Canada*, 187–217.

56 Chant Robertson, "My Child Is Too Fat," 10–14; News Brief, "The Emotional Obese," *CD* 14, no. 3 (March 1948): 92.

57 For the American study, see "Editorial: Obesity and Anorexia," *CMAJ* 73, no. 5 (1 September 1955): 408. For Bruch, see Laski, "The Overnourished and the Undernourished Child," 21; Martel, "Preludin (Phenmetrazine) in the Treatment of Obesity," 119; Dorothy Sangster, "The Tragedy of the Fat Child," *Maclean's* 72, no. 16 (1 August 1959): 37.

58 For culture, see D.A. Hill, "A Wetzel Grid Survey in Toronto," *CJPH* 44, no. 8 (August 1953): 286.

59 Daniel Cappon, "Review Article, Obesity," *CMAJ* 79, no. 7 (1 October 1958): 571–2. For Cappon, see Sangster, "The Tragedy of the Fat Child," 35.

60 Sheila Kieran, "What Diets Fail," *Chatelaine* 39, no. 12 (December 1966): 16.

61 For the literature on psychology, see Bryans, "Childhood Obesity," 487–8; Gilder, "The Fat Child," 1068; Becker, "Medicine Discovers the Teenagers," 42; Myres and Yeung, "Obesity in Infants," 116. Maurice Jetté, William Barry, and Lyon Pearlman, "The Effects of an Extracurricular Physical Activity Program in Obese Adolescents," *CJPH* 68, no. 1 (January/February 1977): 39.

62 Mrs Ruth Mowat, "Letter – Dieting the Doctor's Way," *Chatelaine* 41, no. 1 (January 1968): 68; Adelaide Daniels, "Word to the Wise: 'Let's Stop Being Our Own Worst Enemy,'" *Health* 39, no. 1 (Spring 1973): 26.

63 For ignorance, see Royer, "Problems in Infant Feeding," 992. For frustration, etc., see F. Gerard Allison, "Modern Treatment of Obesity," *ManMR* 40, no. 7 (August–September 1960): 509.

64 Laski, "The Overnourished and the Undernourished Child," 21. For rates of heredity, see Lucien Dubreuil, "L'obésité," *UMC* 81, no. 6 (juin 1952): 707; W.W. Hawkins, "Some Medical and Biological Aspects of Obesity," *CJPH* 54, no. 10 (October 1963): 479; see also Elizabeth Chant Robertson, "How to Help the Overweight Child," *Chatelaine* 34, no. 11 (November 1961): 127.

65 For heredity, see Gilder, "The Fat Child," 1068; Pierre Philippe, "Letter to Editor," *CMAJ* 117, no. 11 (3 December 1977): 1249; Frankle, "When Is a Child a Good Eater?" 13; Simeon Margolis and Dean H. Lockwood, "Obesity," in *The Principles and Practice of Medicine*, 18th ed., ed. A. McGehee Harvey et al. (New York: Appleton-Century Crofts, 1972), 920; Kindl and Brown, "A Programme to Treat Childhood Obesity," 662.

66 For the pituitary gland, see Thomas McCrae, ed., *The Principles and Practice of Medicine*, 10th ed. (New York: D. Appleton and Co., 1925), 445. See also Hugh Grant Rowell, "Weighty Matters," *Maclean's* 48, no. 15 (1 August 1935): 32. It seems that Froelich's syndrome was looked for more often in the United States than in Canada. For the United States, see Dawes, *Childhood Obesity in America*, 91–3.

67 Hilde Bruch, *The Importance of Overweight* (New York: W.W. Norton & Company, 1957), 7, 8; on Bruch, see Paula Saukko, "Fat Boys and Goody Girls: Hilde Bruch's Work on Eating Disorders and the American Anxiety about Democracy, 1930–1960," in *Weighty Issues: Fatness and Thinness as Social Problems*, ed. Jeffrey Sobal and Doanna Maurer (New York: Aldine de Gruyter, 1999), 31–49. One estimate suggested that 78 per cent of obesity in children was not caused by endocrine problems. R. Boucher, "Analyses de quelques travaux récents," *UMC* 54, no. 11 (novembre 1925): 732. For support of the endocrine cause, see Lamont, "Fatigue in Children," 48;

Chatelaine 11, no. 5 (May 1938): 22, advertisement for the Metropolitan Life Insurance Co.
68 Lindsay, "The Overweight Child," 504.
69 Laski, "The Overnourished and the Undernourished Child," 21; *CMAJ* 78, no. 6 (15 March 1958): 70, advertisement for Probese.
70 Gilder, "The Fat Child," 1068; "Review of *Adolescent Nutrition and Growth*, edited by Felix P. Heald, New York: Appleton-Century-Crofts, 1969," *CMAJ* 102, no. 3 (28 February 1970): 433. For hyperinsulinema, see Gilder, "The Fat Child," 1068.
71 Brown, *The Normal Child* (1923), 194–5, 41; "As the Twig Is Bent," *CHJ* 34, no. 7 (November 1937): 48. For teens, see Ian Eisehardt, "Keeping Fit the B.C. Way," *Health* 5, no. 4 (December 1937): 100.
72 For Percival, see John C. Scott, "Keep Fit, Work Hard, Play Fair, Live Clean," *Health* 16, no. 6 (November/December 1948): 14; Brown and Chant Robertson, *The Normal Child* (1948), 151; Elizabeth Chant Robertson, "We Are Shortchanging Our Children on Fitness," *Chatelaine* 31, no. 9 (September 1958): 122. For fitness statistics, see "Are Women the Fitter Sex?" *Health* 24, no. 2 (March/April 1956): 13, for a breakdown of boys and girls.
73 For CAHPER, see Deborah McPhail, *Contours of the Nation: Making Obesity and Imagining Canada, 1945–1970* (Toronto: University of Toronto Press, 2017), 84. For concern about lack of exercise, see "Teens Have Heart Worries," *Chatelaine* 38, no. 9 (September 1965): 17; Becker, "Medicine Discovers the Teen-agers," 26; Beaton, "Energy Balance and Obesity," 481; Carla Rice, "How Big Girls Become Fat Girls: The Cultural Production of Problem Eating and Physical Inactivity," in *Critical Feminist Approaches to Eating Dis/orders*, ed. Helen Malson and Maree Burns (London: Routledge, 2009), 103 for interviews.
74 For ParticipACTION, see Lisa McDermott, "A Critical Interrogation of Contemporary Discourses of Physical (In)Activity amongst Canadian Children: Back to the Future," *Journal of Canadian Studies* 42, no. 2 (Spring 2008): 5–42, especially 11–12, 15. For the boy, see Mark Sarner, "Growing Up Old," *CN* (3 June 1978): 3. For citizenship, see Goldbloom, "Pediatrics," 139. For lack of fitness, see Don Bailey, "Participaction: Childhood Development," *BCMJ* 16, no. 1 (January 1974): 7.
75 For not walking, see Abby Hoffman, "Canadian Kids: C – Fitness," *Chatelaine* 53, no. 11 (November 1980): 248; and Kindl and Brown, "A Programme to Treat Childhood Obesity," 663. For TV watching, see Bailey, "Physical Activity Vital for All Children," 10.
76 Myres, "Obesity," 74; Bryans, "Childhood Obesity," 488.

77 For self-image, see Jon Robison, "Kids, Eating, Weight & Health: Helping without Harming." *Absolute Advantage* 7, no. 1 (2007): 12, 14. For more on the significance of self-esteem in "treatment," see Pamela Rose Ward, "Exploring the Role of Discourse in the Emerging Identities of Children Enrolled in an Obesity Treatment Program" (PhD diss., Memorial University, 2012), 19. On surgery, see Carly Weeks, "Surgery More Effective for Treating Obese Teens," *Globe and Mail*, 10 February 2010, accessed 26 April 2010, https://www.theglobeandmail.com/life/parenting/surgery-more-effective-for-treating-obese-teens/article571664/. However, Dr Arya Sharma fears "there are risks that bariatric surgery could become too common for young people as well as adults."
78 Lindsay, "The Overweight Child," 505.
79 For not dieting, see Edward H. Mason, "The Treatment of Obesity," *CMAJ* 14, no. 11 (November 1924): 1052; Walter R. Campbell, "Obesity and Its Treatment," *CMAJ* 34, no. 1 (January 1936): 42. For Dafoe, see Kerry Segrave, *Obesity in America, 1850–1939: A History of Social Attitudes and Treatment* (Jefferson, NC: McFarland & Co., 2008), 162; Lindsay, "The Overweight Child," 505; Chant Robertson, "My Child Is Too Fat," 11. See also Chant Robertson, "The Tragedy of the Fat Child," 46.
80 Adele White, "Try *This* for *That*," *Chatelaine* 19, no. 9 (September 1946): 54–5. For Oslo breakfast, see B.L. Frank, "De l'importance d'une alimentation appropriée dans la grossesse et la lactation, dans la croissance et le développement des enfants, et dans les états débilitants et la sénilité," *UMC* 83, no. 3 (mars 1954): 296. For low calorie food, see L.S. White, "Weight Watchers Brighten Meals with Special Diet Fruit," *Health* 27, no. 1 (January/February 1959): 12. For educating mothers, see Laski, "The Overnourished and the Undernourished Child," 21.
81 For difficulty of a diet for the young, see Beaton, "Energy Balance and Obesity," 480.
82 Library and Archives Canada, Department of Health, Record Group 29 (RG 29), Nutrition Division, 1921–1971, vol. 934, file 386, 5–4, part 1, Nutrition Services, Foods, Request for Special Dietary Foods, Aug. 1956–63, letter from Mrs S. from Côte Saint-Luc, Montreal, to Department of Nutrition, 22 October 1962; response from J.E. Monagle, Chief, Nutrition Division, 30 October 1962. For teens, see Eveleen Dollery, "Your Diet That Lets You Eat Your Cake and Look Slim, Too," *Chatelaine* 33, no. 3 (March 1960): 102. See also a list of the food teens loved. "Diet Therapy Pointers for Young Athletes," *CFP* 23, no. 5 (May 1977): 128. According to Dawes, American doctors put children on reducing diets more often than British

doctors. It appears that Canadians doctors also didn't put children on diets as often as American doctors. Dawes, *Childhood Obesity in America*, 134, 142.

83 For Simeons' diet, see "Obesity in Children Equally Intractable," 350. For saccharin, see A.B. Morrison, "Editorial: Sugar Substitutes," *CMAJ* 129, no. 5 (17 March 1979): 634. For more on concern about dieting, see "Diet Therapy Pointers for Young Athletes," 128.

84 "Hypertension: Pediatric Hypertension," 33.

85 Gilder, "The Fat Child," 1068. For family, see Kindl and Brown, "A Programme to Treat Childhood Obesity," 662.

86 For Wolfish, see Becker, "Medicine Discovers the Teen-agers," 44. For behaviour modification for youth, see Barbara A. Davis and Daniel A.K. Roncari, "Behavioural Treatment of Obesity," *CMAJ* 119, no. 12 (23 December 1978): 1423. For self-acceptance, see "Obesity in Children Equally Intractable," 350. Behaviour modifaction and psychiatry/psychology were used more often in the United States; see Dawes, *Childhood Obesity in America*, 121–6.

87 Mason, "The Treatment of Obesity," 1052. For the United States, see Dawes, *Childhood Obesity in America*, chapter 2, "The Enduring Promise: The Continued Search for a Pharmaceutical Remedy," 100–14.

88 Lindsay, "The Overweight Child," 506; Leonora Hawirko and P.H. Sprague, "Treatment of Obesity by Appetite-Depressing Drugs," *CMAJ* 54, no. 1 (January 1946): 29.

89 Bruch, *The Importance of Overweight*, 358; Martel, "Preludin (Phenmetrazine) in the Treatment of Obesity," 117–20; *MMC* 11, no. 10 (October 1956): 166, advertisement for Obedrin, *CMAJ* 78, no. 6 (15 March 1958): 70, advertisement for Probese; *CD* 24, no. 5 (May 1958): 18, advertisement for Dexedrine.

90 *CD* 32, no. 11 (November 1966): 6, advertisement for Ambar. For dangers, see *CMAJ* 91, no. 21 (21 November 1964): 46, advertisement for Durabolan.

91 *Chatelaine* 42, no. 10 (October 1969): 8, advertisement for Ayds. Similar to Marmola, Ayds, "the largest selling weight reducing plan in the U.S.," could be purchased from pharmacies without a prescription. With active ingredients benzocaine (a topical pain reliever) and later phenylpropanolamine (PPA, a psychoactive drug), Ayds was a "candy" that supposedly inhibited appetite. Advertisements for Ayds in the 1950s and 1960s were often seen in the popular magazines such as *Chatelaine* with endorsements from well-known actresses and dancers. Phenylpropanolamine was structured very close to amphetamine, and eventually there was concern about it in the United States. See Rasmussen,

On Speed, 241, concerning PPA. For Ayds advertisements, see *Chatelaine* 29, no. 10 (October 1956): 118; *Chatelaine* 29, no. 12 (December 1956): 6; *Chatelaine* 31, no. 10 (October 1958): 107; *CHJ* 53, no. 5 (September 1956): 10. For more on Ayds, see Peter Wyden, *The Overweight Society: An Authoritative, Entertaining Investigation into the Facts and Follies of Girth Control* (New York: William Morrow & Co., 1965), 246. Teen use of Ayds wasn't discussed in Dawes's book *Childhood Obesity in America*.

92 For drug use by teens, see David Lloyd, "Drug Misuse in Teenagers," *CN* 66, no. 9 (September 1970): 48–9. For Pondimin, see *CMAJ* 107, no. 12 (23 December 1972): 1154, advertisement. For the teenage girl, see *CMAJ* 105, no. 3 (7 August 1971): 302–3, advertisement for Pondimin. Dawes notes that the use of amphetamine for children's diets was decreasing in the 1970s in the United States; see Dawes, *Childhood Obesity in America*, 108.

93 For support for HCG, see "Obesity in Children Equally Intractable," 350; see also "Controversies in Medicine Fanned during Association Scientific Meeting," *CMAJ* 113, no. 1 (12 July 1975): 64.

94 Mason, "The Treatment of Obesity," 1052; Lindsay, "The Overweight Child," 506. For exercise as a treatment for obesity, see D.T. Fraser, "Review of *Exercise in Education and Medicine* by R. Tait McKenzie," *PHJ* 19, no. 5 (May 1928): 249. For girls, see Annabelle Lee, "Your Beauty Problem," *Chatelaine* 6, no. 10 (October 1933): 43; and Grace Garner, "Every Girl Her Own Girdle: Teens and Twenties Indoors Winter Sports – for a Super Figure," *CHJ* 41, no. 9 (January 1945): 16.

95 For exercise, see "More Exercise, More Food," *Chatelaine* 40, no. 4 (April 1967): 20; Becker, "Medicine Discovers the Teen-agers," 44. For Goldbloom, see Earl Dumude, "Fat Children," *Chatelaine* 41, no. 9 (September 1968): 14.

96 For team sports, see Jetté, Barry, and Pearlman, "The Effects of an Extracurricular Physical Activity Program," 39. For separate programs for the obese young, see Judith Banning, "A Personal Commitment to Fitness Results in Healthier Client," *CN* 76, no. 5 (May 1980): 40.

97 Lindsay, "The Overweight Child," 506; for 20 per cent treatment success and Wolfish, see "Obesity in Children Equally Intractable," 350.

Chapter 7

1 John T. Powell, "Need for Optimal Activity in Middle Age," *CAHPER* 36, no. 5 (May/June 1970): 18.

2 For different cultures and times, see Sander L. Gilman, *Fat: A Cultural History of Obesity* (Cambridge: Polity Press, 2008), 3. See also Joyce Huff, "A 'Horror of Corpulence': Interrogating Bantigism

382   Notes to pages 208–9

and Mid-Nineteenth-Century Fat-Phobia," in *Bodies Out of Bounds: Fatness and Transgression*, ed. Jana Evans Braziel and Kathleen LeBesco (Berkeley: University of California Press 2001), 319–59; Carole Spitzack, *Confessing Excess: Women and the Politics of Body Reduction* (Albany, NY: State University of New York Press, 1990), 36; Jeffery Sobal and Donna Maurer, "Preface," in *Interpreting Weight: The Social Management of Fatness and Thinness*, ed. Jeffery Sobal and Donna Maurer (New York: Aldine de Gruyter, 1999), vii; Stephen Gundle, *Glamour: A History* (Oxford: Oxford University Press, 2008). For Canada and the media, see Wendy Mitchinson, "The Media and the Ideal and Fat Body: An Examination of Embodiment and Affect in a Canadian Context," in *Reclaiming Canadian Bodies: Visual Media and Representation*, ed. Lynda Mannick and Karen McGarry (Waterloo, ON: Wilfrid Laurier University Press, 2015), 5–32.

3 See Mitchinson, "The Media and the Ideal and Fat Body," 5–32.
4 Joanne Entwistle, "Fashion and the Fleshy Body: Dress as Embodied Practice," *Fashion Theory* 4, no. 3 (2000): 323, 326, 335.
5 For fashions, see Charlotte M. Storey, "Minimizing One's Size: By Wearing Just the Right Clothes," *CHJ* 16, no. 10 (February 1920): 37. For women reaching forty, see Eva Nagel Wolf, "Looking Forty in the Face," *CHJ* 30, no. 10 (February 1934): 22, 39; Annabelle Lee, "Work-a-Day Beauty," *Chatelaine* 6, no. 11 (November 1933): 32; Constance Templeton, "Be Fair to Forty," *Maclean's* 45, no. 22 (15 November 1932): 53. For limiting exercise at forty, see George S. Young, "The Relations between Periodic Health Examinations and Improper Living Habits," *OMR* 2, no. 2 (March 1935): 43.
6 For Bissell, see *CHJ* 33, no. 6 (October 1936): 98, advertisement.
7 For quote, see MAB, "Getting Back to Normal after Summer," *Chatelaine* 3, no. 9 (September 1930): 33. For women who work at a desk, see Janet Lane and Ruth Chandler Moore, "Watch for the Trademark," *CHJ* 33, no. 6 (October 1936): 20, 47, 49. For walking as exercise, see "The Tale of the Years," *CHJ* 34, no. 10 (February 1938): 32.
8 For negative description of a fat woman, see Basil G. Partridge, "Platitoodinous Hooey," *Maclean's* 42, no. 16 (15 August 1929): 14–15, 76–8. In David William Belbeck, "Fat Girl," *Chatelaine* 5, no. 6 (June 1932): 12–13, 30, 32, the "fat girl" didn't get her man, but then the thin woman didn't either. For the dieting woman getting her man, see Pauline J. Labbe, "Slimming a Debutante," *Chatelaine* 6, no. 9 (September 1933): 7–9, 44–6; Frank Perret, "Heavenly Body," *Chatelaine* 24, no. 4 (April 1951): 30–1, 70–5, 86–7. A fat woman had her fat man in Thelma Rudge, "A Sugar-Cured Ham," *Maclean's* 45, no. 1 (1 January 1932): 7–8, 48–9. For the motherly

woman, see W.A. Fraser, "The Lost Stirrup," *Maclean's* 35, no. 9 (1 May 1922): 13–15, 51–5.
9   For photo of police, see Vancouver Archives, AM1535-: CVA 99–1022, 1923.
10 For muscle, see *Eaton's Catalogue*, Spring/Summer 1932, 161, advertisement for Robeleine. For other bodybuilding products, see *Maclean's* 49, no. 2 (15 February 1936): 46, advertisement for Kelpamalt. For exercise equipment, see *Eaton's Catalogue*, Fall/Winter 1932–33, 296. For Canada Dry, see *CHJ* 26, no. 12 (April 1930): 77, advertisement.
11 Martha Banning Thomas, "Ginger Ale and Pop," *The Chatelaine* 4, no. 8 (August 1931): 3–5, 32–3; and *The Chatelaine* 4, no. 9 (September 1931): 12, 28, 30, 32, 35 (part two).
12 For sedentary life, see Hugh Grant Rowell, "Me-Athlete," *Maclean's* 46, no. 18 (15 September 1933): 10, 39–40. For a medical article about limiting exercise at forty, see Young, "The Relations between Periodic Health Examinations and Improper Living Habits," 43.
13 For Mrs Grange, see J. Morton Lewis, "At Seven O'Clock," *CHJ* 19, no. 5 (September 1922): 21, 23. For benign fat men, see E.G. Bayne, "Mr. Fiegenbaum's Find," *CHJ* 26, no. 2 (June 1929): 24, 87–8. For a story of a maimed hero and his villain boss, see Archie P. Mckishnie, "Quits," *Maclean's* 38, no. 19 (1 October 1925): 52–4, 56, 59–63. For a salesman who used his experience to help, see Arthur H. Deute, "Old Plump," *Maclean's* 39, no. 9 (15 April 1926): 20, 53–7. For the portly man, see Ellis Parker Butler, "The Hemmerstich-Beckstar Feud," *Maclean's* 44, no. 9 (1 May 1931): 14–15, 64–6.
14 For the young man, see Dorothy Thomas, "Sweet Summer," *CHJ* 38, no. 7 (December 1941): 8–9, 34, 36, 38. For Mannering, see Benge Atlee, "The Last Armada," *CHJ* 38, no. 9 (February 1942): 5–7, 19, 20, 22.
15 For sedentary work, see Eva Nagel Wolf, "In Self Defence," *CHJ* 38, no. 7 (November 1941): 62.
16 For women, see Jean Alexander, "Keeping Fit for the Job," *Chatelaine* 15, no. 9 (September 1942): 30.
17 "Teens' Routines," *Chatelaine* 16, no. 9 (September 1943): 33.
18 Mark McKague, "Male and Female Body Image in Canada: 1955–1965" (unpublished student paper, University of Waterloo, 2008), 4. For chest spander, see *Eaton's Catalogue*, Spring/Summer 1950, 467. For emphasis on shoulders, chest, and arms for men, see Josephine Lowman, "Why Grow Old? Hubby Hollow Chested? He May Need Exercise," *Globe and Mail*, 8 July 1952, 11. For fear of losing manhood, see Christopher J. Greig, "The Idea of Boyhood in Postwar Ontario, 1945–1960" (PhD diss., University of Western Ontario, 2008), 70.

19 On middle-aged men in stories, see Velda Johnston, "Triangle," *CHJ* 50, no. 7 (November 1953): 9, 33–5, 44, 46–7. See also Josephine Lowman, "Tubby Hubby: Women Prefer Slim Males to Those Who Add Weight," *Globe and Mail*, 28 September 1953, 12; and Lowman, "Why Grow Old?" 15.

20 For men, see Sidney Katz, "Those Middle-Age Blues," *Maclean's* 62, no. 20 (15 October 1949): 15, 36.

21 For staying the same weight as at age twenty-five, see Josephine Lowman, "Tubby Hubby Diet: Obesity Top Killer, Watch Your Weight," *Globe and Mail*, 1 October 1953, 10. For men and age forty, see Robert Thomas Allen, "What It's Like to be Forty," *Maclean's* 65, no. 10 (15 May 1952): 10–11.

22 For airlines, see Patrizia Gentile, "Queen of the Maple Leaf: A History of Beauty Contests in Twentieth Century Canada" (PhD diss., Queen's University, 2006), 118. For the United States, see Eileen Boris, "Desirable Dress: Rosies, Sky Girls, and the Politics of Appearance," *International Labor and Working-Class History* 69 (Spring 2006): 132.

23 For honesty about bulges, see Rosemary Boxer, "Memo from Rosemary," *Chatelaine* 25, no. 4 (April 1952): 5. For hips, see Patricia Skinner, "Stenographer's Spread," *CHJ* 46, no. 10 (February 1950): 38–9. For ugliness, see Kae McColl, "TOPS...To Take Off Pounds," *CHJ* 54, no. 7 (November 1957): 24. For fat as dangerous, see Reva Gerstein, "How to Stay on Your Diet," *Chatelaine* 29, no. 10 (October 1956): 6. For age, see *CHJ* 54, no. 8 (December 1957): 49, advertisement for S.O.S.

24 For "beauty defect," see Eva Nagel Wolf, "Danger Signals," *CHJ* 42, no. 10 (February 1946): 63. For "Top Heavy," see Adele White, "Belittling Tricks," *Chatelaine* 20, no. 9 (September 1947): 10–11. For more on legs and thighs, see Adele White, "Out in the Open," *Chatelaine* 19, no. 6 (June 1946): 56.

25 Yves Theriault, "The Bequest," *Maclean's* 70, no. 14 (6 July 1957): 26–7, 38–9.

26 For beauty contests, see David M. Garner et al., "Cultural Expectations of Thinness in Women," *Psychological Reports* 47, no. 2 (1980): 489. For York University, see Anthony Synnott, "Truth and Goodness, Mirrors and Masks – part I: A Sociology of Beauty and the Face," *British Journal of Sociology* 40, no. 4 (1989): 609. For Thyer, see Kaspars Dzeguze, "A Lean and Hungry Look," *Maclean's* 91, no. 15 (24 July 1978): 29.

27 For Callwood, see Gwen Beattie, "Staying Thin: How the Beautiful People Do It," *Chatelaine* 42, no. 4 (April 1969): 56.

28 Mary Jane Rolfs, "The Cleverest Christmas," *Chatelaine* 35, no. 12 (December 1962): 36–7, 54–6, 58.

29 McKague, "Male and Female Body Image in Canada," 23. For men's need to lose weight, see Marjorie Harris, "Fashion," *Maclean's* 81, no. 9

(September 1968): 85. For looking twenty-five, see W. Schweisheimer, "Your Waistline Is Biggest Health Hazard," *Executive* 7 (April 1965): 60. For Waxman, see Dzeguze, "A Lean and Hungry Look," 29.

30 Dorothy Sangster, "The Trouble with Middle-Aged Men," *Maclean's* 73, no. 12 (4 June 1960): 43. For the boomers and middle-age flab, see John Hofsess, "How to Survive Middle Age," *Maclean's* 86, no. 10 (October 1973): 36.

31 For seventy seconds of exercising, see *Maclean's* 81, no. 11 (November 1968): 62, advertisement for Bullworker exercise. For the seven minute exercise, see *Maclean's* 91, no. 5 (6 March 1978): 45, advertisement for synometrics. For bodybuilding equipment, see *Eaton's Catalogue*, Spring/Summer 1976, 133. For Weider's tablets, see *Eaton's Catalogue*, Spring/Summer 1962, 304, advertisement. For more on Weider, see Mordecai Richler, "You Too Can Have a Body Beautiful," *Maclean's* 73, no. 25 (3 December 1960): 3–31, 44–6. For posture, see Library and Archives Canada, Metropolitan Life Insurance Company, Ac. 901, C3, Pt. 610 no. 680, "Metropolitan's Life's Exercise Guide for Men and Women," 1966, 1.

32 *Maclean's* 92, no. 20 (14 May 1979): 6–7, advertisement for Honda.

33 Bonnie Cornell, "Chatelaine's FAB Diet," *Chatelaine* 48, no. 1 (January 1975): 46.

34 Alexandra Palmer, ed., *Fashion: A Canadian Perspective* (Toronto: University of Toronto Press, 2004).

35 *Eaton's Catalogue*, Spring/Summer 1938, 148.

36 In researching sizing, Carol Cooper noted: "One might query whether men's measurements as stated in the catalogue were even used in filling orders or if the suggestion of a broader chest tapering to a narrow waist was merely an appeal to their vanity. It was probably not the case, but it certainly raises some doubts about the reliability of such measurements."

37 Sears's sizing chart from Christmas 2009 shows men's big fit extending to size 68 (as opposed to 54 or so in Eaton's 1976 catalogue). Researched by Carol Cooper.

38 *Eaton's Catalogue*, Spring/Summer 1947, 190, items 029–150. For diverse ages, see *Eaton's Catalogue*, Spring/Summer 1941, 151. For men who stay young, see *Eaton's Catalogue*, Fall/Winter 1947–48, 242, item 029–134. For shoulders, see *Eatons' Catalogue*, Spring/Summer 1959, 222.

39 For trousers, see *Eaton's Catalogue*, Spring/Summer 1962, 199. For suit shoulders, see *Eaton's Catalogue*, Spring/Summer 1965, 201. For slacks, see *Eaton's Catalogue*, Spring/Summer 1965, 183. For leisure suits in the 1970s, see *Eaton's Catalogue*, Spring/Summer 1976, 238. For flared pants,

see *Eaton's Catalogue*, Spring/Summer 1971, 31. For the mature man, see *Eaton's Catalogue*, Spring/Summer 1974, 200.
40 *Eaton's Catalogue*, Fall/Winter 1920–21, 288. For comfort and fit, see *Eaton's Catalogue*, Spring/Summer 1920, 218; and *Eaton's Catalogue*, Spring/Summer 1935, 131.
41 *Eaton's Catalogue*, Fall/Winter 1920–21, 241. For the "stout appearance," see *Eaton's Catalogue*, Spring/Summer 1923, 204.
42 *Eaton's Catalogue*, Spring/Summer 1923, 210–11; *Eaton's Catalogue*, Spring/Summer 1932, 114, items 44–884, 44–885, 44–850.
43 *Eaton's Catalogue*, Spring/Summer 1944, 167.
44 For photos, see *Eaton's Catalogue*, Spring/Summer 1947, 198, item 29–474; and *Eaton's Catalogue*, Fall/Winter 1947–48, 242, item 029–136. For age, see *Eaton's Catalogue*, Spring/Summer 1950, 241, item 029–1054. For profile, see *Eaton's Catalogue*, Spring/Summer 1953, 239, item 029–1054.
45 For work clothes, see *Eaton's Catalogue*, Spring/Summer 1950, 263, item 28–4009. For shirts, see *Eaton's Catalogue*, Spring/Summer 1956, 240, item 29-G-2474 for robust and item 29-G-2469 for generous cut.
46 *Eaton's Catalogue*, Spring/Summer 1968, 264, 266.
47 *Eaton's Catalogue*, Spring/Summer 1971, 308; *Eaton's Catalogue*, Spring/Summer 1974, 368. For the two models, see *Eaton's Catalogue*, Spring/Summer 1975, 220.
48 For use of the word "husky," see *Eaton's Catalogue*, Spring/Summer 1950, 160. For boys playing, see *Eaton's Catalogue*, Spring/Summer 1956, 181. For the "build," see *Eaton's Catalogue*, Spring/Summer 1959, 181, item 32-K-3173.
49 For husky, see *Eaton's Catalogue*, Spring/Summer 1968, 237. For drawings, see *Eaton's Catalogue*, Spring/Summer 1971, 255.
50 *Eaton's Catalogue*, Spring/Summer 1926, 200.
51 For the Bracer, see *Eaton's Catalogue*, Fall//Winter 1938–39, 305, item 02–1827; *Maclean's* 50, no. 13 (1 July 1937): 45, advertisement; *Maclean's* 52, no. 7 (1 April 1939): 49, advertisement.
52 *Eaton's Catalogue*, Fall/Winter 1947–48, 271, item 12–584 Holdrite.
53 For Harvey Woods, see *Eaton's Catalogue*, Spring/Summer 1965, 215, item 28-A-9208A. For the brief, see *Eaton's Catalogue*, Spring/Summer 1974, 356.
54 *Eaton's Catalogue*, Fall/Winter 1920–21, 58. For hems, see *Eaton's Catalogue*, Spring/Summer 1920, 24, item 84–242. For the end of the 1920s and the 1930s, see *Eaton's Catalogue*, Spring/Summer, 1929, 20; *Eaton's Catalogue*, Spring/Summer 1938, 18. For slenderizing, see *Eaton's Catalogue*, Spring/Summer 1929, 22, items 58–230 and 58–232. For misses sizes, see *Eaton's*

Catalogue, Spring/Summer 1935, 7. See also *Eaton's Catalogue*, Spring/Summer 1935, 5 with junior size.
55 For the hourglass figure, see *Eaton's Catalogue*, Spring/Summer 1941, 5. For slim, see *Eaton's Catalogue*, Spring/Summer 1941, 6, item 58–61; and *Eaton's Catalogue*, Spring/Summer 1947, 91, item G. For Dior, see *Eaton's Catalogue*, Fall/Winter 1947, 12, item C. For sack dress, see Vivian Wilcox, "Everyone's Asking about THE SACK," *Chatelaine* 31, no. 2 (February 1958): 21. For slacks, see *Eaton's Catalogue*, Spring/Summer 1950, 14, 72. For aging, see *Eaton's Catalogue*, Spring/Summer 1953, 92.
56 *Eaton's Catalogue*, Spring/Summer 1962, 5, 3.
57 *Eaton's Catalogue*, Spring/Summer 1968, 91. Mark Tran, "Twiggy, Face of 1966, Reveals She Hated How She Looked," *The Guardian*, 14 February 2016, https://www.theguardian.com/fashion/2016/feb/14/twiggy-face-of-1966-reveals-she-hated-her-looks.
58 *Eaton's Catalogue*, Spring/Summer 1971, 13, 19, 185.
59 Charity Mitchell Johnson, "Would You Prefer to Look Like a Lamp-Shade or Like a Table Bell," *Maclean's* 36, no. 3 (1 February 1923): 60–1.
60 For style, see *Eaton's Catalogue*, Fall/Winter 1926–27, 42, item 58–423. For slimming, see *Eaton's Catalogue*, Fall/Winter 1923–24, 23, item 82–231.
61 For larger women and their double chins, see *Eaton's Catalogue*, Spring/Summer 1926, 79. For coats and the text, see *Eaton's Catalogue*, Spring/Summer 1932, page N.
62 *Eaton's Catalogue*, Spring/Summer 1938, 20, 21.
63 For a dignified frock, see *Eaton's Catalogue*, Fall/Winter 1935–36, 19, item 58–190. For graceful, see *Eaton's Catalogue*, Spring/Summer 1923, 16, item 82–161; *Eaton's Catalogue*, Spring/Summer 1935, 33. For matronly, see *Eaton's Catalogue*, Spring/Summer 1926, 16, item 58–153; and Fall/Winter 1926–27, 7, item 82–401. For ample proportions, see *Eaton's Catalogue*, Fall/Winter 1926–27, 42, item 58–423. For stylish stout, see *Eaton's Catalogue*, Fall/Winter 1926–27, 42, item 58–421. For above average size, see *Eaton's Catalogue*, Spring/Summer 1920, 14, item 58–1403. For large dimensions, see *Eaton's Catalogue*, Spring/Summer 1920, 55.
64 *Eaton's Catalogue*, Spring/Summer 1944, 33.
65 *Eaton's Catalogue*, Spring/Summer 1947, 27, items K and F.
66 For slendering, see *Eaton's Catalogue*, Spring/Summer 1959, 20–2, for costly dresses; 30–1, for housedresses.
67 *Eaton's Catalogue*, Fall/Winter 1944, 14, for maturity; and *Eaton's Catalogue*, Spring/Summer 1944, 22–3, for maturity and dignity.
68 *Eaton's Catalogue*, Spring/Summer 1956, 20, item C, for "not so tall"; and *Eaton's Catalogue*, Spring/Summer 1956, 20, item E, for "average" and "not so-slim."

69 *Eaton's Catalogue*, Spring/Summer 1959, 141.
70 *Eaton's Catalogue*, Spring/Summer 1962, 173; *Eaton's Catalogue*, Spring/Summer 1965, 151–2.
71 Story from Carol Cooper, 30 May 2009.
72 *Eaton's Catalogue*, Spring/Summer 1965, 19, 25–6, items 7 and 9.
73 *Eaton's Catalogue*, Fall/Winter 1962, 60, caption. For Dressler, see *Eaton's Catalogue*, Spring/Summer 1962, 30–1, items 9 and 10; for Dressler earlier, see *Eaton's Catalogue*, Spring/Summer 1944, 26–7, items G and Q.
74 *Eaton's Catalogue*, Fall/Winter 1968, 12.
75 *Eaton's Catalogue*, Fall/Winter 1974–75, 65, item E, for model as slimming. For day dresses, see *Eaton's Catalogue*, Spring/Summer, 65.
76 *Eaton's Catalogue*, Fall/Winter 1974, 67; *Eaton's Catalogue*, Spring/Summer 1975, 62–3; and plus size examples from *Sears Catalogue*, Spring/Summer 2009, 228–31.
77 *Eaton's Catalogue*, Spring/Summer 1923, 84.
78 *Eaton's Catalogue*, Spring/Summer 1920, 149, items 98–1504 and 98–1507. For youth, see Suzanne Marchand, *Rouge à lèvres et pantalon: Des pratiques esthétiques féminines controversées au Québec, 1920–1939* (Montréal: Les Éditions Hurtubise HMH, 1997), 130, and for quotes from women who started to wear corsets at the ages of ten, eleven, and twelve.
79 *CHJ* 19, no. 5 (September 1922): 49, advertisement for Gossard Corsetry.
80 *Eaton's Catalogue*, Spring/Summer 1920, 152 (see various items on the page).
81 For reduction rubber girdle, see *Eaton's Catalogue*, Spring/Summer 1938, 55. For disaster, see "New Sculptured Models," *CHJ* 30, no. 11 (March 1934): 36. For bulging, see *Eaton's Catalogue*, Spring/Summer 1920, 150, items 98–1542 and 98–1536. For the thighs, see *Eaton's Catalogue*, Fall/Winter 1926, 1926–27, 111.
82 For control, see *Eaton's Catalogue*, Spring/Summer 1941, 51, 53, 55; Carolyn Damon, "Foundation for Action," *Chatelaine* 15, no. 4 (April 1942): 45. For the proportional drawing, see *Eaton's Catalogue*, Spring/Summer 1941, 51.
83 *Eaton's Catalogue*, Fall/Winter 1947, 106; and *Eaton's Catalogue*, Spring/Summer 1947, 131.
84 For age eight, see *Eaton's Catalogue*, Spring/Summer 1947, 99, item G. For slim girls wearing girdles and bras, see "For That Willowy Young Look," *Eaton's Catalogue*, Spring/Summer 1947, 125.
85 For nylon, see "Personal Planning," *Chatelaine* 23, no. 10 (October 1950): 79. For control, see *Eaton's Catalogue*, Spring/Summer 1950, 109. For Warner's, see McKague, "Male and Female Body Image in Canada," 9.
86 *Eaton's Catalogue*, Spring/Summer 1955, 102.

87 *Eaton's Catalogue*, Spring/Summer 1965, 97, 99, 7.
88 For Hanes, see *Maclean's* 82, no. 2 (February 1969): 9, advertisement. For the Original Subtract, see *Eaton's Catalogue*, Spring/Summer 1974, 128. For Miss Mary, see *Eaton's Catalogue*, Spring/Summer 1974, 129–30.
89 *Eaton's Catalogue*, Spring/Summer 1974, 119, 126, 128–30.

Chapter 8

1 Eveleen Dollery, "Take It Off! Take It Off!" *Chatelaine* 43, no. 4 (April 1970): 48.
2 Katherine Ashenburg, "Critical Mass," *The Walrus* (January/February 2013): 28–31, 33, 35, 37. See also Terry Poulton, *No Fat Chicks: How Women Are Brainwashed to Hate Their Bodies and Spend Their Money* (Toronto: Key Porter, 1996).
3 For using voices, see Joan Sangster, "Invoking Experience as Evidence," *Canadian Historical Review* 92, no. 1 (March 2011): 135–61. For the voices of those who are fat, see Allyson Mitchell, "Corporeographies of Size: Fat Women in Urban Spaces" (PhD diss., York University, 2006); Moss Edward Norman, "Living in the Shadow of an 'Obesity Epidemic': The Discursive Construction of Boys and Their Bodies" (PhD diss., University of Toronto, 2009); Jenny Ellison, "'Stop Postponing Your Life Until You Lose Weight and Start Living Now': Vancouver's Large as Life Action Group, 1979–1985," *Journal of the Canadian Historical Association* 18, no. 1 (2007): 241–65; Jenny Ellison, "Large as Life: Self-Acceptance and the Fat Body in Canada, 1977–2000" (PhD diss., York University 2010). For films of people who are obese, see *Fat Chance*, directed by Jeff McKay (National Film Board, 1994); and *A Matter of Fat*, directed by William Weintraub (National Film Board, 1969).
4 *The Chatelaine* 1, no. 2 (April 1928): 72, advertisement for Marmola.
5 For Mrs P., see *The Chatelaine* 5, no. 2 (February 1932): 52, advertisement for Kruschen Salts. For the husband, see *Maclean's* 46, no. 18 (15 September 1933): 40, advertisement for Kruschen Salts.
6 *Chatelaine* 15, no. 2 (February 1942): 31, advertisement for DuBarry course.
7 *Chatelaine* 31, no. 10 (October 1958): 99, advertisement for Knox diet.
8 For Ayds narratives, see advertisements in *Chatelaine* 42, no. 10 (October 1969): 8; *Chatelaine* 43, no. 11 (November 1970): 18; *Chatelaine* 47, no. 4 (April 1974): 6; *Chatelaine* 47, no. 2 (February 1974): 4.
9 *Chatelaine* 34, no. 1 (January 1961): 78–9, advertisement for Metrecal.
10 Nita M. Ward, "How I Lost Thirty Pounds," *Chatelaine* 10, no. 10 (October 1937), 52, 58. For another narrative, see E. Christie Anderson, "Of Course You Can Be Slender," *Chatelaine* 12, no. 11 (November 1939): 16, 37–9.

11 James Bannerman (pseudonym for John Charles Kirkpatrick McNaught), "They Used to Call Me Fatty," *Maclean's* 62, no. 4 (15 February 1949): 22, 30–2.
12 Rosemary Boxer, "How *Chatelaine* Planned New Futures for Three Women," *Chatelaine* 25, no. 11 (November 1952): 12–13, 96–7; see pages 13 and 97 for Mildred Bennett.
13 Bob Blackburn, "Eat, Drink...and Feel Smug," *Maclean's* 79, no. 5 (5 March 1966): 22, 40. For another man, see Eric Hutton, "The One Weight-Control System That Works Every Time," *Maclean's* 74, no. 14 (15 July 1961): 7–10, 37–8.
14 For an example of what dieters had eaten, see Eveleen Dollery, "How Ruth Borley Lost Over 100 Pounds in Less Than a Year," *Chatelaine* 40, no. 4 (April 1967): 41–3.
15 Eveleen Dollery, "3 Dazzling Diet Successes," *Chatelaine* 36, no. 4 (April 1963): 40–5.
16 See Eveleen Dollery, "Three Diet Winners Discover New Beauty," *Chatelaine* 37, no. 4 (April 1964): 30–5; and Eveleen Dollery, "Diet to Beauty," *Chatelaine* 38, no. 4 (April 1965): 40–3.
17 For Bodnar, see Dollery, "Diet to Beauty," 40–3. For Ayds advertisement, see *Chatelaine* 40, no. 2 (February 1967): 10.
18 As examples, see Margaret A. Wood, "The Slob Diet & Exercise Program," *Chatelaine* 50, no. 7 (July 1977): 22, 78–9; Val Ross, "Beautiful Losers: Her Story," *Chatelaine* 51, no. 7 (July 1978): 38, 108–9; June Engel with Elizabeth Parr, "Obesity: The Losing Battle That Can Sometime Be Won," *Chatelaine* 53, no. 1 (November 1980): 61, 172–4; Eveleen Dollery, "Fat to Slim," *Chatelaine* 49, no. 4 (April 1976): 53–6; Eveleen Dollery and Donna Alexander Zaica, "How 5 Biggies Became 5 Thinnies," *Chatelaine* 53, no. 4 (April 1980): 52–7; Kaspars Dzeguze, "A Lean and Hungry Look," *Maclean's* 91, no. 15 (July 1978): 29.
19 Dollery, "Take It Off! Take It Off!," 48–51.
20 Alexander Ross, "The Remaking of Mike Crowe," *Financial Post*, February 1973, 6, 8. For another male narrative, see Bill Gladstone, "Beautiful Loser: His Story," *Chatelaine* 51, no. 7 (July 1978): 111.
21 Whitteker (told to Robert Olson), "I Like Being Fat...And Here Are My Reasons," *Maclean's* 70, no. 1 (26 October 1957): 26, 68–73.
22 Ethel Gillingham, "Who Says *Anyone* Can Lose Weight?" *Chatelaine* 34, no. 6 (June 1961): 38–9, 69.
23 On interviews, see Mona Gleason, "'Lost Voices, Lost Bodies'? Doctors and the Embodiment of Children and Youth in English Canada from 1900 to the 1940s, in *Lost Kids, Vulnerable Children and Youth in Twentieth-Century*

Notes to page 248   391

Canada and the United States, ed. Mona Gleason et al. (Vancouver, BC: UBC Press, 2010), 137.
24 Interview participants.

#	Alias	Year of Birth	Age	Date Interviewed	From
1	Mary	1934	75	4 May 2009	Vancouver
2	Heather	1948	61	5 May 2009	Vancouver
3	Jane	1945	64	22 May 2009	Crediton
4	Harry	1965	44	2 June 2009	Waterloo
5	Tina	1945	64	9 June 2009	London
6	Nicole	1952	57	10 June 2009	Guelph
7	Tammy	1945	64	29 June 2009	Amherstburg
8	Sara	1937	72	29 June 2009	Harrow
9	Fran	1967	42	7 July 2009	Waterloo
10	Julie	1962	47	15 July 2009	Brantford
11	Stephanie	1957	52	17 July 2009	London
12	Laura	1958	51	23 July 2009	Burlington
13	Grace	1965	44	27 July 2009	Guelph
14	Lucy	1970	39	28 July 2009	North York
15	Olive	1959	67	28 July 2009	Toronto
16	Doris	1942	67	30 July 2009	Guelph
17	Randy	1962	47	30 July 2009	Guelph
18	Bonnie	1956	52	31 July 2009	Waterloo
19	Leona	1962	47	2 Aug. 2009	Niagara Falls
20	Aileen	1958	51	3 Aug. 2009	Niagara Falls
21	Alice	1935	74	12 Aug. 2009	Mitchell
22	William	1947	62	13 Aug. 2009	Brantford
23	Frank	1946	63	20 Aug. 2009	Toronto
24	Glen	1959	50	1 Sept. 2009	Kitchener
25	Gail	1961	48	3 Sept. 2009	London
26	Nina	1957	52	3 Sept. 2009	London
27	Rose	1952	57	27 Oct. 2009	Waterloo
28	Sasha	1954	55	11 May 2010	Kitchener
29	Irene	1957	53	14 May 2010	Ottawa
30	Connie	1969	41	9 July 2010	Toronto

25 Fortunately, other scholars have interviewed individuals, and a few of them fit the criteria of this study: being overweight by 1980. These voices

have been integrated into this volume where they are appropriate. Carla Rice, in a study of obese women, made a concerted effort to include women of colour and women with disabilities. See Carla Rice, "Becoming 'The Fat Girl': Acquisition of an Unfit Identity," *Women's Studies International Forum* 30 (2007): 158–74, based on interviews with eighteen women. The thesis by Leanne Joanisse also had Canadians interviewed, many from Quebec and from the period of interest for this study. See Leanne Joanisse, "Reducing and Revisioning the Body: Women's Experiences of Weight Loss Surgery" (PhD diss., McMaster University, 2003).

26 For the history of meat and potatoes in the United States, see Harvey A. Levenstein, *Revolution at the Table: The Transformation of the American Diet* (Berkeley: University of California Press, 2003), 21.

27 For a similar situation in the United States (drinking more soda than milk), see Eric Schlosser, *Fast Food Nation: The Dark Side of the All-American Meal* (New York: Harper Perennial, 2005), 54.

28 For Tang history, see Michael Moss, *Salt Sugar Fat: How the Food Giants Hooked Us* (New York: Random House, 2013), 57–9, 127–8, 140.

29 For another example of the impact of World War II, see "Moe" in Heather Sykes (and Deborah McPhail), *Queer Bodies: Sexualities, Genders, and Fatness in Physical Education* (New York: Peter Lang, 2011), 57.

30 See Sykes (and McPhail), *Queer Bodies*, 62, for the problem of weighing children at school by "Starburst."

31 Joanisse, "Reducing and Revisioning the Body," 114, notes that her interviewees seemed to see their fathers as unsupportive; for some, however, it appeared to be their mothers who didn't support them.

32 Rice, "Becoming 'The Fat Girl,'" 169.

33 Ibid., 170.

34 Michele Henry, "Canada's Youth Face Obesity Epidemic," *Waterloo Region Record* 20 June 2011, B6.

35 Dr Bailey remembered a husband who smuggled food to his wife when she was in the hospital for bariatric surgery. "He preferred her to stay fat."

36 For clothing the large body, see Rachel Colls, "Outsize/Outside: Bodily Bignesses and the Emotional Experiences of British Women Shopping for Clothes," *Gender, Place & Culture* 13, no. 5 (October 2006): 529–45; Daiane Scaraboto and Eileen Fischer, "Frustrated Fatshionistas: An Institutional Theory Perspective on Consumer Quests for Greater Choice in Mainstream Markets," *Journal of Consumer Research* 39 (April 2013), 5, doi:10.1086/668298; Celesta "Dolly Dimples" Geyer, *Diet or Die: The Dolly Dimples Weight Reducing Plan* (New York: Frederick Fell, 1968 [published in Canada by George J. McLeod, Toronto]), 79.

37 For a contemporary description, see Henry, "Canada's Youth Face Obesity Epidemic."
38 For first awareness, see also those interviewed in Mitchell, "Corporeographies of Size," 160–5.
39 For a narrative about the impact of pregnancy, see Aaron Derfel, "The War against Obesity," *Montreal Gazette*, 26 March 2011, accessed 9 August 2011, https://www.pressreader.com/canada/montreal-gazette/20110326/292590353334364. See also interviews 5, 7, 8, 10, 11, 19, 28.
40 For disrespect from doctors, see Leanne Joanisse and Anthony Synnott, "Fighting Back: Reactions and Resistance to the Stigma of Obesity," in *Interpreting Weight: The Social Management of Fatness and Thinness*, ed. Jeffery Sobal and Donna Maurer (New York: Aldine de Gruyter, 1999), 57. See also Suzanne in Joanisse, "Reducing and Revisioning the Body," 136.
41 For the story of Poulton, see Joanisse, "Reducing and Revisioning the Body," 34.
42 Joanisse, "Reducing and Revisioning the Body," 35.
43 For liquid diets, see A. Frank, C. Graham, and S. Frank, "Fatalities on the Liquid-Protein Diet: An Analysis of Possible Causes," *International Journal of Obesity* 5, no. 3 (1981): 243–8, https://www.ncbi.nlm.nih.gov/pubmed/7275462.
44 For more on drugs given to children and teens, see Joanisse and Synnott, "Fighting Back," 60; see also Joanisse, "Reducing and Revisioning the Body," 139.
45 See Lee F. Monaghan, *Men and the War on Obesity: A Sociological Study* (London: Routledge, 2008).
46 For a memory of going to Weight Watchers as a teenager, see Ellison, "Large as Life," and her description of Sue Masterton, who felt the whole experience was "shameful," 1.
47 Laura Dawes, *Childhood Obesity in America: Biography of an Epidemic* (Cambridge, MA: Harvard University Press, 2014), chapter 9, "Summer Slimming: Fat Camps as a Diet-and-Exercise Obesity Treatment," 159–69.
48 See Ellison, "Large as Life," 100.
49 For athletics, see Rice, "Becoming 'The Fat Girl,'" 165–6.
50 Rice, "Becoming 'The Fat Girl,'" 164.
51 Mitchell, "Corporeographies of Size," 171, 182, 203. For importance of family, see Alyshia D. Bestard, "Weighted Discourse: Understanding the Lives of Overweight Women" (unpublished Honours BA thesis, University of Western Ontario, 2002), 44.
52 For learning, see Mitchell, "Corporeographies of Size," 309, 318.

Epilogue

1 Antoinette Burton, "Introduction: Archive Fever, Archive Stories," in *Archive Stories: Fact, Fictions, and the Writing of History*, ed. Antoinette Burton (Durham, NC: Duke University Press, 2005), 7–8, quoted in Deborah McPhail, "Canada Weighs In: Gender, Race, and the Making of 'Obesity,' 1945–1970" (PhD diss., York University, 2009), 26.
2 For parenting and mother blaming, see April Michelle Herndon, "Mommy Made Me Do It: Mothering Fat Children in the Midst of the Obesity Epidemic," *Food, Culture & Society* 13, no. 2 (2010): 331–49; Paula J. Caplan and Ian Hall-McCorquodale, "Mother-Blaming in Major Clinical Journals," *American Journal of Orthopsychiatry* 55, no. 3 (July 1985): 345–53. For disadvantaged mothers, see Kirsten Bell, Darlene McNaughton, and Amy Salmon, "Medicine, Morality and Mothering: Public Health Discourses on Foetal Alcohol Exposure, Smoking around Children and Childhood Overnutrition," *Critical Public Health* 19, no. 2 (June 2009): 163.
3 For puberty age of the mother, see Ken K. Ong et al., "Earlier Mother's Age at Menarche Predicts Rapid Infancy Growth and Childhood Obesity," *PLoS Medicine* 4, no. 4 (April 2007): e132, https://www.ncbi.nlm.nih.gov/pmc/articles/PMC1876410/. For weight-loss surgery and pregnancy, see André Picard, "Why Mom's Weight-Loss Surgery Is Good for Baby," *Globe and Mail*, 29 October 2012, accessed 24 January 2016, https://www.theglobeandmail.com/life/health-and-fitness/health/why-moms-weight-loss-surgery-is-good-for-baby/article4699181/.
4 For fruit and vegetables, see Laura Jakul, "The Effect of Anti-Obesity Media on Body Image and Antifat Attitudes" (MA thesis, University of Manitoba, 2005), 28. For how Canadians regard their eating, see CBC News, "Doctor Urges New View of Obesity," 3 January 2011, accessed 5 January 2011, http://www.cbc.ca/news/doctor-urges-new-view-of-obesity-1.984436.
5 CBC News, "Vitamins from A to Zinc: A Reality Check," 17 August 2015, accessed 21 August 2015, http://www.cbc.ca/news/health/vitamins-from-a-to-zinc-a-reality-check-1.3191305.
6 CBC News, "WHO Report Says Processed Meat Causes Cancer, Confusion Follows," 31 October 2015, accessed 8 November 2015, http://www.cbc.ca/news/health/cancer-meat-red-processed-iarc-1.3293541.
7 For milk, see Alissa Hamilton, *Got Milked: What You Don't Know about Dairy, the Truth about Calcium, and Why You'll Thrive without Milk* (New York: HarperCollins, 2015). For a critic of Hamilton's book, see Anne Kingston, "Have We Been Milked by the Dairy Industry?" *Maclean's*, 22

April 2015, accessed 21 August 2015, http://www.macleans.ca/society/health/have-we-been-milked-by-the-dairy-industry/. For saturated fat, see Nina Teicholz, *The Big Fat Surprise: Why Butter and Cheese Belong in a Healthy Diet* (Toronto: Simon & Schuster Canada, 2015).

8 Christoper Labos, "Don't Be Fooled by Big Fat Surprises, Fat Is Still Bad for You," CBC News, 2 March 2015, accessed 21 August 2015, http://www.cbc.ca/news/health/don-t-be-fooled-by-big-fat-surprises-fat-is-still-bad-for-you-1.2965140; CBC News, "'Cut the Crap,' Get Back to Nutritional Basics, Heart and Stroke Foundation Advises," 24 September 2015, accessed 8 November 2015, http://www.cbc.ca/news/health/heart-stroke-saturated-fat-1.3241001.

9 CBC News, "Low-Fat Diets No Help for Weight Loss in Long Run, Review Shows," 29 October 2015, accessed 8 November 2015, http://www.cbc.ca/news/health/low-fat-diets-1.3294853.

10 Gary Taubes, *The Case Against Sugar* (New York and Toronto: Alfred A. Knopf, 2016). For reviews, see Daniel Engber, "The Sugar Wars," *The Atlantic*, January/February 2017, accessed 17 January 2017, https://www.theatlantic.com/magazine/archive/2017/01/the-sugar-wars/508751/; Dan Barber, "What Not to Eat: 'The Case Against Sugar,'" *New York Times*, 2 January 2017, accessed 17 January 2017, https://www.nytimes.com/2017/01/02/books/review/case-against-sugar-gary-taubes.html.

11 Carolyn de la Peña, *Empty Pleasures: The Story of Artificial Sweeteners from Saccharin to Splenda* (Chapel Hill, NC: University of North Carolina Press, 2010), 224.

12 Gilles Plourde and Denis Prud'homme, "Managing Obesity in Adults in Primary Care," *CMAJ* 184, no. 9 (12 June 2012): 1039–44, accessed 8 November 2015, http://www.cmaj.ca/content/184/9/1039.

13 Harriet Brown, "The Obesity Paradox: Scientists Now Think That Being Overweight Can Protect Your Health," *Quartz*, 17 November 2015, accessed 16 January 2017, https://qz.com/550527/obesity-paradox-scientists-now-think-that-being-overweight-is-sometimes-good-for-your-health/; Arya M. Sharma, "Fitness, Fatness and Health," Dr. Sharma's Obesity Notes, 15 September 2009, accessed 17 January 2017, http://www.drsharma.ca/obesity-fitness-fatness-and-health.

14 CBC News, "Brisk Walking: Is It Better Than Vigorous Exercise for Losing Weight?," 7 November 2015, accessed 8 November 2015, http://www.cbc.ca/news/canada/british-columbia/brisk-walking-is-it-better-than-vigorous-exercise-for-losing-weight-1.3309458.

15 Labos, "Don't Be Fooled by Big Fat Surprises."

16 Plourde and Prud'homme, "Managing Obesity in Adults in Primary Care," 1039–44.

Notes on Sources

1 University of Cambridge, Faculty of History, "What Are Historical Sources?," accessed 27 March 2015, https://www.hist.cam.ac.uk/prospective-undergrads/virtual-classroom/historical-sources-what.
2 For an excellent description of statistics today, see Michael Gard, "Hearing Noises and Noticing Silence: Towards a Critical Engagement with Canadian Body Weight Statistics," in *Obesity in Canada: Critical Perspectives*, ed. Jenny Ellison, Deborah McPhail, and Wendy Mitchinson (Toronto: University of Toronto Press, 2016), 44–6.
3 For an overview of print culture and advertising, see Jackson Lears, *Fables of Abundance: A Cultural History of Advertising in America* (New York: Basic Books, 1994), quotes on 1, 4; Judith Williamson, *Decoding Advertisements: Ideology and Meaning in Advertising* (London: Marion Boyars Publishers, 2005 [1978]); Russell T. Johnson, *Selling Themselves: The Emergence of Canadian Advertising* (Toronto: University of Toronto Press, 2001); Roland Marchand, *Advertising the American Dream: Making Way for Modernity, 1920–1940* (Berkeley: University of California Press, 1986); Stephanie C. Roy, Guy Faulkner, and Sara-Jane Finlay, "Fit to Print: A Natural History of Obesity Research in the Canadian News Media," *Canadian Journal of Communication* 32, nos. 3/4 (2007): 575–94.
4 Peter Burke, *Eyewitnessing: The Uses of Images as Historical Evidence* (Ithaca, NY: Cornell University Press, 2001), 95, 126
5 For the modern period, see Deborah Lupton, "The Construction of Patienthood in Medical Advertising," *International Journal of Health Services* 23, no. 4 (1993): 805–19, accessed 20 August 2009, https://www.ncbi.nlm.nih.gov/pubmed/7506237; Tim Scott, Neil Stanford, and David R. Thompson, "Killing Me Softly: Myth in Pharmaceutical Advertising," *British Medical Journal* 329 (18 December 2004): 1484–7, accessed 20 August 2009, http://www.bmj.com/content/bmj/329/7480/1484.full.pdf. For a historical look, see Heather Molyneaux, "In Sickness and in Health: Representations of Women in Pharmaceutical Advertisement in the *Canadian Medical Association Journal*, 1950–1970" (PhD diss., University of New Brunswick, 2009), chapter 1, "Advertising the Female Form: Historians and the Visual," 33–57.
6 See *CD* 13, no. 4 (April 1947): 101, advertisement for Dexedrine; *CD* 41, no. 2 (February 1975): 80–2, advertisement for Sanorex.

7 Michelle Denise Smith, "Model Nation: Identity and Citizenship in Canadian Women's Mass-Market Magazines, 1928–1945" (PhD diss., University of Alberta, 2008), 122–3. Other statistics for *CHJ* and *Chatelaine* are as follows: 1929: 102,279 and 57,053; 1930: 114,987 and 74,278; 1935: 206,961 and 215,353; 1940: 260,715 and 260,133, respectively.
8 Valerie Korinek, *Roughing It in the Suburbs: Reading Chatelaine Magazine in the Fifties and Sixties* (Toronto: University of Toronto Press, 2000), 66.
9 Williamson, *Decoding Advertisements*, 31, 38.
10 See Donica Belisle, *Retail Nation: Department Stores and the Making of Modern Canada* (Vancouver, BC: UBC Press, 2011), 148–51; Korinek, *Roughing It in the Suburbs*, 37.
11 Korinek, *Roughing It in the Suburbs*, 14.
12 Belisle, *Retail Nation*, 27; see also Lorraine Frances O'Donnell, "Visualising the History of Women at Eaton's, 1869 to 1976" (PhD diss., McGill University, 2002).
13 For the richness of catalogues, see Shirley Lavertu, "Catalogues and Women's Fashion," in *Before E-Commerce: A History of Canadian Mail-order Catalogues*, online exhibition, Canadian Museum of History, accessed 25 May 2009, http://www.historymuseum.ca/cmc/exhibitions/cpm/catalog/cat2103e.shtml.
14 O'Donnell, "Visualising the History of Women at Eaton's," 340, 342, 348.
15 Sizing information was gathered once a decade between 1920 and 1950. Formal size charts were offered in 1920, but ceased until 1950. For the intervening years, measurements were supplied with particular styles. However, at times these styles lacked certain measurements, for example, a bust and waist might be supplied but no hip size. After 1950, formal size charts were available.
16 Anne Hayward, "Mail-Order Catalogues: Research Tools for Material History," *Alberta Museums Review* (Fall 1987): 9.
17 See Joy Parr, "'Don't Speak for Me': Practicing Oral History amidst the Legacies of Conflict," *Journal of the Canadian Historical Association* n.s. 21, no. 1 (2010): 1–12; Joan Sangster, "Invoking Experience as Evidence," *Canadian Historical Review* 92, no. 1 (March 2011): 135–61; Pierre Nora, "Between Memory and History: Les Lieux de Mémoire," *Representations* 26 (Spring 1989): 7–24; Kerwin Lee Klein, "On the Emergence of Memory in Historical Discourse," *Representation* 69 (Winter 2000): 127–50
18 Mona Gleason, *Small Matters: Canadian Children in Sickness and Health* (Montreal and Kingston: McGill-Queen's University Press, 2013), 15.

Index

Abbott Laboratories, 50, 267
Aboriginal children. *See* Indigenous children
Aboriginal peoples. *See* Indigenous people
acupuncture, 117, 262
Adelaide Daniels Enterprises, 139
Adjudets, 168
Adulteration Act, 27
advertising/advertisements: "before" and "after," 275; body image and, 49; for chocolate, 49; during Depression, 51; fat babies in, 178–9; fat narratives in, 239–41; food, and environmental theory, 6; and food choices, 32; for food products, 48–9, 57; gender and, 48–9, 208; ideal body in, 215; images of children eating, 43–4; in medical journals, 48, 50; men in, 212; and nutritional knowledge, 48; overweight in, 207; pharmaceutical companies and, 50; in popular media, 48, 274–5; of products for infants, 180; on psychological issues, 133; regulations, 30; during World War II, 49. *See also* pharmaceutical advertisements; *and under titles of periodicals*
age: and body image, 23; and chubbiness of girls, 230; and dieting, 129; and exercise, 105, 113, 268; and fashionableness, 23; and fat men, 221; and fatness, 58, 72–3, 208–9; gender and, in Eaton's catalogues, 216–17; and ideal weight measurement, 62; and idealized body, 207–8; of men in Eaton's catalogues, 218–19; of models in Eaton's catalogues, 226–7; and obesity, 66–7; and obesity statistics, 5; and overweight, 69, 209; and physical activity, 112; and unchanging eating habits, 83; and weight, in men's clothing, 220, 223; and weight, in women's clothing, 229–30, 231; and weight gain, 79; and weight maintenance, 61, 64f; and women's employment, 213; and youthful styles in women's clothing, 226

agency: lack in children/teenagers, 174; obesogenic society and, 5–6
Agnew, G. Harvey, 146
Albertan, The, on Danilowich family Christmas dinner, 68f
Allison, Dr, 107
Ambar #2 Extentabs, 151, 203
American Medical Association (AMA): Code of Ethics, 143; on HCG, 150. See also *Journal of the American Medical Association (JAMA)*
Amobarbital, 166
amphetamines, 147–50, 154, 156, 157, 164
Angel, A., 89, 102, 103, 188
Anglo-French Drug Company, 146
anorexia nervosa, 91, 95, 190
appearance: centrality of, 206; and womanhood, 236. See also body image
appetite: appestat, 95; control, 21, 164, 165f; heredity and, 96; mechanisms of, 122. See also eating
appetite suppressants: as adjunct to dieting, 140, 141; advertisements for, 76, 273; amphetamines as, 149; for child/teen obesity, 202–4; Leith on, 152; during pregnancy, 178; as reflection of proliferation/power of pharmaceutical companies, 141; sedatives/tranquilizers added, 152; surgery vs, 170, 171; in teen obesity, 260. See also drugs
Armstrong, John B., 107
Ashenburg, Katherine, 237
Atkins, Robert/Atkins diet, 126, 130
attractiveness: and employed women, 213–14; and employment, 106; exercise and, 113, 197; fat and, 66; fatness and, 58; fitness and, 268; slenderness and, 3; weight loss and, 113; women and, 22, 212
Ayds, 203–4, 240, 244–5, 380n91
Ayerst Laboratories, 151

babies. See infants
baby boom/boomers, 44, 188, 215
Bakery Foods Foundation of Canada, 123
Baldock, Donald, 178
Bamadex, 151
Bannerman, James, 120, 242, 243
bariatric surgery, 171–2, 392n35
Barry, William, 193–4
Bascobert, Jeannette, 240
Bauer, W.W., 62
Beasley Reducing Corset, 115
Beaton, John R., "Energy Balance and Obesity," 191
Becoming Women: The Embodied Self in Image Culture (Rice), 10
Beef Information Centre, 33
behavioural therapy, 131, 135–6, 140, 202, 260
Belchetz, Brett, 268
Belisle, Donica, 275
Bell, Gordon, 135, 157
Bennett, Mildred, 242–3
benzedrine, 147–9
"Bequest, The" (Theriault), 213
Berton, Pierre, 155
biological theory, 8–9
biopower, 21
Biphetamine, 133, 153, 160, 161–3
Blackburn, Bob, 124, 243
blaming: for food intake, 109; heredity vs, 266; of housewives on relief for food choices, 40; of individual, 20, 32, 265; for

lack of exercise, 109; of mother (*see* mother-blaming); of women, for eating habits, 37–8
Boas, Franz, 34
Bodies Out of Bounds, 16
Bodnar, Willa, 244–5
body image(s): and advertisements, 49; age and, 23; centrality of, 206, 207, 264; children and, 198; class and, 22–3; clothes and, 208, 216; as construct, 236; and eating habits, 198; in Eaton's catalogues, 24–5, 276; elderly and, 23; exercise and, 209; and fatness, 207; gender and, 22, 235–6; and health, 207; medical experts and, 236; men and, 209–13; sizes of clothes and, 216; standard, as middle class/white, 22; weight and, 23; weight and height together in, 20; women and, 208, 226; World War II and, 211–12; youthfulness in, 235. *See also* idealized body image
body mass index (BMI), 12, 13, 19, 58–9, 184, 267, 268
body/-ies: acceptance of, 95; control over own, 10; ectomorphic, 63; endomorphic, 63; frames, and weight/height, 61; history of, 20; ideal vs normal types, 206; and identity, 20; as machines, 59; measurement of, 21; measurements and health, 207; mesomorphic, 63; shapes, 63; standardization of, 59; weight, and aesthetic tracking of, 21–2
Boigny, Maurice, 112
Borden Company, 49
Bovril, 127
Bowen, R.C., 172

Boxer, Rosemary, 242–3
boys: build vs weight, 222; clothing for, 218, 221–2, 256; "husky," 218, 221–2, 256; and slenderness, 219. *See also* teenage boys
Bracer underwear, 222, 223
brain, larger brain theory, 13
Breitman, Kenneth, 134
Brosin, Henry W., 129
Brown, Alan, 34–5, 196, 197; *The Normal Child*, 51, 178, 180, 187, 191
Bruch, Hilde, 70, 91, 188, 192–3, 195; *The Importance of Overweight*, 97, 203
Bryans, A.M., 191, 198
Burgess, Beverley A., 137

Callwood, June, 214
Calorie Counters, 194, 261, 262
calories, 87f; charts, 201; decreasing, 129; elderly cutting back on, 45; expenditure in exercise, 107; fad diets vs, 124; gender, and needs, 42; intake, as cause of obesity, 84; intake needs, 37, 38; intake of overweight vs average weight people, 114; low-calorie diets, 152, 201, 237, 244, 246, 262; medical diets and intake, 118; reduction of needs, 32; as underlying dieting, 120; usage in metabolism, 103
Camp Slim-Teen, 199f
Camp Support girdle, 115
Campbell, Walter R., 60, 83, 108–9, 119, 128, 146, 200; "Obesity and Its Treatment," 132, 171
Canada Dry advertisements, 209–10
"Canada Weighs In: Gender, Race, and the Making of 'Obesity'" (McPhail), 18–19

Canada's Food Rules/Guide, 33, 53, 55, 137, 191, 201
Canadian Association of Health, Physical Education and Recreation (CAHPER), 197
Canadian Association of Health, Physical Education and Recreation (CAHPER) journal: Fairbanks on Canadian lifestyle, 107; Landa article on teenage obesity, 189–90
Canadian Association of Organizations for Weight Watchers, 139
Canadian Calorie Counters, 137
Canadian Consumer, on eating habits, 33
Canadian Council on Nutrition (CCN): creation of, 29; dietary standards, 29, 35, 42, 182; dietary surveys of cities, 35–6; existence under review, 36; and nutrient needs of Canadian vs European women, 37; and Official Food Rules, 32–3
Canadian Dietetic Association, 51, 79, 130
Canadian Doctor, The (*CD*): advertisements in, 273; Camp Support girdle advertised in, 115; cartoon on nonparticipation in sports/exercise, 117; dieting humour in, 123; Probese advertising, 161; Stephen on physicians and food, 54; on weight loss, 113
Canadian Family Physician: on diets, 121; HCG in, 150–1; Kenshole on fenfluramine in, 157–8; psychological case study in, 94
Canadian Health Measures survey, 184
Canadian Heart Foundation, 71–2
Canadian Home Economics Association, 51
Canadian Home Fitness Test, 4
Canadian Home Journal (*CHJ*), 274; articles about drugs, 145; children's exercises in, 196–7; Gossard Corsetry advertisements, 232; and ideal body, 207; "Minimizing One's Size: By Wearing Just the Right Clothes," 208; Phillips on men's waist measurement, 76; on Preludin and Levenor, 156; on thinness in daughters, 42
Canadian Journal of Public Health (*CJPH*): Beaton on energy balance and obesity, 191; Bryans on food production/distribution and childhood eating, 191; on children's weight vs health, 186; Keir on exercise for weight loss, 114; Myres/Yeung on infant obesity, 182–3; on nutrition, 30; on obesity, 30, 58; on obesity vs overweight, 65
Canadian Lancet and Practitioner, The, "What We Eat and Why," 83
Canadian Magazine, The: Lea on Mayo Brothers' 18-day diet, 122–3; on proper diet, 28; on spinach fast, 123
Canadian Medical Association (CMA): Cathcart paper on children's weight, 189; Committee on Pharmacy, 152; on drug restriction, 157; on threshold weight of overweight/obesity, 63; on vitamins, 53
Canadian Medical Association Journal (*CMAJ*): advertisements in, 273;

on American obese children, 192–3; on caloric intake, 84–5; on Canada's Food Guide, 33; on children's use of saccharin, 201; Dexedrine advertising in, 153–4, 159–60; on dieting, 125f; drug advertisements in, 159; on drug therapy, 155; on emotional instability linkage with anorexia/obesity, 91; exercise in, 113; on family histories of obesity, 98; Frosst's Blaud Capsules advertisement in, 48; Garn on heredity and children's growth, 187; on HCG injections, 201; on heredity and appetite, 96; Hollenberg on heredity and obesity, 99; Iodesin advertising in, 146; Lindsay on overweight child, 187; Morrison on appetite suppressants, 157; on obesity, 57, 70; on obesity–coronary disease connection, 77; overvitaminization in, 53; on overweight, 78; Prelutal advertisement in, 150; and psychological view of obesity, 92; on race/heredity and obesity, 96; on ranges of obesity weights, 63; self-help groups in, 137–8; on Simeons' 500-calorie diet, 201; surgery in, 171–2

Canadian National Exhibition (CNE), and fat people as "freaks," 238f

Canadian Nurse, The (CN): about, 272; on childhood weight, 186; on diets, 119; on eating as cause of childhood obesity, 190–1; Farmer's Wife (milk) advertisement, 50; on food prices vs doctors ordering expensive diets for patients, 52; on mania/depression linked to appearance, 77; on overweight/overeating vs exercise, 106; Spencer Body and Breast Supports advertised in, 115; on weight gain during pregnancy, 178

Canadian Nurses Association, and physical fitness at 1974 convention, 79

Canadian Obesity Network (CON), 11, 111, 118

Canadian Paediatric Society Nutrition Committee, 183

Canadian Psychiatric Association, 132

Canadian Public Health Association: Child Hygiene section, 51; Nutrition Committee, 54

Canadian Weight-Height Survey, 19

Cappon, Daniel: on Bruch's work, 193; *Eating, Loving and Dying: A Psychology of Appetites*, 67, 95; on eating references in vocabulary, 84; on family dynamics, 98; on girls' overeating, 91; on heredity, 97; on methods of measuring fat, 63; on psychotherapy, 132; Sangster and, 92; on therapists' competence, 134; on weight as aspect of modernity, 90

carbohydrates, 83, 86, 124, 126, 130, 243, 245, 261

cardiovascular disease, 72, 184

Care of the Child, The (Goldbloom), 180

Carnation: Instant Breakfast, 51; Milk, 179, 180–1

Carney, M.J., 179

Case Against Sugar, The, 267

Cass, Elie, 117

Cathcart, E.P., 189
CBC Radio, *Sports College*, 106
CBC TV, *Newsmagazine*, 106
Centre for Human Metamorphosis, 137
cereals, 50
Chandler, A., 179
Chant Robertson, Elizabeth: on Bruch's views, 192; on children's eating problems, 41–2; on children's food habits, 200; on dangers of dieting, 129; on determination of fatness in children, 187; on exercise as health vs weight issue, 197; on fats in diet, 70–1; on increased consumption of fat, 52–3; *The Normal Child*, 178, 191; on teenagers and exercise, 197
Chatelaine: advertisements in, 275; Ayds advertisement in, 203–4; Baby Clinic, 180; on behaviour therapy for dieting, 136; Callwood on overweight, 214; Carnation Milk advertisement in, 179; Chant Robertson on children's never having learned to eat properly, 192; Chant Robertson on determination of fatness in children, 187; Chant Robertson on teenagers and exercise, 197; "The Cleverest Christmas," 214; diets in, 124, 126; drug articles, 145; Dubarry Success course advertisement in, 240; on eating habits, 32; exercise in, 106; fat narratives in articles vs advertisements, 241–5, 246–7; on food designations, 54; on genetics and obesity, 99; on hand-me-down notions about food, 31; on HCG, 150; on heredity, 97; on honesty regarding women's bodies, 213; on housework as exercise, 105; and ideal body, 207, 209, 212; on immigrants' eating practices, 67; James on hereditary obesity, 98; Kieran on food as mother's substitute for love of children, 193; Kieran on gender differences in emotion and overeating, 93; Kieran's exposé of diet physicians, 158; Kruschen Salts advertisement in, 239–40; Marmola advertising in, 145–6, 159; McCullough on drugs for weight loss, 154–5; McCullough on lack of appetite in children, 40; "Miss C.'s Diet Book," 188; mother's letter re children of families on relief, 40; numbers of readers/subscribers, 274; nutrition articles, 51; and Poulton, 237–8; Preludin article, 156; on psychological causation, 94; on psychological tricks in dieting, 135; on shift from hand to electric typewriters, 107; on Slim Jym device, 113; staplepuncture in, 117; surgery in, 171; Swift's Premium "franks" advertisement in, 44; Vita-Thin advertisement in, 127; on weight, 60–1, 62; on weight maintenance, 106; White on teenage girls with weight problem, 200; "Your Diet That Lets You Eat Your Cake and Look Slim, Too," 201
child obesity: and adult obesity, 184; and anorexia nervosa, 190; causes, 190–8, 205; and changing food habits, 200–1; and citizenship,

197; and clothing, 264; complexity of, 198; counselling for, 198; and dieting, 198, 200, 201–2, 259, 261–2; drug treatment for, 202–4; eating habits and, 190–1; emotional reaction to, 205; endocrine system and, 195–6; energy equation and, 204–5; and exercise, 196–8, 262; family and, 263–4; in fat narratives, 248–57; fitness for, 204–5; growing rate of, 195; and health, 184–5, 188–9; heredity and, 194–5; historiography, 186; hypertension and, 201; Indigenous children and, 184; infant obesity vs, 183; measurement of, 184, 187, 188; in medical journals, 192–3; metabolism and, 195, 196; mother-blaming for, 190, 205, 257–8; mother's age at puberty and, 266; overeating and, 185; overweight parents, and, 333n62; and physical activity, 189; physical causes, 195–6; physicians and, 258–9; poverty and, 184; as precursor to adolescent/adult obesity, 189–90; psychological causes, 192–4; and psychological health, 184–5, 189; psychotherapy for, 202; self-awareness, 263; treatment of, 198–205, 206; weight as measurement for, 188. *See also* infant obesity; teen obesity
Child Welfare, Division of, 28, 177
Child Welfare Council of Canada, 51
Childhood Obesity in America (Dawes), 186
children: advertisements and, 49; and body image, 198; Bruch on heredity and behaviour, 97; and candies/sweets, 191–2; chubby image, 38, 42, 43, 44, 188–9; fitness in, 197–8; and food as reward, 193; food choices, 42, 44, 185f; Indigenous, in residential schools, 46; individual growth patterns, 186–7; lack of agency, 174; malnutrition, 40, 41, 43; marketing of images, 43–4; measurement/surveys of, 34–5; mortality, 176f; nutrition, 38, 41–4, 49; with obese parents, 188; overnourishment, 188; overweight, 38, 44; psychological relationship with mothers, 192; and saccharin, 201; sedentariness, 198; thinness in, 176f; treatment of, 174; undernourishment of, 4; underweight, 44; walking vs riding to school, 197–8; weight charts for, 186; weight vs health in, 186–7; weight/height charts, 34–5, 187
chocolate, 49
cholesterol, 50–1, 70, 71–2, 303n46
Christian, Henry A., *The Principles and Practice of Medicine*, 83
Christie, Helen, 78
Christie, W.F., 76, 100, 101, 112–13; *Ideal Weight*, 66; *Obesity*, 56, 66, 70
citizenship: child/teen obesity and, 197; men's suits and, 219; obesity and, 77; overweight and, 22
Clarkotabs, 147
"Cleverest Christmas, The" (*Chatelaine*), 214
clothes: and body image, 216; for boys, 218, 219, 221–2, 256; for children, 264; for girls, 222, 255–7; ready-made, 208; significance

of, 208; teen obesity and, 255–7; thinness and, 208; youth culture and, 255–6. *See also* men's clothing; women's clothing
clothing sizes, 217–18; and body image, 216; for boys, 218; for "chubby" girls, 226, 230; in Eaton's catalogues, 216; of girls, 224, 226; measurements for, 216; measurements for men's, 217–18; measurements for women's, 224; in Sears catalogues, 385n37; standard, 216; and standardization of bodies, 276; stout men, 217, 221; for stout women, 224; teen, 224, 230; women's, 224; women's as slimming, 224
Cochrane, W.A., 181
Cold War, 77, 113, 197
Collett, Elaine, 71
Collyer, James A., "The Unhappy Fat Woman," 65
consumerism: in Canada vs US, 19; diet product, 241; and eating habits, 32; food, 241; in US vs France, 17
Contours of the Nation: Making Obesity and Imagining Canada (McPhail), 18–19
Cooper, Carol, 385n36
Cormier, Auréa, 122
coronary heart disease, 72, 77
Corporation professionnelle des diétistes au Québec, 122
"Corporeographies of Size: Fat Women in Urban Spaces" (Mitchell), 10
cosmetic surgery, 171
counselling. *See* psychological treatment

Cram, D.M., 63
Cramer, H.I., 101, 120, 129
Cranfield, John, 19
Croft, Barbara, "LP (Liquid Program) Diet," 126
Crowe, Mike, 245–6
culture: and child/teen obesity, 193; dieting and, 118, 123; eating and, 84; heredity vs, 97
Cunliffe, Alison, 34

Dafoe, Dr, 200
Dairy Industry Act, 27
Daniels, Adelaide, 138, 139, 194
Danilowich families, 68f
Darlene Slenderizing Glamour Salon Device, 116f
Davis, Barbara A., 135–6
Davis, G. Albert, 34–5
Dawes, Laura, 379n82; *Childhood Obesity in America*, 186
Deabutal Gradumet, 151
deaths. *See* mortality
Decoding Advertisements (Williamson), 274–5
Dekrysil, 155
"Deliberating Man's Appearance in the Year 2000" (CBC Radio), 106
Demers-Desrosiers, Louise A., 172
depression, 90, 95
Depression: Aboriginal peoples and, 45, 47f; advertising during, 51; blaming of housewives on relief for food choices, 40; blaming of mothers for nutritional deficiencies, 41; and eating habits, 251–2; and food availability, 83; food scarcity during, 41f; and infants, 177; men's loss of employment during, 210;

nutrition during, 3–4, 23, 29; and overeating, 86
Desoxyn, 151
Dexamyl, 153–4, 166, 168
Dexedrine, 147, 149, 152–4, 157, 159–60, 163, 166, 167f, 203; Spansule, 149, 164, 165f, 168
Dexobese, 168
diabetes: blaming of individual for, 259; child/teen obesity and, 184; drugs for diabetics, 151; effect on foetus, 174; in elderly, 76; in Indigenous groups, 13; obesity and, 74, 76, 77, 78; overweight and, 77; and pregnancy, 178; sugar and, 267
Diagnostic and Statistical Manual of Mental Disorders (DSM), 89, 94
Dickens, Charles, *The Pickwick Papers*, 18
dieting: adjuncts to, 111, 131, 133, 140, 141, 263; age and, 129; appetite suppressants and, 140, 141; calories underlying, 120; child obesity and, 198, 200, 201–2, 259, 261–2; as control device, 118; culture and, 118, 123; as cycle, 246; determining goal of, 121; eating habits and, 121, 123; efficacy of, 12, 16, 111; exercise and, 110, 140, 263; gender and, 124; hospitalization and, 120; inefficacy of, 246; institutional, 119; and nutrition, 118, 129, 130; pharmaceuticals and, 21, 90, 129, 133, 152–3; physicians and, 119, 120–1, 259–60; psychological treatment and, 131, 133, 140; and slowing of metabolism, 238; stages of, 118; successful, 242, 244, 245–6;
surgery as admission of failure of, 140; teen obesity and, 198, 200, 201–2, 259; as treatment, 118–31; trends, 267; and weight loss, 120, 237–8, 263; and weight regain, 118; yo-yo, 129
diets, 125f; accompanying passive "exercise" methods, 117; Atkins, 126, 130; Ayds Vitamins and Mineral Candy Reducing Plan, 244–5; banana, 130, 261; choice of, 110; crash, 130; Dr Gold's liquid, 126; Drinking Man's, 124, 130, 243; D-Zerta, 128; 18-day, 122–3, 128; fad, 111, 122–6, 131; families and, 118–19; grapefruit, 122–3, 130, 261; Hay diet, 123; Knox Eat-and-Reduce Plan, 240; liquid, 127, 129–30, 237, 242, 259, 260–1; low-calorie, 152, 237, 244, 246, 262; low-fat, 267; maintenance of, 120, 121; medical, 110–11, 118–22; Metrecal, 240–1; orange-juice-Knox-gelatine, 123–4; Pennington, 126; product, 111, 127–8; product consumerism, 241; safety of, 111, 128–31; Simeons' 500-calorie, 201; Stillman, 129, 261; Vita-Thin, 127
Dimson, Colleen, 241
dinitrocresol, 155
dinitrophenol, 155
Dionne quintuplets, 200
Dior, Christian, 226
disease(s): and causation, 74; fat reserves and, 76; relationship with obesity, 4, 76, 78, 173
DNA, thrifty gene theory, 8
doctors. *See* physicians
Dollery, Eveleen, 244, 245
Dominion grocery stores, 31

Donsky, Marla, 245
Dressler, Marie, 231
Drinking Man's Diet (DMD), 124, 130, 243
Drug Advisory Committee, 144–5
drugs: about, 142–70; for child/teen obesity, 202–4, 206; combinations of, 151; diet aids, 133; efficacy, 151–3; ethical, 143; federal government and, 144–5; gender and, 159–63; for health problems, 155–6; history of use, 21; increasing specialization of, 151; integration into medicine, 141; lack of efficacy, 263; legislation, 142–5; marketing of, 145; medical partnership with, 163–70; mood-altering, 90; non-medical use, 153–4, 204; and obesity, 94–5; patent, 143, 144; patient consent, 145; patient understanding of, 158; and psychological problems, 141; safety concerns, 154–5, 163, 166; sales percentage increases, 142; Schedule F, 144–5; Schedule G, 157; scientific experiments, 148–9; in teen obesity, 260; thyroid, 145–7; trust in, 153; types of, 145–51; warnings, 155–8; and weight loss, 141, 155. *See also* appetite suppressants
DuBarry Success course, 240, 241
Dubé, J.E., 44–5
Dubreuil, Lucien, 102; "L'obésité," 97
Dumas, Paul, 172
Durabolin, 203
Dzeguze, Kaspars, 130
D-Zerta, 128

eating: control over, 164, 165f; culture and, 84; measurement/surveys, 34–7; Pett on, 30; post–World War II economy and, 84; psychological factors, 91, 94, 132–3; stages of process, 135–6; types of eaters, 95; urge for, 86; vocabulary references to, 84; women and, 91. *See also* appetite; food; overeating
Eating, Loving and Dying: A Psychology of Appetites (Cappon), 67, 95
eating habits: age and, 83; body image and, 198; changing, 200–1; child/teen obesity, and changing, 200; and child/teen obesity, 190–1; Depression and, 251–2; dieting and, 121, 123; and eating "well," 22, 50, 266; eating well vs badly, 28; elderly and, 88–9; families and, 201–2, 266; in France vs US, 17, 373n32; heredity vs, 96, 249–52; of men, 44–5; mood and, 93; mothers and, 201; numbers of meals, 121; nutrition education vs, 252; as solving problem of obesity, 122; teenage girls and, 200; teenagers and, 201, 205; in US vs France, 17; and weight, 88, 243–4; World War II and, 252; young women, 37
Eaton's: and steam baths, 115; Stout Man's Shop, 221
Eaton's catalogues: about, 24–5, 275–6; body image in, 24–5; boys in, 218, 219, 221–2; clothing sizes in, 216; drawings vs photographs in, 216; exercise equipment in, 105; fat bodies in, 24–5; fat men in, 219–20; and fat people, 216; gender, and age spectrum in, 217;

and ideal body, 207; idealized body in, 216; Marie Dressler Slender Stouts, 231; men in, 216–17, 217–23; older men vs women in, 216–17; women in, 216, 223–35; young men in, 219

economy: obesity and, 5; post– World War II, 31, 84

Edmonton: dietary surveys, 36; Grads, 66; nutritional survey, 40; Obesity Staging System, 11

elderly: and body image, 23; eating habits, 88–9; and exercise, 105; men, and nutrition, 45; metabolism in, 103; nutrition of, 45; obesity and associated health issues, 76; women as non-existent in Eaton's catalogues, 217

electricity treatment, 114

electroshock treatment, 133, 134

Elizabeth II, Queen, 124

Elliott, Charlene D., 30

Ellison, Jenny, 18

emotional obesity, 91, 92

employed mothers: and child/teen obesity, 193; and malnutrition, 43

employed women: age and, 213; attractiveness and, 213–14; health of, 30; slenderness and, 213–14; during World War II, 30, 212

employment: attractiveness and, 106; men's loss of, during Depression, 210

endocrine system, 100, 101–3, 145–7, 151, 195–6

endogenous obesity, 70, 102, 146, 187, 195

energy: and body in balance, 103; efficient utilization of food energy, 103; exercise and intake of, 111; fat and, 70; metabolism and, 99

"Energy Balance and Obesity" (Beaton), 191

energy equation: attitudes towards, 81; and child/teen obesity, 204–5; and complexity of obesity, 83; energy expenditure in, 104; and five causes of obesity, 82; and obesity, 81, 89; overeating and, 82; physical activity and, 106–7; as underlying theory of weight, 103; weight and, 326n2

energy expenditure: in energy equation, 104; exercise and, 104, 111; four different types of, 73; obesogenic environment and, 7; and obesogenic environment theory, 8; thyroid extract and, 202; voluntary vs involuntary, 110; weight loss as reducing, 111

Entwistle, Joanne, 20, 208

environmental theory, 5–7

epidemiology, 74

Eskatrol Spansule, 151

estrogen, 67, 77, 102

ethnicity/race: and dietary fat, 70–1; and endocrine system, 100; and heredity, 96; nutrition and stereotyping, 23; obesity statistics, 5; and obesity theories, 8; thrifty gene theory and, 13; weight as cultural vs genetic, 97; and weight/height charts, 59; white skin colour as standard body, 22

eugenics movement, 96

exercise: about, 268; as adjunct to diet, 263; advantages of, 12; age and, 105, 112, 113, 268; amount of, 268; and attractiveness, 113, 197;

and BMI, 268; and body image, 209; and caloric expenditure, 107; as cause of obesity, 268; child obesity and, 189, 262; and child/teen obesity, 196–8; cold temperatures and, 117; decline in, 7; dieting vs, 110; effective vs ineffective, 111–14; and energy equation, 106–7; and energy expenditure, 104, 111; fat men and, 221; fatness and lack of, 105; and fitness, 117; gender and, 105; and health, 114, 205, 268; housework as form of, 105; lack as cause of obesity, 104–7; lack as global pandemic, 111; for men, 215; in middle age, 105; in older people, 105; and overweight, 197; passive, 114–18; percentage not engaging in, 106; physical education, 7; physicians and, 113; as preventative, 114; psychological treatment vs, 140; in schools, 197, 204; sedentariness vs, 263; spas, 113; teenage girls and, 199f; as treatment for obesity, 111–18; as weak partner to dieting, 140; and weight gain, 12, 112; and weight loss, 112–13, 114, 117, 205, 237, 242, 262, 263; and weight loss vs health, 113; and weight maintenance, 114; Weight Watchers and, 139; women and, 111–12. *See also* fitness
"Exercise is the Bunk – Relax" (Hunt), 113
Exercycle (Automatic Exerciser), 117
exogenous obesity, 70, 102, 187, 195
expensive tissue hypothesis, 8
Ezrin, Calvin, *Your Fat Can Make You Thin*, 259–60

Fairbanks, Bert L., 107, 114, 122
families: and child obesity, 263–4; dieting and, 118–19; eating habits, 96, 201–2, 249–52, 266; food and, 194, 249–52; immigrant, 250; psychology, 193; siblings, 249; situations as cause of obesity, 257–8; teasing and, 253; teen obesity and, 205, 263–4. *See also* heredity
Family Allowance, creation of, 30
Farmer's Wife (milk) advertisement, 50
Farquharson, R.F., 190
Farrell, Amy Erdman, *Fat Shame: Stigma and the Fat Body in American Culture*, 16
fasting, 119, 121, 129, 261, 262; feasting vs, 8
fat, body: abdominal, 318n56; active vs inert, 70; age and, 72–3, 208–9; "baby fat," 186; belly, 69; and bodily organs, 75; brown, 70, 73, 103–4, 318n56; burning of, 158; cells, 70, 72–3, 182, 183, 191, 205; diseases and reserves of, 76; and energy, 70; fitness and, 79; free vs fixed, 70; HCG and, 150; health concerns regarding, 73; heredity and storage of, 96; inner vs subcutaneous, 72; locations of, 102; mobilization/transportation of, 158; need for, 66; negative aspects, 71–3; and obesity, 56; obesity vs, 65; positive aspects, 69–71; subcutaneous, 318n56; types of, 69–71; as unattractive, 66; visceral, 318n56; white, 318n56
Fat: A Cultural History of Obesity (Gilman), 17
fat babies. *See under* infants

fat bodies. *See* fatness
Fat Boys: A Slim Book (Gilman), 17
"Fat" Female Body, The (Murray), 10
Fat History (Stearns), 16–17, 373n32
Fat Is a Feminist Issue (Orbach), 95
fat measurement: ponderal index, 62; skinfold/calipers, 62, 63, 184, 188; somatyping and, 63; and threshold for obesity, 63, 65; X-rays and, 63
fat men: described as "stout," 219; fat women as outliers, vs, 236; history of, 17; "jolly fat man" image, 242; "king size" and, 221; as sedentary, 221; in stories, 211. *See also* stout men
fat narratives: about, 239, 263–4; in advertising, 239–41; "before and after," 239–41, 247; child obesity in, 248–57; early years families, 248–52; interviews, 248–63; in media, 248; in periodicals, 241–7, 275; in popular press, 239–47; social life, 252–7; teen obesity in, 252–7; third-person use in, 242–3; weight causes/treatments, 257–63. *See also* interviews
Fat Shame: Stigma and the Fat Body in American Culture (Farrell), 16
fat women: as outliers, vs fat men, 236; stigmatization of, 16, 237
fatness: age and, 58, 207–8; and attractiveness, 58; as beauty defect, 213; body image and, 207; eating as cause of, 83; in Eaton's catalogues, 24–5, 216; and "fat" as word of acceptance, 20; fat people as "freaks," 238f; fat phobia and, 11, 173; fat studies, 9–11, 16; gender and, 66, 68; history of

concern regarding, 14, 16; and idealized body, 207–8; and lack of exercise, 105; in magazine articles, 57; in media, 208; modernity and, 86; and obesity, 3; obesity vs, 9; overeating and, 89; positive views of, 9; statistics and fixation on, 58; stigmatization of, 9, 11, 73, 215, 238f, 269; as stressful, 269; women and, 9

fatness activism: emergence of, 138; fat studies and, 16; and feminism, 9; positive view of fatness, 9; rejection of word "obese," 20; themes, 16; and weight loss, 11

fat(s), dietary: about, 52–3, 69–73; calories, 319n58; consumption of, 84; in dieting, 124; percentages in food consumption, 73; questioning whether problematic, 88; reduction of consumption, 72; saturated, 308n98; saturated vs unsaturated, 72; three types of, 150; types of food, 69

Federal Food, Drug and Cosmetics Act (US), 143

Federal Trade Commission, 143

feminism: fatness activism and, 9; and overweight, 95; and slenderness, 9, 95

Fen-Phen, 157

fiction: fat men in, 211; gender in, 209; ideal body in, 215; middle-aged men in, 212; older women in, 214; World War II, 212

Financial Post, fat narratives in, 245–6

First Nations. *See* Indigenous people

Firstbrook, Dr, 114

fitness: and attractiveness, 268; BMI and, 268; body fat and, 79;

in children, 197–8; for child/teen obesity, 204–5; and democracy, 77; exercise and, 117; and health, 4, 268; low levels of, 4; men and, 106; popularity of, 113–14; sedentary life and, 105–6; women and, 106, 112f. *See also* exercise
Fleischmann: Oil, 50–1; Yeast, 49
Fleming, Grant, 101
foetus, 174, 177
food: access to, 29; advertisements, and environmental theory, 6; advertisements for products, 48–9, 57; balance of, 267; canning, 28; centrality of, 6; changing environment, and heredity, 98; children and, 185f; consumerism, 241; convenience, 6, 31, 84, 85–6; Depression and, 83, 251–2; emotional relationship with, 89, 90; enrichment of, 52; faddism, 32, 52; families, 194, 249–52; health claims for, 29; health food stores, 54; helping size, 191; and history of obesity, 22; immigrants and, 31, 250; intake matching metabolism, 97; knowledge regarding intake, 191–2; low-calorie, 200; and nutrition, 266; Pett on, 30; post–World War II economy and, 84; price control, 30; psychological factors, 132–3; public beliefs about, 31; as reward, 193; risk estimates, 267; in schools, 33–4, 191; slow/local movement, 6; as substitute for love, 193; surveillance, 29; taste/tasting of, 8, 13, 252; tasting of, 8, 13; teens and, 185f; traditional immigrant, 67; variety of, 267. *See also* calories; eating
Food and Drug Administration (FDA; US), 143, 144
Food and Drug Directorate, 157
Food and Drugs Act, 28, 144, 157
food choices: advertising and, 32; blaming of individual for, 32; children making own, 42, 44; difficulties in, 266–7; income and, 6; teenage girls making own, 42; and weight, 83
food industry: advertising to physicians, 50; efficiency of production, 31; as market-driven, and nutrition, 6; products for infants, 181; removal of nutrients vs shelf life, 29
Foods without Fads (McHenry), 32
FORCE cereal, 48
Forth, Christopher E., 281n2
Foucault, Michel, 21
Fowler, E., 128
Framingham study, 71
France: eating habits compared to US, 17, 373n32; US compared to, 16–17
Fraser Institute, 5
Freedhoff, Yoni, 267
French Canadians: English Canadians compared to, 67. *See also* Quebec (province)
Freud, Sigmund, 193
Friedman, Abraham I., *How Sex Can Keep You Slim*, 117
Froelich, Alfred/Froelich's syndrome, 195, 196, 202
Frosst's Blaud Capsules, 48
"Fun and Fitness" (Cochrane clinic), 205

Galton, Lawrence, 150, 156
Gard, Michael, 12, 173; *The Obesity Epidemic: Science, Morality and Ideology*, 14, 104
Gariépy, L.-Henry, 155
Garn, Stanley M., 187
Geekie, D.A., 157
gender: advertisements and, 48–9; and age spectrum in Eaton's catalogues, 216–17; and body image, 22, 235–6; and caloric needs, 42; and cause of overweight, 160–1; in clothing styles, 234; and dependence, 93; and dieting, 124; and drug treatment, 159–63; in Eaton's catalogue visuals, 216, 234; and exercise, 105; and fat, 66, 68, 211; fiction and, 209; and fitness, 106; and "husky" boys vs "chubby" girls, 221–2; and ideal body image, 208; in locations of body fat, 102; and made-to-measure clothing, 217, 229; and measurement, 62–3; and media use of bodies to sell products, 208; and obesity, 66, 67–9; and obesity rates/statistics, 5, 13–14, 22, 91; and obesity theories, 8; in older men vs women in Eaton's catalogues, 216–17; in perceptions of overweight, 211; pharmaceutical advertising and, 159–63; in psychological reasons for obesity, 93–4; and psychological stress, 91; and reactions to weight loss, 242, 243; and seeking help for problems with weight, 69; and silhouettes, 276; and social class/socioeconomic status, 69; and stigmatization, 16; and surgery, 170; and teenage nutrition, 38–9; and variations in bodies, 214–15; and weight concerns, 17; and weight loss, 122, 363n80; and weight/height charts, 59
General Foods, 63
general practitioners. *See* physicians
genetics: hardwired theory, 8, 96; and obesity theories, 8–9; thrifty gene theory, 8, 13, 19. *See also* heredity
Gifford-Jones, W., 79
Gilder, S.S.B., 196, 201
Gillingham, Ethel, 246–7
Gilman, Sander L., 73, 373n32; *Fat: A Cultural History of Obesity*, 17; *Fat Boys: A Slim Book*, 17; *Obesity: The Biography*, 17–18
"Ginger Ale and Pop" (Canada Dry), 209–10
girls: as "chubbies," 222, 226, 230; clothes, 222, 255–7; clothing sizes, 224, 226; health as employees in World War II industries, 30; pyjama party, 185f; undergarments, 233
Gleason, Mona, *Small Matters: Canadian Children in Sickness and Health*, 277–8
Globe and Mail: Lowman on emotional obesity, 92; "Tubby Hubby Diet" column, 84; on weight loss and loss of identity, 140
Gold, Dr, liquid diet, 126
Goldbloom, Alton, 42, 44, 50, 187; *The Care of the Child*, 180
Goldbloom, Richard, 204
gonads, 100, 102
Good Health (Phair and Speirs), 70

Goodeve, Mildred D., 40
Gossard Corsetry, 232
government(s): drug legislation, 144–5; and food prices, 30; and health of children/youth, 42; national nutritional survey, 36–7
Grignon, Jean, 189
group therapy, 132, 134. *See also* self-help groups

Haig, G.T., 42–3; "Suppose Tommy Won't Eat," 42
Halifax: dietary surveys, 36; nutritional survey, 41
Hancock, T., 182
Hanes' Panty Pair, 234
Hanley, F.W., 134, 186–7
hardwired theory, 8, 96
Harris, Marjorie, 33
Harrowsmith, on overweight and mortality, 78
Harvard University, 72
Harvey, William, 73
Harvey Woods 5BX Reducers, 223
Hattie, William H., 40
Hawirko, Leonora, 90, 147–9, 203
Hawkins, W.W., 195
Hay, William Howard, 123
health: BMI and, 58–9, 268; body image and, 207; body measurements and, 207; child obesity and, 184–5, 188–9; exercise and, 205, 268; fat and, 73; of fat babies, 180–1; in fat studies, 11; fitness and, 4, 268; of girls/women working in World War II industries, 30; healthism, 21; and healthy living vouchers, 7; malnourishment and, 189; obesity and, 4, 74–80, 130; obesity panic and, 12–13; overweight and, 22, 74, 259; teen obesity and, 184–5, 188–90; weight and, 186, 268; weight loss and, 12–13; of World War I recruits, 3, 26, 27–8; of World War II recruits, 30
Health: cartoon on fat in, 72; Johnson on nutritional information for mothers, 43; Laski on overnourished child, 188; liquid protein diets in, 129; Weight Watchers in, 138; White on cyclamates, 128
Health, Department of, creation of, 28
Health and Unemployment (Marsh), 35
Health and Welfare Canada: on diets, 130; on energy equation, 81; on fat percentage in diet, 73
health premiums, obesity and size of, 5
Health Protection Branch, 145
Hector, Richard I., 133
Heineck, Aimé-Paul, 170–1
Heinz, 179, 181
Henry, Sarah, 137
heredity: adopted children and, 98; and appetite, 96; as biological vs social, 97; blame vs, 266; and "build" of body, 222; as cause of obesity, 96–9, 249; and children's growth patterns, 187; and child/teen obesity, 194–5; culture vs, 97; environmental factors vs, 98; family eating habits vs, 96, 249; and fat storage, 96; growing rate of obesity vs, 98; in medical journals, 97; and metabolism, 96, 97, 99, 103; physicians and, 97, 98, 195; in popular media, 97, 98; and prognosis, 96–7; and race/ethnic

groups, 96, 97; statistics and, 96, 97, 195; and weight loss, 96. *See also* families; genetics
Hermiston, Alana, 49
Hill, Donald E., 53, 181–2
Himms-Hagen, Jean, 73, 103–4
Hippocrates, 14, 17
Hirsch, Doris L., 92–3
Historicizing Fat in Anglo-American Culture (Levy-Navarro), 9–10
Hofsess, John, 215
Holdrite underwear, 222–3
Hollenberg, Charles H., 99, 130
Honda Accord, 215
hormones, 103; human chorionic gonadotropin (HCG), 150–1, 201, 204, 237
Housewives Association of Canada, 51
Housewives Consumer Association, 30
housework, 105, 106
How Sex Can Keep You Slim (Friedman), 117
Hunt, Morton, "Exercise is the Bunk – Relax," 113
Hutton, Eric, 124
hydrotherapy, 114
Hyland, H.H., 190
hyperinsulinemia, 196
hypertension, 74, 201, 267
hypnosis, 133–4, 260–1, 262
hypothalamus, 101–2, 103

Ideal Weight (Christie), 66
idealized body image: in advertisements, 215; in Eaton's catalogues, 216, 276; fatness/age vs, 215; in fiction, 209; gender and, 208; illusion and, 216; impossibility of, 215; in popular media, 207; post–World War I, 208; as stigma, 236; unreality of, 235. *See also* body image
identity: body and, 20; in historiography, 22–3; weight and, 23; weight loss, and loss of, 140
"I'm Reducing" (Sinclair), 120
immigrants: and eating well, 68f; and food, 31, 250; mothers, 192; post–World War II, 31; traditional foods, 67
Importance of Overweight, The (Bruch), 97, 203
income. *See under* social class
Indigenous children: and diabetes, 184; and obesity, 184
Indigenous people: age, and overweight, 69; assimilation of, 19; attitude towards government nutritional guides, 46; Canadian racism and, 19; Depression and, 45, 47f; diabetes in, 13; malnutrition, 45–6; obesity rates, 19; obesity statistics, 5; southern diet and, 23, 67; and white paper (1969), 46; women's nutrition, 36; youth in residential schools, 46. *See also* Inuit
infant feeding: bottle, 177, 179, 182, 183, 192; breast, 66, 100, 177, 179, 180, 181, 183–4, 248, 249; food products for, 181; formulas, 177, 179, 181, 183–4, 249; habits, 177, 182, 183–4; and overeating, 180, 181; weaning, 180, 182, 183
infant obesity: about, 174–84; adolescent obesity vs, 183; causes, 182–3, 205; child obesity vs, 183; connection with adult obesity, 183; emotional reaction to, 205; food

416　Index

products for, 181; measurement of, 181; in medical journals, 182–3; overweight vs, 183; timing of diagnosis, 181–2; treatment for, 205–6. *See also* child obesity
infants: advertising of products for, 178–9, 180; baby-scales, 179; born before mother's surgery, 266; chubby image, 175f, 177, 178–9; Depression and, 177; fat as healthy, 180–1; influenza epidemic and, 177; maternal mortality and, 37; mortality, 3, 38, 176f, 177, 178; overweight, 180; sleeping habits, 177; thinness in, 176f; weak, 178; weight gain, 180–1, 183
influenza epidemic, 28, 177
insurance companies: and mortality rates/studies, 61, 75–6; on overeating, 84; and weight, 59, 61
International Agency for Research on Cancer (IARC), 266–7
International Obesity Task Force, 184
interviews, 248–63; about, 247, 248, 263, 277–8; Aileen, 251, 254, 261; Alice, 251; Connie, 252, 255, 262; Doris, 250, 255, 258, 259–60, 262; Frank, 257, 261; Grace, 249, 250, 251, 253, 254, 261; Heather, 254, 257; Irene, 252, 254, 261, 262; Jane, 249, 254, 255, 256–7, 258, 260, 262; Julie, 251, 256, 259, 262; Laura, 251, 252, 254, 255, 256, 257, 258, 260, 262, 269; Leona, 250, 252–3, 256, 258; Lucy, 250, 251, 253, 255, 261; Mary, 254, 257, 261, 262; Nicole, 256; Nina, 249, 251–2, 254, 255, 258, 264, 269; Olive, 250, 251, 259, 260–1, 262–3, 264; Randy, 253, 256, 257, 258–9, 269; Rose, 251, 253, 254, 261, 264; Sasha, 253, 254; Stephanie, 248–9, 254, 257, 258, 260, 269; Sylvie, 253; Tammy, 250, 251, 258, 261; Tina, 262; William, 252, 254, 260, 261, 262. *See also* fat narratives
Inuit: age, and overweight, 69; Canadian racism and, 19; changing food intake environment as changing children's bodies of, 98; decline of fitness among, 106; nutrition, 36; southern diet and, 23, 67; and sugar, 86. *See also* Indigenous people
Inuit women: nutrition, 36; weight gain, 67
Inwood, Kris, 19
Iodesin (Iodobesin), 146
Ionamin, 133, 160, 161–3, 162f
i-sometric-isotonic method, 117

James, Florence, 98
Jeffrey, Bill, 55
jejunoileal bypass (shunt) surgery, 171, 172
Jensen, Trudy, 127
Jetté, Maurice, 193–4
Jewish children, and obesity, 193
Joanisse, Leanne, 392n25
Johnson, Catherine Ann, 240
Johnson, R.H., 43
Jones, Stefanie A., 10
Journal of the American Medical Association (JAMA): advertising revenue, 144; Hay diet in, 123; on safety of Dexedrine, 166

Kahan, Scott, 9
Katz, Sidney, 113, 124, 135, 156, 157, 212

Katzmarzyk, Peter T., 19
Keenberg, A., 132
Kefauver-Harris Drug Amendments, 143
Keir, Sandy, 114
Kenshole, Anne B., 157–8
ketones, 86
Keys, Ancel, 71, 122
Kieran, Sheila, 93, 158, 159, 193
Kilpatrick, Blanche, 242
King of Kensington (TV show), 214
Kisby, Russ, 106
Knox gelatine: Knox Eat-and-Reduce Plan, 240, 241; orange-juice-Knox-gelatine diet, 123–4
Kruschen Salts, 127, 239–40, 241
Kulczcki, L.L., 180–1
Kwong, Edward, 130

Labos, Christopher, 268
Lalonde, Marc, 58, 113
Lambert, Daniel, 15f
Lancet, The, on obesity, 57
Landa, Sam, 189–90
Large as Life self-help group, 254
Laski, Bernard, 188, 195, 196
le Riche, W. Harding, 54, 107, 152
Lea, Virginia, 122–3
League of Nations: Mixed Committee on the Problem of Nutrition, 29; optimal nutritional standards, 35, 37
leanness. *See* slenderness
Lears, Jackson, 273
LeBesco, Kathleen, *Revolting Bodies? The Struggle to Redefine Fat Identity*, 11
Lee, Annabelle, 61
Lee, Peggy, 247f
Leith, Dr Wilfred, 121, 126, 152
Levenor, 156

Levenstein, Harvey A., 82, 373n32; *Paradox of Plenties*, 17; *Revolution at the Table*, 17
Levy-Navarro, Elena, *Historicizing Fat in Anglo-American Culture*, 10
Lexchin, Joel, *The Real Pushers: A Cultural Analysis of the Canadian Drug Industry*, 168
life expectancy/longevity, 61, 74
lifestyle choices, 5
Lindsay, Lionel, 189, 190, 195–6, 198, 200, 202–3, 204, 206; "The Overweight Child," 187
liposuction, 171
literature: challenging fatness/obesity, 9–14; fat studies, 9–11, 16; historical studies, 14–19; on nutrition, 51. *See also* fiction; media; medical journals/literature
Little, Alick, 71
Little Corporal Belt, 115
London School of Economics, 268
Longhurst, Robyn, 10
Lowman, Josephine, 92, 113
"LP (Liquid Program) Diet" (Croft), 126
Luciani, Patrick, *XXL: Obesity and the Limits of Shame*, 7

MacDonald, Janine, 130
Maclean's: articles on nutrition, 51; Berton on drug therapy, 155; on body fat and risk to organs, 75; on clothing for stout women, 227; diets in, 124; Dzeguze on liquid diets, 130; fat narratives in articles, 242, 243, 246; Fleischmann's Yeast advertisement, 49; Fleming on glands, 101; Gifford-Jones on overweight/weight gain, 79; humour section on limitations

of fat persons, 105; Hunt on exercise, 113; and ideal body, 207; Katz interview with Bell on drugs, 157; Katz on behaviour therapy, 135; Katz on diet pills, 156; Katz on testosterone, and men's body image, 212; Kruschen Salts advertisement in, 239–40; Little Corporal Belt promoted in, 115; McCoy's Cod Liver Extract Tablets advertisement, 48; men's support underwear advertised in, 222; on normal weight, 62; numbers of readers/subscribers, 274; on obesity, 57, 62; Paupst on psychiatrists and overeating, 94; on psychodietetics, 91–2; on rejection rates of World War II recruits, 4; Robertson on fitness, 117; Rowell's story "Me-Athlete," 210; Sangster on health problems of middle-aged men, 214; Westinghouse oven advertisement in, 83; Whitteker on heredity, 98; on women's nutritional deficiencies, 37–8

magazines: about, 274–5; advertisements in, 274–5; dieting in, 119; dieting vs food in, 84; ideal body in, 207; nutrition in, 51, 54; and nutritional knowledge, 48; on overweight, 57; pharmaceutical articles in, 145. See also media; medical journals/literature; *and specific titles*

Magic Controller, 233

malnutrition: Aboriginal peoples and, 45–6; causes, 47; of children in Quebec, 43; chubby children and, 189; fat babies and, 181; health consequences, 189; mother-blaming for, 192; mothers' employment and, 43; obesity and, 32, 56; overnutrition as, 30, 32; overweight and, 26, 35, 56; poverty and, 29, 35; pregnant women, 38; of school children, 34–5; southern diet and, 67; surveys, 37; thin bodies and, 3; undernutrition of children, 4; undernutrition vs overnutrition, 57; underweight and, 26, 35, 43, 177; and weight/height charts, 60. See also nutrition

"Managing Obesity in Adults in Primary Care" (Plourde and Prud'homme), 268

Manitoba, underweight in, 36

Manitoba Medical Review: Desoxyn advertisement, 83; Keenberg on motive to lose weight, 132

Manshanden, Maria, 244

March, Janet, 52

Maritimes, overweight in, 67

Marliss, Dr, 131

Marmola tablets, 145–6, 159, 239, 241

Marsh, Leonard C., 29; *Health and Unemployment*, 35

Marshall, Benjamin, 15f

Martel, Antonio, 67, 149–50, 203

Mason, Edward H., 56–7, 70, 75, 100, 119, 128, 132, 204

massage, 114, 115, 117

Mayo Brothers' 18-day diet, 122–3

Mayo Clinic Diet, 130

McCoy's Cod Liver Extract Tablets, 48

McCrae, Thomas, 96, 99–100; *The Principles and Practice of Medicine* (1925 ed.), 119

McCullough, John W.S., 35, 38, 40, 154–5
McFetridge, J. Grant, 84–5, 91
McHenry, E.W., 30, 31, 34, 37, 58, 71, 124; *Foods without Fads*, 32
McLaren, Barbara, 32, 62–3
McPhail, Deborah, 106; "Canada Weighs In: Gender, Race, and the Making of 'Obesity,'" 18–19; *Contours of the Nation: Making Obesity and Imagining Canada*, 18–19
measurement(s): about, 21, 34–7, 59; of body, 21; of child/teen obesity, 184, 187, 188; for clothing sizes, 216; computer analyses and, 63; of eating/nutrition, 34–7; of fat men, 220; gender and, 62–3; and girls' clothing sizes, 224, 226; for infant obesity, 181; mathematical equations for, 62–3; for men's clothing sizes, 217–18; methods, and statistics, 69; of obesity, as changing, 21; of obesity, as obvious, 56; ponderal index, 62; problems of, 265; of school children, 34–5; somatyping and, 63; and teen clothing sizes, 224; weight as, 21–2; in weight charts for children/teens, 186; and women's clothing sizes, 224; X-rays, 63. *See also* clothing sizes; fat measurement; weight
Meat and Canned Foods Act, 27
"Me-Athlete" (Rowell), 210
media: advertisements in, 48; drug advertising in, 157; drug safety concerns in, 154–5; fat bodies in, 208; fat narratives in, 239–47, 248; on heredity, 98; heredity in, 97; on psychological causes of obesity, 91–2; slenderness in, 207, 208; understanding of obesity, 265. *See also* literature; magazines
Medical Care Act, 78
medical journals/literature: about, 271–3; advertisements in, 48, 50, 152–3; Bruch's work in child/teen obesity in, 192–3; fat men as sedentary in, 221; heredity in, 97; infant obesity in, 182–3; obesity in, 56, 57; pharmaceutical advertisements in, 142, 144, 145, 204; pharmaceutical companies and, 273; social class in, 77; surgery in, 170–1. *See also specific titles*
medicalization, 4, 20–1, 50, 56, 205
medicine: history of view of obesity, 17–18; and science, 269
men: in advertisements, 212; age and weight, 220; ages in Eaton's catalogues, 218–19; body image, 209–13; body profile, 217–18; bodybuilding, 210f, 215; clothing sizes, 217–18; eating habits, 44–5; in Eaton's catalogues, 216–23; emotional reactions to weight, 245–6; and exercise, 215; faces in Eaton's catalogues, 217, 218; and fitness, 106; hair in Eaton's catalogues, 217; obesity statistic, 5; overweight as sign of importance in, 22; psychological associations with eating, 91; and self-help groups, 138; silhouettes, 218, 219; and slenderness, 3, 119, 216, 218–19, 220; social class and obesity, 67; social class in Eaton's catalogues, 220; support underwear, 222–3;

weightlifters, 209, 210f; and weight-loss groups, 261. *See also* fat men; stout men; young men

menopause: estrogen and, 67, 77, 102; and obesity, 66, 101

men's clothing: quality of, 221; silhouettes, 218, 219; slimness in, 236; styles for stout men, 220–1; suits, 218, 219, 220, 221, 223, 229, 236, 276

mental illness, obesity as, 4, 89–90

metabolic/endocrine factor: as cause of obesity, 100, 101, 102–3; thyroid and, 93. *See also* endocrine system

metabolism: basal rate (BMR), 100, 101, 122, 146, 151–2, 202; and calorie usage, 103; as cause of obesity, 99–101; and child/teen obesity, 195, 196; dieting, and slowing of, 238; dinitrophenol and, 155; efficiency, 103; in elderly, 103; endocrine system and, 100; energy equation and, 83; food intake vs, 97; heredity and, 96, 97, 99, 103; resting rate, 99; three components of, 99; varying rates of, 99–100

Metrecal, 240–1, 261

Metropolitan Life Insurance Company, 60, 61, 84, 154, 155–6

microbe hypothesis, 6–7

middle age: and exercise, 105; and fitness, 106; "middle-aged spread," 212

middle class: children's nutrition, 43; standard body as, 22

middle-aged men: aging bodies, 212–13; and fashionableness, 23; in fiction, 212; and weight, 214–15

middle-aged women: and fashionableness, 23; and overweight, 214

milk: and calcium, 267; Carnation, 179, 180; cereals and, 50; children and, 38, 39; days, 119, 123; in food standards, 46; Indigenous people and, 46; teenagers and, 39, 44. *See also* infant feeding

Mil-ko, 181

Mills, E.S., 96, 97

"Minimizing One's Size: By Wearing Just the Right Clothes" (*Canadian Home Journal* [*CHJ*]), 208

"Miss C.'s Diet Book" (*Chatelaine*), 188

Miss Mary/Lady Mary of Sweden, 234

Mitchell, Allyson, 263; "Corporeographies of Size: Fat Women in Urban Spaces," 10

modernity: and fatness, 86; and obesity, 7; obesity as metaphor for, 5; and weight, 90

Molyneaux, Heather, 160

Monagle, J.E., 53, 191, 201

moral panic, 11, 14

morbid obesity, 17

morbidity: mortality vs, 323n87; obesity and, 75; from surgery, 171–2

Morrison, A.B., 157

Morse, W.I., 92–3

mortality: child, 176f; infant, 3, 176f, 177, 178; insurance companies and rates of, 61; maternal, 4, 37; of metabolically healthy obese vs other causes, 13; morbidity vs, 323n87; obesity and rates of, 77–9; obesity as risk factor, 74–5; overweight and rates of, 75–6, 77; from post–World War I influenza,

28; use of studies, 75–6; weight and, 61; during World War I, 27–8
Mosby, Ian, 23, 45–6
mother-blaming: for children's malnutrition, 41, 192; for child/teen obesity, 190, 205, 257–8; for lack of nutritional knowledge, 194; for nutrition, 266; physicians and, 193; stigmatization and, 16
mothers: age at puberty and child obesity, 266; and changing family eating habits, 202; and children's eating habits, 201; children's psychological relationship with, 192; and food as substitute for love, 193; immigrant, 192; infants born before surgery of, 266; knowledge of nutrition, 38; maternal mortality, 4, 37; nutrition, 6, 37, 40, 178; obesity in, and overweight babies, 177; as responsible for family nutrition, 44; sympathy for, 43. *See also* employed mothers
Mowat, Ruth, 194
Murray, Samantha, 11; *The "Fat" Female Body*, 10; *Queering Fat Embodiment*, 10
Myres, Anthony W., 182, 198; "Obesity in Infants," 182–3

National Population Health Survey, 74–5
Neilson chocolate advertising, 49
Nembutal, 151
Nemo Corsets, 232
Nestle, Marion, 72
Never Satisfied: A Cultural History of Diets, Fantasies and Fat (Schwartz), 16
New England Journal of Medicine, 72

New Image (Toronto), 137
New Tenuate, 151
Nicolson, Malcolm, 51
No Fat Chicks (Poulton), 238–9
Normal Child, The (Brown), 51, 180, 187
Normal Child, The (Brown and Chant Robertson), 178, 191
Norman, Moss, 184–5
Nujol salad dressing, 127
Nutri-Bio, 51
nutrition: advertisements and knowledge of, 48; blaming of individual for choices, 32; of children, 38, 42–4, 49; contested nature of study of, 26; and controlling of body, 51; during Depression, 3–4, 23, 29; dieting and, 129, 130; eating well and, 50, 266; education, 6, 28, 48, 51–4, 122, 191, 252; of elderly, 45; food and, 266; history of, 22, 26, 27–34; Indigenous people and, 23; Inuit and, 23; knowledge about, 84; lack of knowledge about, 6; literature regarding, 51; in magazines, 48, 51, 54; market-driven food industry and, 6; measurement/surveys, 34–7; medical diets and, 118; mother-blaming for, 194, 266; of mothers, 37; mothers and, 6, 38, 40; nursing mothers and, 178; physicians and, 28, 48, 52, 53–4; in pregnancy, 177–8; in public health literature, 272; and racial stereotyping, 23; specific nutrients vs overall picture, 53; supplementary nutrients, 50; surveys, 22, 26–7, 38, 45, 46, 69, 114; teenage girls,

53; of women, 37–8. *See also* malnutrition
Nutrition Canada, 58
Nutrition Division, National Health and Welfare, 44

Obedrin, 203
"obese": fat activists' rejection of word, 20; medical practitioners and, 20
"L'obésité" (Dubreuil), 97
"L'obésité" (Verdy), 172
obesity: anti-obesity products, 58; causes of, 82, 108–9, 146–7, 257–8; challenges to all viewpoints on, 265; as clinical, 72; definition of, 65; as a disease, 73; exogenous vs endogenous factors, 70, 102, 146, 187, 195; groups at risk for, 56; health problems linked to, 74, 76, 77–8; history of rise of interest in, 56–8; lack of consensus on, 265; as medical term implying sickness, 65; medicalization of, 4; multifactorial nature of, 109; origins of word, 20; overweight vs, 183; as pathological, 73; psychological problems and, 89–95; scientists and, 265; "types," 319n59; as vicious circle, 190
Obesity (Christie), 56, 66, 70
"Obesity and Its Treatment" (Campbell), 132, 171
Obesity and Leanness (Rony), 101
obesity epidemic, 4, 11–12, 13–14, 57–8, 73
Obesity Epidemic: Science, Morality and Ideology, The (Gard and Wright), 14, 104

Obesity in Canada: Critical Perspectives, 11–12
"Obesity in Infants" (Myres and Yeung), 182–3
Obesity: The Biography (Gilman), 17–18
O'Day, Patsy, 242
Offer, Avner, 289n52
l'Office de la protection du consommateur du Québec, 138
Official Food Rules, 29, 32–3. *See also* Canada's Food Rules/Guide
Ogilvie, G.F., 61, 80
Oliver, H.D., 63
Olympic Games: 1928, 66; 1976, Montreal, 113
Ontario, statistics on weight in, 37
Ontario Dietetic Association, 33
Ontario Health Association, 33
Ontario Health Insurance Plan (OHIP), 151
Ontario Medical Association (OMA): and diet manual, 33; and drugs to treat obesity, 151; on obesity, 58, 78; Salmon on shunt surgery, 171
Ontario Medical Review, review of Bruch on children's weight, 188
Orbach, Susie, *Fat Is a Feminist Issue*, 95
organotherapy, 145
Original Subtract advertisement, 234
Osler, William, 65–6, 111. *See also Principles and Practice of Medicine, The*
Oslo breakfast, 200
Osmos, 114–15
Ovaltine, 48, 49
Overeaters Anonymous (OA), 137, 138
overeating: about, 82–9; as cause of obesity, 109, 266; causes, 91; children and, 188; and child/teen

obesity, 185, 190–1; complexity of reasons for, 89; culture and, 84–6; and fat cells, 191; fatness and, 89; food production/distribution and, 191; hunger "mechanism" and, 83–4; importance of food and, 85–6; infants and, 180, 181; life insurance companies on, 84; psychological/psychiatric approach, 93–4; psychology of, 90; reasons for, 82, 83, 109; undernutrition vs, 57; underweight vs, 188; and weight gain, 237, 244

overweight: in advertisements, 207; age and, 69, 209; boys, 221–2; children, 38, 44, 187, 196; and citizenship, 22; co-morbidities, 166; and diabetes, 77; exercise and, 197; feminism and, 95; in fiction, 209; gender and cause of, 160–1; gender in perceptions of, 211; and health, 12, 22, 74, 259; infants, 177, 180, 183; as lifelong, 121; magazine articles on, 57; malnutrition and, 26, 35, 56; middle-aged women and, 214; and mortality rates, 75–6, 77; obesity vs, 65, 183; parents, and child obesity, 333n62; population percentages as, 58, 69; and psychological problems, 94, 246; regional rates, 67; and risk, 21; sedentariness and, 105; as sign of importance in men, 22; smoking compared, 78; underweight vs, 62

"Overweight Child, The" (Lindsay), 187

Pacific National Exhibition (PNE): "Better Babies Contest," 175f; Darlene Slenderizing Glamour Salon Device at, 116f; Honey-O concession, 87f

Paradox of Plenties (Levenstein), 17

ParticipACTION, 113, 197

Paupst, James, 94

Pausé, Cat, *Queering Fat Embodiment*, 10

Pearlman, Lyon, 193–4

Pennington, Alfred/Pennington Diet, 126

Pennington's clothing store, 256

Penny Light, Tracy, 22

Pensions and National Health: Drug Advisory Committee and, 144–5; on saccharin pills, 127–8

Percival, Lloyd, 197

Percy, Lloyd, 106

Pett, L. Bradley: on 1970 national nutrition survey, 36–7; on body frames in weight/height charts, 80; on endocrine origin of obesity, 147; on fat intake and heart disease, 71; on modern Canadian living, 32; on psychological associations between men and eating, 91; and size of babies, 181; on societal importance of food, 85; summary of dietary habits at end of 1940s, 30; on weight charts, 61, 62; on weight charts for children/teens, 186–7; on yo-yo dieting, 129

Phair, J.T., *Good Health*, 70

Pharmaceutical Advertising Advisory Board (PAAB), 145

pharmaceutical advertising/advertisements: about, 273–4; for appetite suppressants, 273; for child/teen obesity drugs, 204; detail included in, 156, 170; gender and, 159–63; as mediator between researchers and practitioners, 170; in medical journals, 142, 144, 145, 152–3, 204; physicians and, 143–4, 163–70, 274; in popular press, 157; as primers on specific drug use, 170; on psychological issues, 133; to public, 143–4, 145; science in, 166, 168, 274; side effects listed in, 156–7; and teen obesity, 203–4; US history of, 143–4

pharmaceutical companies: advertising by, 50; appetite suppressants as reflection of proliferation/power of, 141; claims declining over time, 154; competition among, 147; and medical journals, 273; ownership, 142; relationship with physicians, 53, 141, 142, 144, 168, 170, 274; and temptation of food in advertisements, 83

Pharmaceutical Manufacturers Association of Canada (PMAC), 145

pharmaceuticals. *See* drugs

phendimetrazine, 157

phenmetrazine, 149–50, 157

Philip, Prince, 4

Phillips, Alan, 71

Phillips, Joan, "Watch Your Husband's Waistline," 76

physical activity. *See* exercise

Physical Work Capacity test, 197

physicians: and child obesity, 258–9; and clinical inspection for obesity, 61–2; counselling child patients, 202; and dieting, 119, 120–1, 122, 123, 259–60; and drug safety, 166; and exercise, 113; and fat patients, 58; food company advertising to, 50; goals vs those of insurance company charts, 62; and heredity, 97, 98, 195; and international literature/meetings, 19–20; in interviews, 258–60; lack of expertise in obesity, 268; and medical journals, 272; and mother-blaming, 193; and nutrition, 28, 48, 52, 53–4; obesity education for, 57; on PAAB, 145; pharmaceutical advertising and, 163–70, 274; and pharmaceutical advertising to public, 143–4; pharmaceutical companies and, 53, 141, 142, 144, 168, 170, 274; and physical causes of child/teen obesity, 195–6; practices devoted to obesity, 313n12; and psychological treatment, 131–6; and psychology, 90, 94, 96; and psychology of children/teens, 193–4; on puberty/menopause as adding fat, 22; social class and, 77; social/cultural perceptions, 11; teen obesity and consulting of, 189; and treatment, 173; use of "obese," 20; and weight loss, 268; Weight Watchers and, 138–9; and weight/height charts, 60; and weight-loss drugs, 155

Pickwick Papers, The (Dickens), 18

pituitary gland, 101, 102, 195

"Platitoodinous Hooey" (short story), 209

Plourde, Gilles, "Managing Obesity in Adults in Primary Care," 268

Ponderal, 154

Pondimin, 157–8, 204

popular media. *See* media

Poser, Ernest G., 136, 260

Poulton, Terry, 237–9, 259; *No Fat Chicks*, 238–9
poverty: and childhood obesity, 184; and malnutrition, 29, 35
Prairies, overweight in, 67
pregnancy: appetite suppressants during, 178; as cause of obesity, 257, 263; diabetes and, 178; effect of older mothers on foetus, 174, 177; fantasies, 91; and malnutrition, 38; nutrition in, 177–8; and obesity, 66, 100, 101; weight gain during, 74, 177–8, 257
Preludin, 149–50, 152, 156, 157, 164, 166, 191, 203
Prelutal, 150, 156
Pre-Sate, 154
Price, Eileen, 84–5, 91
Principles and Practice of Medicine, The, 103, 271–2; 1893 ed., 66, 75, 99, 104, 111, 118, 187; 1912 ed., 66, 96, 99–100, 111, 187; 1925 ed., 66, 96, 119; 1938 ed., 146, 155; 1947 ed., 66, 83, 96–7, 123; 1976 ed., 121; 1980 ed., 109, 172
Probese, 147, 152, 157, 161, 164, 168, 169f, 203
Probesil, 151
protein, 124, 129–30, 178, 185, 215, 261
Prud'homme, Denis, "Managing Obesity in Adults in Primary Care," 268
psychiatry, 132, 133, 202
psychoanalysis, 132
psychodietetics, 91–2
psychological problems: about, 89–95; child/teen obesity and, 184–5, 189; gender and, 91; and lessening of problems, 131; and overweight, 246; pharmaceuticals and, 141

psychological treatment: about, 131–40; as adjunct to dieting, 111, 131, 133; behaviour modification vs, 135; for child/teen obesity, 198, 202; as fallback position, 140; lack of permanent success of, 139
psychology: and child obesity, 192–4; emergence as discipline, 90; family, 193; of obesity, 90; of overeating, 90; physicians and, 90, 96, 131–6; self-help groups, 136–40; and teen obesity, 193–4; of weight gain, 90
puberty: as cause of obesity, 263; as complicating treatment, 206; early, in mother and children, 266; impact of, 257; obesity as retarding, 189; physicians and connection with weight, 22; and sedentariness, 66; and sexual attraction, 255; thyroid extracts at, 202; and weight gain, 196
Public Health Journal, The, children's eating habits in, 190
public health periodicals, 272
Pure Food and Drugs Act (US), 143

Quaker Oats Company, 127
Quebec (province): children's dietary deficiencies in, 43; culture and eating in, 84; English compared to French Canadians of, 67; overweight in, 67; reduction of fat consumption in, 72
Quebec City: dietary surveys, 35–6; nutritional survey, 41
queer studies, fat studies and, 10
Queering Fat Embodiment (Pausé, Wykes, and Murray), 10

Rabinowitch, I.M., 77
race. *See* ethnicity/race
Real Pushers: A Cultural Analysis of the Canadian Drug Industry, The (Lexchin), 168
Recreation Canada fitness test, 79
Red Cross Society, 51
Regina Rural Health Region, 54
Reichert, Beverley, 34
Relax-A-Cisor, 115
Renulife Violet Ray, 114
Revicaps, 168
Revolting Bodies? The Struggle to Redefine Fat Identity (LeBesco), 11
Revolution at the Table (Levenstein), 17
Rice, Carla, 253, 392n25; *Becoming Women: The Embodied Self in Image Culture*, 10
risk(s): causation vs, 74; changing meaning of, 73–4; epidemiology and, 74; estimates regarding food, 267; insurance companies and, 59; obesity and, 5; overweight and, 21; statistics and, 73
R.J. Strasenburgh, 163
Robertson, John, "You Know the 60-Year-Old Swede Who's Fitter Than a 30-Year-Old Canadian?," 117
Robillard, Rosario, 77
Rodger, D.E., 84–5, 91
Roncari, Daniel A.K., 135–6
Rony, Hugo, 102; *Obesity and Leanness*, 101
Ross, J. Andrew, 19
Rothstein, William, 73–4
Rowell, Hugh Grant, "Me-Athlete," 210
Royal Canadian Air Force (RCAF): exercise programs, 107, 113; health of recruits, 30

Royal College of Physicians and Surgeons of Canada, and HCG, 150–1

saccharin, 119, 127–8, 201
Sackett, David, 65
Salmon, P.A., 171
salyrgan, 148
Sangster, Dorothy, 92, 214
Saturday Night, March on nutrition, 52
schools: children walking vs riding to, 197–8; exercise in, 197, 204; food in, 33–4, 191; hatred of, 254; Indigenous children in residential, 46; malnourishment in, 34–5, 43; nutrition experiment in, 53; teasing at, 252–3; violence, 253; weight scales in, 35
Schwartz, Hillel, *Never Satisfied: A Cultural History of Diets, Fantasies and Fat*, 16
science: experiments, and drugs, 148–9; and medicine, 269; and obesity, 265; in pharmaceutical advertisements, 166, 168, 274; and statistics, 269
Sears catalogues, 256, 385n37
sedentariness: active overeaters vs, 160; of activities, 7; and advantages of exercise, 12; in children/teenagers, 198; exercise vs, 263; and fat men, 221; and overweight/weight gain, 105; and passive activity, 118; post–World War II, 31; puberty and, 66; and search for fitness, 105–6
Seeman, Neil, *XXL: Obesity and the Limits of Shame*, 7
Segall, Howard N., 61
self-acceptance, 139, 202, 238–9

self-awareness, 134–5, 263
self-help groups, 136–40, 171, 254, 261–2
seniors. *See* elderly
set-point weight hypothesis, 13, 89
Shadow on a Tightrope: Writings by Women on Fat Oppression, 9
Sharma, Arya, 11, 111, 118, 326n2
Sheldon, William Herbert, 63
Shepel, L., 172
Shephard, R.J., 88
Shepherd, R.W., 65
silhouettes: gender and, 276; as illusion, 276; of men, 218, 219; of women, 223, 226; women's clothing, 226
Simeons, Albert T.W., 150; 500-calorie diet, 201
Simpson, J.C., 29–30
Sinclair, Gordon, 115; "I'm Reducing," 120
SK&F (Smith Kline & French), 153–4
slenderness: and attractive body, 3; boys and, 219; dominance in media, 208; emergence as dominant image, 119; and employed women, 213–14; feminism and, 95; and idealized body image, 235; and image of stout women, 229; media use of, 207; men and, 3, 119, 216, 218–19, 220; men's clothing and, 216, 234, 236; of models for stout women, 231; teenage girls and, 42; thinness vs, 235f; in women's clothing, 224, 225f, 226, 234, 236; and women's employment, 213; young women and, 3, 211f. *See also* thinness
Slim Jym, 113

Small Matters: Canadian Children in Sickness and Health (Gleason), 277–8
Smith, David, 51
social class: age-weight connection in Eaton's catalogue visuals, 217; and body images, 22–3; and Depression malnutrition, 23; and ease of weight loss, 241; gender as factor within, 69; and health problems, 76–7; income, and food choices, 6; income and obesity statistics, 5; medical literature and, 77; of men in Eaton's catalogues, 220; and obesity in men, 67; obesity statistics, 5; physicians and, 77; and psychiatric counselling, 92–3; and suits, 218; and weight/height charts, 59; and women's weight, 69
social construction: of attitudes towards obesity, 14; of body image, 236
society, as obesogenic, 5–6
Speirs, N.R., *Good Health*, 70
Spencer Body and Breast Supports, 115
Sports College, 197
Sports College (CBC Radio), 106
Sprague, P.H., 90, 147–9, 203
Standard Brands bread for dieting, 127
standardization, 59
statistics: conflation of overweight with obesity, 13; correlations, 73, 78, 269; gender and, 22; growing rate of obesity and, 98; heredity, 96; and heredity, 97, 195; history of collection of, 12; history of trajectory of, 19; inaccuracy of, 58; Indigenous child obesity, 184;

measurement methods and, 69; in mortality studies, 75–6; on obesity rates, 69; problems of, 265, 272; and risk, 73–4; science and, 269; worldwide, 5. *See also* measurement(s)
Statistics Canada, on food, 6
steam baths, 115
Stearns, Peter, 186; *Fat History*, 16–17, 373n32
Stefansson, Vilhjalmur, 28
Stennett, R.G., 63
Stephen, Irmin, 54
Stettner, Shannon, 22
stigma/stigmatization: and fat women, 16, 237; of fatness, 9, 11, 215, 238f, 269; gender and, 16; idealized body as, 236; and mother-blaming, 16
Stillman diet, 129, 261
stout men: age and, 221; clothes sizing for, 217, 221; clothing compared to stout women's, 227, 229; clothing styles for, 220–1; in Eaton's catalogues, 217, 219–20, 223; fat men described as, 219; measurements for, 220; and physical activity, 221; replaced by "king size," 221. *See also* fat men
stout women, 228f; age and, 229–30; clothes sizing for, 224; clothing for, 227, 229; correction of appearance, 229; in Eaton's catalogues, 224, 227, 229; foundation garments for, 231–4; illusion creation, 229; images in Eaton's catalogues, 229, 231; and made-to-measure clothing, 229; models as not fitting image, 231; scarcity of clothes for, 231; suits for, 229

Stuart, Richard B., 139
Sucaryl, 128
sugar, 28, 86, 88f, 127, 178, 191–2, 267
Sugar Association, 72
"Suppose Tommy Won't Eat" (Haig), 42
surgery: about, 141–2, 170–2, 263; as admission of failure of dieting, 140; during another surgery, 171; appetite suppressants vs, 170, 171; bariatric, 171–2; cosmetic, 171; failure of dieting and, 141; gastric bypass, 172; gastric restriction/banding, 170; gender and, 170; infants born before mother's, 266; intestinal malabsorption, 170; jejunoileal bypass (shunt), 171, 172; liposuction, 171; in medical journals, 170–1; and morbidity, 171–2; physician reactions to, 170–1; staplepuncture, 117; stomach stapling, 238; in teen obesity, 198; types of, 170
surveys: city dietary, 35–6; malnutrition, 37; of population nutrition, 34–7; of school children, 34–5
Swan Valley, MB, study of infants, 180–1
Swift: Canadian bacon, 180; Premium "franks," 44; Strained Meats, 180

Take Off Pounds Sensibly (TOPS), 136–7, 138, 255, 261
teen obesity: appetite suppressants in, 260; camps, 199f, 263; causes, 190–8, 205; and changing food habits, 200–1; child obesity as precursor to, 189–90; and

citizenship, 197; and clothes, 255–7; complexity of, 198; and dieting, 198, 200, 201–2, 259; drugs and, 202–4, 260; eating habits and, 190–1; emotional reaction to, 205; endocrine system and, 195–6; energy equation and, 204–5; exercise/fitness and, 196–8, 204–5; families and, 263–4; family environment and, 205; growing rate of, 195; and health, 184–5, 188–90; heredity and, 194–5; historiography, 186; infant obesity vs, 183; measurement of, 184, 187, 188; in medical journals, 192–3; mother-blaming for, 190, 205; overeating and, 191; physical causes, 195–6; and physician consulting, 189; psychological causes, 193–4; and psychological health, 184–5; psychotherapy for, 198, 202; puberty and, 255; self-awareness, 263; surgery for, 198; treatment of, 198–205, 206; weight as measurement for, 188. *See also* child obesity

teenage boys: genitalia, 196; poor health of World War II recruits, 29–30; and slenderness, 219; sweet/starch consumption, 191. *See also* boys; young men

teenage girls: and breakfast, 200; clothing sizes, 224, 230; exercise by, 199f; fashions for overweight, 230; fat, 227; making own food choices, 42; nutrition, 38–9, 53; and thinness/slenderness, 42; undergarments, 233; and weight loss, 53. *See also* girls; young women

teenagers: eating habits, 44, 201, 205; and food, 185f; and image vs nutrition, 44; lack of agency, 174; nutrition during World War II, 41–2; nutritional deficiencies, 40; sedentariness in, 198; and self-help groups, 138; treatment of, 174; weight charts for, 186; weight vs health in, 186–7; weight/height charts, 187; and youth culture, 174, 191, 193–4, 205

Tenuate Dospan, 164
Therapeutic Products Directorate, 158
Theriault, Yves, "The Bequest," 213
thinness: and clothes, 208; culture of abundance vs, 16; of fashion models, 227; in infants/children, 176f; and malnutrition, 3; of models in Eaton's catalogues, 216, 226; of mothers and underweight infants, 178; pressure towards, 246; slenderness vs, 235f; teenage girls and, 42. *See also* slenderness
thrifty gene theory, 8, 13, 19
Thyer, Suzanne, 214
thyroid, 93, 100, 102, 103, 145–7; extract, 151–2, 196, 202; hypothyroidism, 101, 146
Tidmarsh, F.W., 39, 60
Tillson's bran, 127
TOPS. *See* Take Off Pounds Sensibly (TOPS)
Toronto: children's dietary study in, 43; dietary surveys, 35–6; nutritional survey, 41
treatment(s): about, 110–11, 140, 172–3; behavioural therapy, 260; of children/teenagers, 174, 198–205, 206; drug, 141, 142–70; hypnosis, 260–1, 262; for infant

obesity, 205–6; interviews, 259–63; as multivaried, 110, 262–3; physicians and, 258–60; self-help groups, 136–40; surgery, 141–2, 170–2; team global approach, 173
Trerice, A. Corinne, 123
"Tubby Hubby Diet" column (*Globe and Mail*), 84
Twiggy (model), 227

underwear: foundation garments, 115, 231–4, 236; for men, 222–3
underweight: adolescent boys, 29–30; children, 44, 187, 188; infants, 177, 178; malnutrition and, 26, 35, 43, 177; overweight vs, 62; women, 212. *See also* thinness
"Unhappy Fat Woman, The" (Collyer), 65
L'Union Médicale du Canada (UMC): Demers-Desrosiers on regulation of eating, 172; Dubé on men's meat consumption, 44–5; Dumas on obesity treatment, 172; on exercise, 112; Heineck on surgery, 170–1; history of, 271; on nutrients, 54; pharmaceutical advertising in, 273; Robillard on obesity-diabetes relationships, 77; Verdy on obesity treatment, 172
United Nations, on caloric needs, 32
United States: Canada compared to, 19; Center for Disease Control and Prevention, 184; children on reducing diets in, 379n82; eating habits compared to France, 17; France compared to, 16–17; French eating habits compared to, 17, 373n32; history of drugs in, 143–4; ownership of pharmaceutical companies, 142; Society of Actuaries, 61; Supreme Court, 143
Université de Montréal, Departement de nutrition, 122
University of Manitoba, study of housebound elderly, 45
University of Toronto, Faculty of Food Sciences, 120, 132–3

Valentti, Rosa, 31
Vancouver Police Mutual Benevolent Association, 209, 210f
Verdy, Maurice, 58; "L'obésité," 172
Victoria General Hospital (Halifax), psychiatric counselling of patients in, 92–3
Victorian Order of Nurses (VON), 51
Virol, 178–9
virus hypothesis, 9
Visiting Homemakers Association, 51
vitamins, 28, 30, 50, 53, 266; D, 52; K, 52
Vita-Thin, 127
Vitou clinic, Port Royal, QC, 259
Vranic, Magda, 79

Ward, Nita, 241–2
Warner's Girdle, 233
"Watch Your Husband's Waistline" (Phillips), 76
Waxman, Al, 214
Weekend Magazine, Atkins diet in, 126
Weider, Ben, 215
weight: in advertisements for food products, 57; and aesthetic tracking of body, 21–2; age and men's clothing, 220, 223; age and women's clothing, 229–30, 231; birth, 248; in BMI, 58; and body image, 23; clinical inspection

for, 61–2; comparing to weight/height chart, 60; eating habits and, 88; and energy equation, 326n2; energy equation as underlying theory of, 103; exercise and maintenance of, 114; fixation on, 12; food choices and, 83; gender differences in seeking help for problems with, 69; and health, 186, 267, 268; with height as body image, 20; and identity, 23; Indigenous people and, 69; insurance companies and, 59, 61; Inuit and, 69; maintenance of youthful, 61, 64f, 106; meaning of, 21; meaning of normal, 65; as measurement, 21–2, 188; middle-aged men and, 214–15; modernity and, 90; mortality and, 61; in Ontario, 37; regional differences in, 67; regulating mechanism, 100; set-point hypothesis, 13, 89; skinfold thickness tests, 62; social class and gender, and, 69; stability over time, 65; threshold for obesity, 63, 65; weighing oneself, 59–60; worldwide change in, 5
weight charts: challenges to, 79; for children/teenagers, 186, 187; weight/height charts, 34–5, 56, 59, 60–1, 62–3, 65, 187; weight-height-age survey, 62
weight gain: age and, 79; death of parent and, 257; eating habits and, 243–4; estrogen and, 67; exercise and, 12, 112; hardwired concept of, 8; by infants, 180–1, 183; lack of exercise and, 104–5; lack of fitness and, 106; obesogenic environment theory and, 8; overeating and, 237, 244; during pregnancy, 74, 177–8, 257; psychology of, 90; at puberty, 196; sedentariness and, 105; stress and, 257; weight loss difficulties following, 263; winter and, 105, 213
weight loss: and attractiveness, 113; avoidance of, 79, 130; bathing, 114–15; belt wearing, 115; Benzedrine and, 147; and continuing health problems, 246; dieting and, 120, 237–8, 263; difficulty following weight gain, 263; drugs and, 141; exercise and, 112–13, 114, 117, 205, 237, 242, 262, 263; exercise vs dieting in, 110; fat activists and, 11; gender and, 122, 242, 243, 363n80; and health, 12–13; heredity and, 96; inability for, 257; inactive methods, 114–15; and leanness, 119; and loss of identity, 140; numbers of meals and, 121; physicians and, 268; and psychological problems, 131; psychology and, 133; as reducing energy expenditure, 111; and slenderness, 119; teenage girls and, 53; and transformation, 242–5, 243; weight maintenance following, 114, 245, 257; and weight regain, 242, 263
Weight Watchers, 137, 138–9, 194, 261, 262, 263
Weight Watchers magazine, Original Subtract advertisement, 234
"What We Eat and Why" (*The Canadian Lancet and Practitioner*), 83
Whetmore, Dr, 28
White, Adele, 200
White, L.S., 128, 200
Whitteker, Byng, 98, 246, 247f

Williamson, Judith, *Decoding Advertisements*, 274–5
Willson, Margaret, 17
Wilson, D.R., 114, 152
Winick, Dr, 79, 98, 130
Wolfish, Martin, 202, 206
women: aging body and, 208–9; and appearance, 236; and attractiveness, 22, 212; blaming, for eating habits, 37–8; and body image, 208; body politics, 22; drawings vs photographs of, 216; and eating, 91; in Eaton's catalogues, 216, 223–35; and emotional obesity, 91; and exercise/sports regime, 111–12; and fatness, 9; and fitness, 106, 112f; as more prone to obesity, 66; nutritional education directed at, 52; nutritional health, 37–8, 40; and obesity, 67–9; obesity statistic, 5; as psychiatric patients, 93; and self-help groups, 138; underweight, 212. *See also* fat women; employed women; mothers; stout women; young women
women's clothing: age and youthful styles in, 226; foundation garments, 231–4, 236; nylon, 233; silhouettes, 223, 226; sizes, 224; slenderness in, 225f, 226, 234, 236; suits, 229; variety of fashions, 223–4; youthfulness in, 224, 226, 229–30, 234, 236
Worker, The, use of word "fat," 57
World Health Organization (WHO): and BMI, 12, 184; IARC, 266; and obesity as global epidemic, 73; on obesity epidemic, 4; on obesity statistics, 5; Task Force on Obesity, 267
World War I: health of potential recruits, 3, 26, 27–8; influenza following, 28, 177
World War II: advertising during, 49; amphetamines during, 147; and body image, 211–12; children's nutrition during, 41–2; and eating habits, 252; employed women during, 212; fiction, 212; health of girls/women working in industries, 30; health of recruits, 4, 29–30; and overeating, 86; postwar economy, 31; rationing, 30
Wright, Jan, 173; *The Obesity Epidemic: Science, Morality and Ideology*, 14, 104
Wykes, Jackie, *Queering Fat Embodiment*, 10

XXL: Obesity and the Limits of Shame (Seeman and Luciani), 7

Yeung, David, 182; "Obesity in Infants," 182–3
York University, study of women workers at, 213–14
"You Know the 60-Year-Old Swede Who's Fitter Than a 30-Year-Old Canadian?" (Robertson), 117
Young, Charlotte M., 63, 67–9, 72, 77
young men: in Eaton's catalogues, 219; and fashionableness, 23; health as World War I recruits, 3, 26, 27–8; health as World War II recruits, 4, 29–30; and income and obesity, 69; and slenderness, 3. *See also* teenage boys

Young Men's Christian Association (YMCA), 51
young women: eating habits, 37; and fashionableness, 23; nutritional levels, 37–8; and slenderness, 3, 211f; and sports, 66. *See also* teenage girls
Young Women's Christian Association (YWCA), exercise in Edmonton gymnasium, 112f

"Your Diet That Lets You Eat Your Cake and Look Slim, Too" (*Chatelaine*), 201
Your Fat Can Make You Thin (Ezrin), 259–60
youth culture, 174, 191, 193–4, 205, 255–6
youth obesity. *See* child obesity; teen obesity

www.ingramcontent.com/pod-product-compliance
Lightning Source LLC
Chambersburg PA
CBHW030259080526
44584CB00012B/368